Rehabilitation from COVID-19

T0332651

Rehabilitation from COVID-19

An Integrated Traditional Chinese and Western Medicine Protocol

Edited by

Wenguang Xia
Xiaolin Huang

Translated by

Chanjuan Zheng

China Press of Traditional Chinese Medicine
Beijing

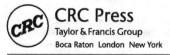

CRC Press
Taylor & Francis Group
Boca Raton London New York

CRC Press is an imprint of the
Taylor & Francis Group, an **informa** business

First edition 2021
CRC Press
6000 Broken Sound Parkway NW, Suite 300, Boca Raton, FL 33487-2742

and by CRC Press
2 Park Square, Milton Park, Abingdon, Oxon, OX14 4RN

Library of Congress Cataloging-in-Publication Data

Names: Xia, Wenguang, editor. | Huang, Xiaolin, editor.
Title: Rehabilitation from COVID-19 : an integrated traditional Chinese and
Western medicine protocol / [edited by] Wenguang Xia, Xiaolin Huang ;
[translated by] Chanjuan Zheng.
Description: Boca Raton : Taylor & Francis, 2021. | Includes
bibliographical references and index.
Identifiers: LCCN 2020058321 (print) | LCCN 2020058322 (ebook) | ISBN
9780367678364 (hardback) | ISBN 9781003143147 (ebook)
Subjects: LCSH: COVID-19 (Disease)--Treatment. | Integrative medicine. |
Medicine, Chinese Traditional.
Classification: LCC RA644.C67 R44 2021 (print) | LCC RA644.C67 (ebook) |
DDC 616.2/414--dc23
LC record available at https://lccn.loc.gov/2020058321
LC ebook record available at https://lccn.loc.gov/2020058322

ISBN: 978-0-367-67836-4 (hbk)
ISBN: 978-0-367-69767-9 (pbk)
ISBN: 978-1-003-14314-7 (ebk)

Typeset in Kepler Std
by Deanta Global Publishing Services, Chennai, India

Contents

Foreword   xix

Preface   xxiii

About the Editors   xxv

Editorial Board of COVID-19 Rehabilitation Diagnosis and
Treatment Guidance of Integrated Traditional Chinese and
Western Medicine   xxvii

1 Clinical Basis of COVID-19   1
   1.1   Etiology   1
   1.2   Epidemiology   2
      1.2.1   Source of Infection   2
      1.2.2   Route of Transmission   2
         1.2.2.1   Respiratory Droplet Transmission   2
         1.2.2.2   Close Contact Transmission   3
         1.2.2.3   Fecal–Oral Transmission   3
         1.2.2.4   Aerosol Transmission   3
         1.2.2.5   Mother-to-Child Transmission   3
      1.2.3   Susceptible Groups   3
      1.2.4   Mortality Rate   4
   1.3   Pathogenesis   4
      1.3.1   Excessive Inflammatory Response and Cytokine Storm   4
      1.3.2   Oxidative Stress (Peroxidation Damage)   5
      1.3.3   Hypoxemia   5
   1.4   Pathology   6
      1.4.1   Lungs   6
      1.4.2   Spleen, Hilar Lymph Nodes, and Bone Marrow   6
      1.4.3   Heart and Blood Vessels   7
      1.4.4   Liver and Gallbladder   7
      1.4.5   Kidney   7
      1.4.6   Other Organs   7
   1.5   Clinical Manifestations   7
      1.5.1   Epidemiological Characteristics   8
      1.5.2   Main Symptoms   8

	1.5.3		Respiratory System Signs	8
	1.5.4		Clinical Outcomes	9
1.6	Laboratory Examination and Imaging Examination			9
	1.6.1		Routine Examination	9
	1.6.2		Virological Testing	9
		1.6.2.1	Virus Nucleic Acid Testing	9
		1.6.2.2	Serological Test	10
	1.6.3		Chest Imaging Examination	11
		1.6.3.1	Chest X-ray	11
		1.6.3.2	Chest CT Examination	11
Bibliography				13

2 Diagnosis and Treatment of COVID-19   15

2.1	Clinical Diagnostic Criteria			15
	2.1.1		Diagnostic Criteria	15
		2.1.1.1	Suspected Cases	15
		2.1.1.2	Confirmed Cases	16
	2.1.2		Clinical Classification	17
		2.1.2.1	Mild	17
		2.1.2.2	Moderate	17
		2.1.2.3	Severe Cases	17
		2.1.2.4	Critically Severe	18
	2.1.3		Warning Signals	18
		2.1.3.1	Adults	19
		2.1.3.2	Children	19
	2.1.4		Auxiliary Examination	19
		2.1.4.1	Laboratory Examination	19
		2.1.4.2	Chest Imaging	20
	2.1.5		Differential Diagnosis	20
		2.1.5.1	Upper Respiratory Disease	20
		2.1.5.2	Other Viral and Mycoplasma Pneumonia	20
		2.1.5.3	Non-Infectious Disease	20
	2.1.6		Reporting and Exclusion System	20
		2.1.6.1	Reporting System	20
		2.1.6.2	Exclusion Criteria	21
2.2	Clinical Treatment			21
	2.2.1		Treatment Place Determination According to the Patient's Condition	21
	2.2.2		General Treatment	22
	2.2.3		Treatment of Severe and Critically Severe Cases	23
		2.2.3.1	Principles of Treatment	23
		2.2.3.2	Respiratory Support	23
		2.2.3.3	Circulation Support	24

		2.2.3.4	Renal Failure and Renal Replacement Therapy	24
		2.2.3.5	Recovered Patients' Plasma Therapy	25
		2.2.3.6	Blood Purification Treatment	25
		2.2.3.7	Immunotherapy	26
		2.2.3.8	Other Treatment Measures	26
		2.2.3.9	Rehabilitation Treatment	26
		2.2.3.10	Psychotherapy	27
	2.2.4	Treatment and Prevention of Complications		28
		2.2.4.1	Prevention of Ventilator-Associated Pneumonia	28
		2.2.4.2	Prevention of Deep Vein Thrombosis	28
		2.2.4.3	Prevention of Catheter-Related Bloodstream Infection	28
		2.2.4.4	Prevention of Stress Ulcers	28
		2.2.4.5	Prevention of ICU-Related Complications	29
	2.2.5	Traditional Chinese Medicine Treatment		29
		2.2.5.1	Medication Observation	29
		2.2.5.2	Clinical Treatment (Confirmed Cases)	29
	2.2.6	Criteria and Precautions after Being Discharged from the Hospital		30
		2.2.6.1	Discharge Criteria	30
		2.2.6.2	Precautions after Being Discharged from the Hospital	30
		2.2.6.3	Re-Positive Nucleic Acid Conversion after Being Discharged from the Hospital	30
Bibliography				31

3 Dysfunctions of COVID-19   **35**
3.1	Respiratory Dysfunction			35
	3.1.1	Dyspnea		35
		3.1.1.1	Definition of Dyspnea	35
		3.1.1.2	Mechanisms That Cause Dyspnea	36
		3.1.1.3	Pathophysiology of Dyspnea	36
	3.1.2	Hypoxemia		38
		3.1.2.1	Hypoventilation	38
		3.1.2.2	Diffusion Impairment	39
		3.1.2.3	Local Ventilation/Blood Flow Disorder	39
		3.1.2.4	Increase of Dead Space	39
		3.1.2.5	Decreased Oxygen-Carrying Capacity	39
	3.1.3	Acute Respiratory Distress Syndrome and Respiratory Failure		40
3.2	Physical Dysfunction			41
	3.2.1	Tachycardias		41
		3.2.1.1	Cause of Tachycardia	41
		3.2.1.2	Heart Rate and Oxygen Uptake	42
	3.2.2	Decreased Exercise Ability and Tolerance		42
		3.2.2.1	Fatigue	43

		3.2.2.2	Immobilization Syndrome	43
3.3	Psychological and Social Dysfunction			44
	3.3.1	Post-Traumatic Stress Disorder (PTSD)		44
		3.3.1.1	Clinical Symptoms of PTSD	45
		3.3.1.2	Prognosis and Influence of PTSD	46
	3.3.2	Adjustment Disorder		46
	3.3.3	Bereavement and Mourning Reaction		47
	3.3.4	Sleep Disorder		47
	3.3.5	Activities of Daily Living Dysfunction		48
	3.3.6	Social Engagement Dysfunction		48
Bibliography				49

4 Assessment for Rehabilitation of COVID-19 — 51

4.1	Assessment for Respiratory Function			51
	4.1.1	Assessment of Respiratory Function		52
		4.1.1.1	Subjective Symptoms	52
		4.1.1.2	Objective Examination	52
	4.1.2	Measurement of Respiratory Muscle Function		54
		4.1.2.1	Measurement of Respiratory Muscle Strength	55
		4.1.2.2	Measurement of Respiratory Muscle Endurance	55
		4.1.2.3	Measurement of Respiratory Muscle Fatigue	55
	4.1.3	Small Airway Function Examination		55
	4.1.4	Common Assessment of Respiratory Function		55
		4.1.4.1	Dyspnea Scale	55
		4.1.4.2	Body-Weight Assessment of Cardiopulmonary Function	56
		4.1.4.3	Cardiopulmonary Exercise Test (CPET)	56
4.2	Assessment of Physical Function			56
	4.2.1	Body-Weight Assessment of Muscle Strength		56
		4.2.1.1	30-Second Chair Standing Test	56
		4.2.1.2	30-Second Arm Curl Test	57
	4.2.2	Assessment of Flexibility		57
		4.2.2.1	Sit-and-Reach Test	57
		4.2.2.2	Improved Twist Test	57
		4.2.2.3	Back-Scratch Test	57
	4.2.3	Assessment of Balance		57
		4.2.3.1	One-Leg Standing Balance Test	57
		4.2.3.2	Functional Reach Test	57
		4.2.3.3	Timed Up and Go Test	57
	4.2.4	Assessment of Pain		57
		4.2.4.1	Single-Dimensional Assessment	57
		4.2.4.2	Multi-Dimensional Assessment	58
4.3	Assessment for Psychosocial Function			58

4.3.1	Assessment of Psychological Function	58
	4.3.1.1 Evaluation of Mental and Psychological State	58
	4.3.1.2 Commonly Used Psychological Assessment Scales	58
4.3.2	Assessment of ADL	59
4.3.3	Health-Related Quality of Life (HRQL) Scale	59
4.3.4	World Health Organization Quality of Life-BREF (WHOQOL-BREF)	60
Bibliography		60

5 Modern Rehabilitation Techniques for COVID-19   61

5.1	Respiratory Rehabilitation Therapy Techniques		62
	5.1.1	Intervention Activities in the Early Stage	62
		5.1.1.1 Respiratory Control Techniques	62
		5.1.1.2 Energy-Saving Techniques	63
	5.1.2	Posture Management	63
		5.1.2.1 For Patients with ARDS	64
		5.1.2.2 For Patients with Sedation or Consciousness Disorders	64
	5.1.3	ACT	64
		5.1.3.1 Effective Cough	65
		5.1.3.2 ACBTs	65
		5.1.3.3 OPEP	67
		5.1.3.4 High-Frequency Chest Wall Oscillation (HFCWO)	67
		5.1.3.5 Postural Drainage Techniques	67
		5.1.3.6 Other Chest Physical Therapy Techniques	67
	5.1.4	Breathing Training	68
		5.1.4.1 Respiratory Pattern Training	69
		5.1.4.2 Relaxation Training	71
		5.1.4.3 Local Dilation Breathing Training	71
	5.1.5	RMT	71
	5.1.6	Breathing Exercises	72
	5.1.7	Respiratory Intervention Techniques	73
		5.1.7.1 Patient's Position	73
		5.1.7.2 Sputum Suction	73
		5.1.7.3 Mechanical/Artificial Dilated Ventilation	73
		5.1.7.4 Precautions in Manual Treatment	74
		5.1.7.5 Precautions for HFCWO	74
		5.1.7.6 Precautions for ACBTs	74
	5.1.8	Principles of Techniques Implementation	74
5.2	Rehabilitation Treatment Techniques for Physical Function		75
	5.2.1	Aerobic Exercise	75
	5.2.2	Strength Training	77
		5.2.2.1 Upper Limbs Strength Training	79

	5.2.2.2	Core Strength Training	81
	5.2.2.3	Lower Limbs Strength Training	81
5.2.3	Balance Training		83
	5.2.3.1	For Patients Who Can't Stand	84
	5.2.3.2	For Patients Who Can Barely Get Up	84
	5.2.3.3	For Patients Who Can Stand on a Flat Surface for a Certain Time	84
5.2.4	Flexibility Training		84
5.2.5	Precautions		85
	5.2.5.1	Pain	85
	5.2.5.2	Fatigue	85
	5.2.5.3	Panting	85
	5.2.5.4	Difficulty in Breathing	85
5.3	Treatment Techniques of Psychosocial Functional Rehabilitation		85
	5.3.1	Activities of Daily Living Training	86
	5.3.1.1	Basic Activities of Daily Living (BADL) Training	86
	5.3.1.2	Instrumental Activities of Daily Living (IADL)	89
	5.3.2	Therapeutic Activities	89
	5.3.2.1	Psychological Therapy	89
	5.3.2.2	Occupational Therapy	90
	5.3.2.3	Social Therapy	90
	5.3.3	Main Techniques and Methods for Psychological Rehabilitation of COVID-19 Patients	90
	5.3.3.1	Supportive Therapy	90
	5.3.3.2	Cognitive Therapy	92
	5.3.4	Behavior Therapy	94
Bibliography			96

6 Traditional Chinese Medicine Rehabilitation Treatment Techniques for COVID-19   **99**
6.1	Treatment with Traditional Chinese Medicine		99
	6.1.1	Principles of Treatment	100
	6.1.2	Treatment Mechanisms	100
	6.1.3	Clinical Manifestations Stage	103
	6.1.3.1	Medical Observation Stage	103
	6.1.3.2	Clinical Treatment Stage	103
6.2	External Treatment Techniques of TCM		107
	6.2.1	Acupuncture Therapy	107
	6.2.1.1	Principles of Treatment	108
	6.2.1.2	Treatment Mechanisms	108
	6.2.1.3	Choice of Acupoints	110
	6.2.1.4	Location of Points	111

6.2.1.5   Operation Method   112
6.2.1.6   Contraindication to Acupuncture   112
6.2.2   Moxibustion Therapy   112
6.2.2.1   Principles of Treatment   112
6.2.2.2   Treatment Mechanism   112
6.2.2.3   Selection of Acupoints   114
6.2.2.4   Operation Method   114
6.2.2.5   Precautions   114
6.2.2.6   Contraindication of Moxibustion   115
6.2.3   Acupoint (Meridian) Massage Therapy   115
6.2.3.1   Principles of Treatment   116
6.2.3.2   Treatment Mechanism   116
6.2.3.3   Selection of Points   116
6.2.3.4   Location of Acupoints   117
6.2.3.5   Operation Method   118
6.2.3.6   Operation Precautions   118
6.2.3.7   Contraindications   118
6.2.4   Acupoint Application Therapy   119
6.2.4.1   Treatment Mechanism   119
6.2.4.2   Operation Method   121
6.2.5   Auricular Acupoint Pressing Therapy   122
6.2.5.1   Treatment Mechanism   122
6.2.5.2   Auricular Point Selection   123
6.2.5.3   Auricular Point Positioning   123
6.2.5.4   Operation Method   124
6.2.5.5   Contraindications   124
6.2.6   Cupping Therapy   124
6.2.6.1   Treatment Mechanism   125
6.2.6.2   Location Selection   126
6.2.6.3   Location   126
6.2.6.4   Operation Methods   126
6.2.6.5   Contraindications   127
6.2.7   Scraping Therapy   127
6.2.7.1   Treatment Mechanism   127
6.2.7.2   Location Selection   128
6.2.7.3   Positioning   128
6.2.7.4   Operation Method   129
6.2.7.5   Contraindications   129
6.2.8   Bloodletting Therapy   129
6.2.8.1   Treatment Mechanism   130
6.2.8.2   Selection of Acupoints   131
6.2.8.3   Location of Acupoints   131

		6.2.8.4 Operation Method	131
		6.2.8.5 Contraindications	132
6.3	Techniques of TCM and Guided Therapy		132
	6.3.1	Baduanjin	132
	6.3.2	Tai Chi Chuan	132
	6.3.3	Five-Animal Exercise	133
	6.3.4	Yi Jin Jing	134
	6.3.5	Liu Zi Jue	134
6.4	Other Therapies		135
	6.4.1	Emotion Therapy of TCM	135
		6.4.1.1 Ancient Chinese Medicine Emotion Therapy	135
		6.4.1.2 Application of Emotion Therapy in Chinese Medicine	138
		6.4.1.3 Precautions	140
	6.4.2	Music Therapy	141
Bibliography			141

7 Diagnosis and Treatment Model of the COVID-19 Rehabilitation Unit   145

7.1	Concept of the COVID-19 Rehabilitation Unit		145
7.2	Role and Significance of the COVID-19 Rehabilitation Unit		147
	7.2.1	Role of the COVID-19 Rehabilitation Unit (CRU)	147
	7.2.2	Significance of Constructing the COVID-19 Rehabilitation Unit	147
		7.2.2.1 Producing Effective Clinical Results	147
		7.2.2.2 Improving the Satisfaction of Patients and Their Families	147
		7.2.2.3 Conducive to Clinical Research on the Rehabilitation of COVID-19	148
7.3	Construction of the COVID-19 Rehabilitation Unit		148
	7.3.1	Types of COVID-19 Rehabilitation Units	148
		7.3.1.1 CRUs in the Ultra-Early Period	148
		7.3.1.2 CRUs in the Early Period	148
		7.3.1.3 CRUs in the Convalescent Period	148
	7.3.2	Conditions for the Establishment of the COVID-19 Rehabilitation Unit	149
		7.3.2.1 Equipment Conditions for Isolation Wards	149
		7.3.2.2 Setting Up Rehabilitation and Treatment Areas	150
		7.3.2.3 Membership of the CRU and Relevant Work	150
7.4	Diagnosis and Treatment Plan for the COVID-19 Rehabilitation Unit		153
	7.4.1	Dysfunction	154
		7.4.1.1 Respiratory Dysfunction	154
		7.4.1.2 Physical Dysfunction	154
		7.4.1.3 Psychological Dysfunction	155

	7.4.1.4	Barriers to Social Participation	155
7.4.2	Work Principles		156
7.4.3	Work Requirements		156
7.4.4	Workflow		156
7.4.5	Diagnosis and Treatment Plan		158
	7.4.5.1	Assess COVID-19 Patients in Detail	158
	7.4.5.2	Hold a CRU Teamwork Group Meeting	158
	7.4.5.3	Contents of Rehabilitation Nursing	158
	7.4.5.4	Treatment Measures	159
	7.4.5.5	Preventing Complications	160
	7.4.5.6	Rehabilitation Therapy	160
	7.4.5.7	TCM Rehabilitation Therapy	160
	7.4.5.8	Extended Rehabilitation Therapy	161

7.5   Common COVID-19 Complications and Their Management   161
    7.5.1   COVID-19 Associated Venous Thromboembolism   161
        7.5.1.1   VTE Risk Factors and Risk Assessment   161
        7.5.1.2   VTE Prevention Advice for Inpatients in the CRU Ward   162
        7.5.1.3   COVID-19 Complicated with DVT   163
    7.5.2   Pressure Ulcers   164
        7.5.2.1   Stages of Pressure Ulcers   164
        7.5.2.2   Treatment of Pressure Ulcers   164
    7.5.3   Urinary Tract Infections   165
    7.5.4   Malnutrition   166
        7.5.4.1   Nutritional Screening and Assessment for COVID-19 Patients   166
        7.5.4.2   Selection of a Nutritional Treatment Plan   166
    7.5.5   Disuse Muscle Weakness and Muscle Atrophy   166
    7.5.6   Joint Contracture   167
    7.5.7   Disuse Osteoporosis   167
Bibliography   168

8 Management of COVID-19 Rehabilitation Nursing   171

8.1   Establishment and Management of the Ward   171
    8.1.1   Establishment of the Rehabilitation Isolation Ward   171
        8.1.1.1   Rational and Scientific Layout   171
        8.1.1.2   Establishment of Nursing Staff   172
    8.1.2   Establishment of the Rehabilitation Isolation Ward   172
        8.1.2.1   Management of Nursing Personnel   172
        8.1.2.2   Disinfection and Isolation Management in the Ward   172
        8.1.2.3   Protection Management of Medical Staff   175
8.2   Rehabilitation Nursing of Chinese and Western Medicine   177
    8.2.1   Objective of Rehabilitation Nursing   177

| | 8.2.2 | Rehabilitation Nursing Assessment | 177 |

8.2.2   Rehabilitation Nursing Assessment   177
   8.2.2.1   Course of Onset and Treatment   178
   8.2.2.2   Psychosocial Data   178
8.2.3   Rehabilitation Nursing Measures   178
   8.2.3.1   Nursing Guidance and Training Techniques for Respiratory Function   179
   8.2.3.2   Nursing Guidance and Training Techniques for Effective Coughing   182
   8.2.3.3   Nursing Guidance and Training Techniques of Postural Drainage   184
   8.2.3.4   Nursing Guidance and Training Techniques for Enhancing Muscle Strength and Endurance   185
   8.2.3.5   Psychological Rehabilitation Nursing   187
8.2.4   TCM Nursing   188
   8.2.4.1   Instructions for Taking TCM Decoctions   188
   8.2.4.2   Appropriate TCM Nursing Techniques   188
   8.2.4.3   Emotion Nursing   190
8.3   Discharge Guidance and Health Education   191
  8.3.1   Attention to Diet   191
  8.3.2   Adherence to Breathing Training and Activities   192
  8.3.3   Disease Prevention   192
Bibliography   192

9   Clinical Rehabilitation of COVID-19   195
9.1   Guiding Principles and Connotations of Rehabilitation Intervention   195
  9.1.1   Guiding Principles of Rehabilitation   195
    9.1.1.1   Adherence to the Whole-Course Psychological Intervention   195
    9.1.1.2   Safe and Effective Improvement of Cardiopulmonary Function   195
    9.1.1.3   Gradual and Steady Improvement of Physical Fitness   196
  9.1.2   Connotations of Rehabilitation Intervention   196
    9.1.2.1   Improvement/Enhancement of Cardiopulmonary Function   196
    9.1.2.2   Enhancement of Activity/Physical Strength   196
    9.1.2.3   Positive Health Education, Rehabilitation Guidance, and Psychological Treatment   196
9.2   Clinical Management of Rehabilitation Diagnosis and Treatment   197
  9.2.1   Relevant Policies and Basis in Rehabilitation Diagnosis and Treatment   197
  9.2.2   Process Management of Rehabilitation Diagnosis and Treatment   197
    9.2.2.1   Working Principles   197

		9.2.2.2	Safety Precautions	198
		9.2.2.3	Overall Objective	198
		9.2.2.4	Job Description	198
		9.2.2.5	Diagnosis and Treatment Procedures	199
		9.2.2.6	Precautions	199
		9.2.2.7	Prerequisites for Intervention	199
		9.2.2.8	Suspension and Withdrawal of Rehabilitation Treatment	202
	9.3	Different Clinical Types and Stages of Rehabilitation Treatment		203
		9.3.1	Rehabilitation for Hospitalized Patients with COVID-19	203
			9.3.1.1 Rehabilitation Treatment for Mild Patients	203
			9.3.1.2 Rehabilitation Treatment for Moderate Patients	205
			9.3.1.3 Rehabilitation Treatment for Severe/Critically Severe Patients	207
		9.3.2	Rehabilitation Treatment of COVID-19 Patients after Being Discharged from the Hospital	209
			9.3.2.1 Rehabilitation Treatment for Mild/Moderate Discharged Patients	210
			9.3.2.2 Rehabilitation Treatment for Discharged Patients with Severe/Critically Severe Disease	211
	Bibliography			214

10	**Psychological Rehabilitation of COVID-19**			**217**
	10.1	Assessment of Psychological Disorders		217
		10.1.1	Role and Purpose of Psychological Disorder Assessments	218
			10.1.1.1 Role of Psychological Disorder Assessments	218
			10.1.1.2 Purpose of Psychological Disorder Assessments	218
		10.1.2	Appropriate Population for Assessment of Psychological Disorders and Their Psychological Characteristics	218
		10.1.3	Psychological Assessment Methods	219
			10.1.3.1 Interview	220
			10.1.3.2 Observation	220
			10.1.3.3 Work Analysis	220
			10.1.3.4 Psychological Tests	220
			10.1.3.5 Medical Tests	221
		10.1.4	Psychological Assessment of COVID-19 Patients	222
			10.1.4.1 Assessment of Emotions and Feelings	222
			10.1.4.2 Assessment of Stress	223
			10.1.4.3 Observation and Medical Testing	225
		10.1.5	Prospects	225
	10.2	Treatment of Psychological Disorders		225
		10.2.1	Objectives of Psychological Rehabilitation	226

10.2.2	Objects of Psychological Rehabilitation	226
10.2.3	Principles of Psychological Rehabilitation Treatment	226
10.2.4	Psychological Rehabilitation Treatment Methods	226
	10.2.4.1 Psychological Support Therapy	226
	10.2.4.2 Focus Solution Mode	227
	10.2.4.3 Music Therapy	228
	10.2.4.4 Cognition Therapy	228
	10.2.4.5 Behavior Modification Therapy	229
	10.2.4.6 Relaxation Therapy	231
	10.2.4.7 Group Psychotherapy	231
	10.2.4.8 Family Psychotherapy	232
	10.2.4.9 Biofeedback Therapy	232
	10.2.4.10 Physical Factor Therapy	233
	10.2.4.11 Exercise Training	233
	10.2.4.12 Occupational Therapy	233
	10.2.4.13 TCM Therapy	233
	10.2.4.14 Traditional Exercise Therapy	234
	10.2.4.15 Pharmacotherapy	234
	10.2.4.16 Health Education	234
10.2.5	Determination of Psychological Rehabilitation Treatment Prescription	234
	10.2.5.1 Confirmed COVID-19 Patients	234
	10.2.5.2 Patients with Respiratory Distress, Extreme Restlessness, and Difficulty in Expression	235
	10.2.5.3 Mild Patients for Home Isolation and Patients with Fever for Treatment	235
	10.2.5.4 Suspected Patients	235
	10.2.5.5 Medical Staff and Related Personnel	236
	10.2.5.6 People Who Are in Close Contact with Patients (Family Members, Colleagues, Friends, etc.)	236
	10.2.5.7 People Who Are Reluctant to Seek Medical Treatment in Public	236
	10.2.5.8 Susceptible Groups and the General Public	236
10.2.6	Forms of Psychological Rehabilitation Counseling	237
Bibliography		237

11	**Assessment and Treatment for Malnutrition of COVID-19 Patients**		**239**
11.1	Overview		239
11.2	Assessment of Malnutrition		241
	11.2.1	Nutrition Risk Screening	241

		11.2.1.1	NRS-2002 Assessment Scale for Reduced Nutritional Status Score and Its Definition	242
		11.2.1.2	NRS-2002 Assessment Scale for the Severity of Disease and Its Definition	242
		11.2.1.3	Relationship between the NRS-2002 Assessment Scale Score Results and Nutrition Risk	242
		11.2.1.4	NRS-2002 Score Significance for COVID-19 Patients	244
	11.2.2	Commonly Used Nutritional Status Evaluation Indicators for Nutritional Assessment		244
		11.2.2.1	Nutrition History	244
		11.2.2.2	Anthropometry	244
		11.2.2.3	Laboratory Investigations	246
11.3	Nutritional Support Therapy			247
	11.3.1	Medical and Nutritional Treatment Recommendations for COVID-19 Patients		248
	11.3.2	Nutritional Treatment Plan for COVID-19 Patients		248
		11.3.2.1	Purpose of Nutritional Therapy	248
		11.3.2.2	General Principles of Nutritional Therapy	249
		11.3.2.3	Nutritional Treatment Approaches for COVID-19 Patients	249
		11.3.2.4	Amount of Nutritional Feeding for COVID-19 Patients	250
		11.3.2.5	Recommended Intake of Special Nutrients for Severe COVID-19 Patients	251
11.4	Dietary Guidance			252
	11.4.1	Dietary Guidance for Different Populations of COVID-19		253
		11.4.1.1	Nutritional Diet for Ordinary or Convalescent Patients	253
		11.4.1.2	Nutritional Treatment for Patients with Severe Syndrome	253
		11.4.1.3	Nutritional Dietary Guidance for Frontline Workers	254
		11.4.1.4	Nutritional Dietary Guidance for Prevention and Control among the General Population	255
	11.4.2	TCM Diet Guidance		256
		11.4.2.1	First Prescription	256
		11.4.2.2	Second Prescription	256
		11.4.2.3	Third Prescription	257
Bibliography				257

12 Community- and Home-Based Rehabilitation of COVID-19 — 259

| 12.1 | Community-Based Rehabilitation | 259 |

12.1.1   Dysfunction Requiring Rehabilitation Treatment   260
          12.1.1.1   Dysfunction of Daily Living Ability and Social
                      Participation   260
          12.1.1.2   Respiratory Dysfunction   260
          12.1.1.3   Physical Dysfunction   260
          12.1.1.4   Psychological Dysfunction   261
12.1.2   Goals of Rehabilitation   261
12.1.3   Process of Rehabilitation   261
12.1.4   Implementation of Rehabilitation Treatment   262
12.1.5   Content of Rehabilitation   262
          12.1.5.1   Rehabilitation Evaluation   262
          12.1.5.2   Rehabilitation Treatment   262
          12.1.5.3   Configuration and Use of Auxiliary Appliances   263
12.2 Home-Based Rehabilitation   264
12.2.1   Traditional Methods   265
          12.2.1.1   Baduanjin   265
          12.2.1.2   Simplified Tai Chi Chuan   269
          12.2.1.3   Five-Animal Exercise   271
          12.2.1.4   Yi Jin Jing   276
12.2.2   Rehabilitation Exercise of Respiratory Function   286
          12.2.2.1   Position Management   286
          12.2.2.2   Airway Clearance Technology   286
          12.2.2.3   Respiratory Muscle Training   287
12.2.3   Physical Function Rehabilitation Exercises   288
          12.2.3.1   Aerobic Exercise   288
          12.2.3.2   Strength Training   289
          12.2.3.3   Flexibility Training   294
          12.2.3.4   Balance Training   294
12.2.4   Oxygen Therapy   294
12.2.5   ADL Intervention   296
12.2.6   Psychological Reconstruction   296
12.2.7   Diet Adjustment   296
12.3 Contraindications and precautions   297
12.3.1   Contraindications   297
12.3.2   Precautions   297
Bibliography   298

Appendices: Related Rating Scales   301

Index   337

Foreword

Since COVID-19 was first diagnosed in Wuhan in December 2019, it has posed a serious threat to public health due to its widespread infectivity and strong pathogenicity. Due to the absence of confirmed targeted drugs and vaccines, the prevention, control and treatment of COVID-19 are extremely difficult. However, under the correct leadership of the Party Central Committee, the medical workers strictly followed the guidance of General Secretary Xi Jinping, including "follow the law of development of TCM [traditional Chinese medicine], inherit the essence, and maintain integrity and innovation", "attach importance to both Chinese and Western medicine", "strengthen the cooperation of Chinese and Western medicine, and establish a joint consultation system for Chinese and Western medicine", to actively carry out antipandemic work, and has achieved world-renowned results. Practice has proven that TCM has played an irreplaceable role in the battle against this major pandemic, complementing and coordinating with the strengths of Western medicine and has achieved good clinical results. In the thousands of years of history of the Chinese nation, pandemics had invaded China repeatedly. The Huangdi Neijing states that "the five pandemics are easily infected, no matter how big or small they are, and all have similar symptoms". When reviewing the history of TCM in fighting against pandemics, TCM has played an important role in respiratory pandemics, especially severe acute respiratory syndrome (SARS) in 2003 and the H1N1 influenza in 2009. COVID-19 is categorized as a "plague" as per Chinese medicine. It is called a "damp toxin pandemic" according to the epidemiological investigation of its characteristics and syndrome elements. Summarizing the clinical experience and prevention policies of the fight against COVID-19, giving full play to the advantages of integrated traditional Chinese and Western medicine, and improving and optimizing treatment programs with Chinese characteristics will contribute to the global fight against the pandemic through the insights and experiences of China.

The lead writing unit of this book is the Integrated Traditional Chinese and Western Medicine Hospital of Hubei Province. It is the first medical institution to report the novel coronavirus pneumonia in Wuhan, and it is also the first unit undertaking the establishment of novel coronavirus pneumonia emergency wartime projects by the Ministry of Science and Technology. During the fight against the pandemic, it is also the first hospital to publish a paper on the treatment of novel coronavirus pneumonia with integrated traditional Chinese and Western medicine. At the same time, they are also the first hospital in the country to establish and operate a COVID-19 rehabilitation ward, which provided the Hubei Provincial headquarters with a COVID-19 integrated traditional Chinese and Western medicine rehabilitation diagnosis and treatment plan, compiled popular science manuals and work manuals for novel coronavirus pneumonia, and accumulated a lot of clinical experience in rehabilitation of integrated Chinese and Western medicine. The main participants in this book are experts from Tongji Hospital Affiliated to Huazhong University of Science and Technology, Union Hospital of Huazhong University of Science and Technology, People's Hospital of Wuhan University, Zhongnan Hospital of Wuhan University, and Beijing Hospital of Traditional Chinese Medicine Affiliated to Capital Medical University, which is rushing to help Wuhan. They participated in the compilation of the book, gave the detailed explanations on the basic theories of traditional Chinese and Western medicine, disease characteristics, epidemiology, clinical treatment, and rehabilitation of integrated traditional Chinese and Western medicine, especially the description of the psychological intervention, home and community rehabilitation guidance, which provides guidance and assistance to medical workers in tertiary hospitals, county and city hospitals, and community health service centers engaged in the diagnosis and treatment of COVID-19. The content of this book covers the whole rehabilitation work guidance for outpatient service, hospitalization, and discharge. This book is based on clinical practice and introduces in detail the TCM rehabilitation technology. It is a pioneering work on the rehabilitation of COVID-19 that concentrates on the essence of Chinese and Western medicine rehabilitation and plays an exemplary role in the rehabilitation guidance for convalescent patients in particular. In summary, the work is highly scientific and practical.

Under the correct leadership and unified deployment of the Party Central Committee with General Secretary Xi Jinping as the core, and under the inspiration of the sincerity and spirit of universal salvation of millions of Chinese and Western doctors, hundreds of millions of soldiers and civilians have united and worked bravely. Wuhan, this heroic city, is about to usher in an all-out victory in this battle. "The mountains and rivers are full of spring, and the family and the country are in good condition". Spring has arrived as scheduled, and the pandemic will eventually subside, but this battle will be recorded in history and be remembered forever. "Dare to forget the suffering of Jiangcheng in two months, and one hundred thousand white armor will fight hard". And our medical workers still have a long way to go!

Boli Zhang (*at Wuhan East Lake*)
Academician of Chinese Academy of Engineering
Honorary Dean of China Academy of Chinese Medical Sciences
President of Tianjin University of Traditional Chinese Medicine

Preface

With the continuous progress of clinical treatment for COVID-19 in China, the number of confirmed cases in Wuhan and other provinces and cities has been cleared up so far, indicating a phased victory in the battle against the pneumonia pandemic. In order to further consolidate the layered and refined management of COVID-19 patients and construct an integrated prevention–treatment–rehabilitation diagnosis and treatment model, the rehabilitation intervention of COVID-19 is of great urgency. In response to this, the Integrated Traditional Chinese and Western Medicine Hospital of Hubei Province, as the first unit in the country to carry out the COVID-19 rehabilitation wards, took the lead in compiling the *Rehabilitation from COVID-19: An Integrated Traditional Chinese and Western Medicine Protocol* to provide timely and individualized rehabilitation treatment for COVID-19 patients with impairments in respiratory, physical, other organ, and psychological functions, which will help COVID-19 patients recover their lung and motor function and the ability of daily living as much as possible as well as shorten the course of disease, reduce sequelae, promote social harmony and progress, and provide reference for the global fight against the pandemic and subsequent response to various major pandemics.

Regarding the rehabilitation of COVID-19, this book explains the integrated traditional Chinese and Western medicine rehabilitation treatment of mild, ordinary, severe, and critical patients in the acute and recovery phases and gives a comprehensive description from the aspects of the rehabilitation goals, rehabilitation assessment, rehabilitation treatment and the guidance for home rehabilitation. The content is informative, in particular, how the early exploration of the COVID-19 rehabilitation unit applied the method of combining theory with practice and provides a reference for the rehabilitation treatment of infectious diseases in our country through a clear rehabilitation flowchart. In terms of rehabilitation evaluation of COVID-19, according to the concept of bio–psycho–social medical model and the needs of rehabilitation medicine, the rehabilitation evaluation method of COVID-19 is introduced in detail. Different rehabilitation plans have been developed for the guidance of outpatient, hospitalization, and home and community rehabilitation. The indications and contraindications of related rehabilitation treatment techniques and various complications associated with the disease are also introduced. The content is extensive and highly practical, therefore this work can be promoted and applied nationwide.

Given the special stage of the pandemic, the limited timeline for writing the book, and multiple organizations and multiple authors, there may be inconsistencies in level and style. However, the book is rich in content and meets the actual needs of the majority of medical workers. Its content ranges from medical, technical, and nursing, to Chinese and Western medicine rehabilitation, thus can provide practical and feasible rehabilitation diagnosis and treatment paths for clinical practice.

Director of World Health Organization Rehabilitation Training and Research Cooperation Center

Vice President of Chinese Association of Rehabilitation Medicine

Director of Rehabilitation Medicine Department of Tongji Hospital Affiliated to Tongji Medical College of Huazhong University of Science and Technology, Doctoral Supervisor

Xiaolin Huang
March 2020 in Wuhan

About the Editors

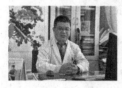**Wenguang Xia**, Doctor of Medicine, Chief Physician, Master's Supervisor, Vice President of Integrated Traditional Chinese and Western Medicine Hospital of Hubei Province, Academic Leader of Rehabilitation Medical Center, Director of Integrated Traditional Chinese and Western Medicine Rehabilitation Clinical Medicine Research Center of Hubei Province, Director of Rehabilitation Medicine of Hubei Association of Integrated Traditional Chinese and Western Medicine, Director of Rehabilitation Medical Education of Hubei Rehabilitation Medical Association, Deputy Director of Physical Medicine and Rehabilitation of Hubei Medical Association, Executive Director and Deputy Secretary General of Hubei Association of Rehabilitation Medicine, Executive Director and Deputy Secretary General of Hubei Association of Integrated Traditional Chinese and Western Medicine, Deputy Leader of the Rehabilitation Group of Physical Medicine and Rehabilitation of Chinese Medical Association, Standing Member of the Rehabilitation Medicine Branch of Chinese Association of Integrated Traditional Chinese and Western Medicine, Member of Rehabilitation Physician Branch of Chinese Physician Association, and Member of Physical Medicine and Rehabilitation Youth Committee of Chinese Medical Association, etc. Wenguang is a visiting scholar at the University of Hong Kong and the State University New York (SUNY) Upstate Medical University in the United States; Wenguang are one of the leading medical talents in Hubei Province and the young and middle-aged medical talents in Wuhan city. Wenguang has published more than 50 papers in the past five years, including eight Science Citation Idex (SCI) papers and three medical monographs as editor-in-chief. Wenguang is an editorial board member of the *Chinese Journal of Physical Medicine and Rehabilitation* and a specially appointed reviewer for *China Rehabilitation*. Wenguang has presided over more than 10 projects for the National Scholarship Fund, National Health Commission, and Provincial Natural Fund, and won the Science and Technology Progress Award of Hubei Province. His main research direction is neurological rehabilitation and severe disease rehabilitation. He specializes in the integration of traditional Chinese and Western medicine to evaluate, diagnose, and treat post-stroke dysfunction.

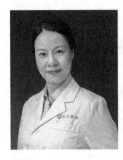

Xiaolin Huang, Professor, Chief Physician, Doctoral Supervisor, Director of Rehabilitation Medicine Teaching and Research Section (Department) of Tongji Hospital Affiliated to Tongji Medical College of Huazhong University of Science and Technology, Director of World Health Organization Rehabilitation Training and Research Cooperation Center, Vice President of Chinese Rehabilitation Medical Association, Vice Chairman of Physical Medicine and Rehabilitation Association of Chinese Medical Association, Vice Chairman of Rehabilitation Medicine Branch of China Medical Care International Exchange Promotion Association, Chairman of Hubei Rehabilitation Medical Association, Director of Hubei Rehabilitation Medical Quality Control Center, etc. Xiaolin is also the chief editor of the *Chinese Journal of Physical Medicine and Rehabilitation*, the chief editor of the *China Rehabilitation* journal, the deputy editor of *Neurological Injury and Functional Reconstruction*, the deputy editor of *Journal of Rehabilitation*, and an editorial board member for *Chinese Journal of Rehabilitation Medicine*. Xiaolin's areas of expertise include, clinical medicine, teaching and scientific research. Her specialties include neurological rehabilitation, rehabilitation of spine, bone, and joint injuries. In recent years, she has presided over the National 863 Program, the National Natural Science Foundation, the National Support Program, the Ministry of Education's Doctoral Fund for Overseas Studies, the International Cooperative Scientific Research Program, and the Key Science and Technology Projects of Hubei Province. She has participated in the key clinical discipline project of medical institutions of the Ministry of Health, the key research project of the "Tenth Five-Year Plan" of the Ministry of Science and Technology, and the major research plan funded by the National Natural Science Foundation of China.

Editorial Board of COVID-19 Rehabilitation Diagnosis and Treatment Guidance of Integrated Traditional Chinese and Western Medicine

Chapter 1
Clinical Basis of COVID-19

COVID-19 is an acute infectious disease caused by the novel coronavirus. It is mainly transmitted by respiratory droplets and can also be transmitted by contact. The clinical symptoms are mainly fever, dry cough, fatigue, and gradual dyspnea. Severe cases may develop into acute respiratory distress syndrome. The World Health Organization (WHO) has officially named the disease COVID-19. This disease is a new infectious and highly contagious disease.

1.1 ETIOLOGY

2019-nCoV is an RNA virus that is widely found in humans and animals. It belongs to the coronavirus family of the nest virus order and belongs to the β genus of coronavirus. The coronavirus genus has an envelope. The particles are round, oval, or pleomorphic, with a diameter of 60 nm–140 nm. Its genetic characteristics are obviously different from those of severe acute respiratory syndrome coronavirus (SARS-CoV) and Middle East respiratory syndrome coronavirus (MERS-CoV). Current research has shown that it is most similar to the bat SARS-like coronavirus (bat-SL-CoVZC45) of the Chinese chrysanthemum bat, with nucleotide homology reaching more than 85%. It shares approximately 78% and 50% homology to SARS virus and MERS virus, respectively, which once brought grave disasters to China.

How does the 2019-nCoV work? The spike protein (S protein) on the surface of the virus enters the host cell by interacting with specific receptors on the cell surface. Then it enters the cell through membrane fusion and releases its genome into the cytoplasm. The virus mainly binds to angiotensin-converting enzyme 2 (ACE2) via the S protein on its surface. During fusion, the S protein undergoes structural rearrangement to fuse the viral membrane with the host cell membrane, thereby infecting human respiratory epithelial cells. It has a higher affinity than SARS-CoV and, therefore, is more infectious.

1

When isolated and cultured *in vitro*, 2019-nCoV can be found in human respiratory epithelial cells in about 96 hours, while it takes about 6 days to isolate and culture in Vero E6 and Huh-7 cell lines.

The physicochemical properties of COVID-19 are mainly understood from studies on SARS-CoV and MERS-CoV. The virus is sensitive to ultraviolet rays and heat and can be effectively inactivated by 56°C for 30 minutes, ethyl ether, 75% ethanol, chlorine-containing disinfectant, peracetic acid, chloroform, and other lipid solvents; however, chlorhexidine cannot kill the virus effectively.

1.2 EPIDEMIOLOGY

1.2.1 Source of Infection

It is currently believed that the source of infection is mainly COVID-19 patients, with an incubation period of 1–14 days, mostly 3–7 days. There are very few cases with an incubation period of more than 14 days, but the longest can even reach 24 days. Infected yet asymptomatic patients and patients who do not show obvious clinical symptoms due to weak immune system stress response or their own physical characteristics do carry the virus and can infect others. Because there are no clinical symptoms, asymptomatic infected persons are not easily detected, and even the patients themselves are not aware of the infection, which is difficult to control and get them isolated in time, thus it could easily cause large-scale transmission.

1.2.2 Route of Transmission

Transmission through respiratory droplets and close contact are the main route of transmission. There is a possibility of aerosol transmission in a relatively closed environment when exposed to high concentrations of aerosols for a long period of time. Because 2019-nCoV can be isolated in feces and urine, attention should be paid to the aerosol or contact transmission caused by feces and urine pollution to the environment. The possibilities of other routes of transmission require further research.

1.2.2.1 Respiratory Droplet Transmission
Respiratory droplet transmission is the main mode of the transmission of 2019-nCoV. The virus is spread through droplets produced when patients cough, sneeze, and talk, and those who are susceptible will be infected after inhalation.

1.2.2.2 Close Contact Transmission

2019-nCoV can also be transmitted through indirect contact with infected patients. Indirect contact transmission means that people come into contact with the droplets containing the virus through touching the surface of objects, and then touch their mouth, nose, eyes, and other mucous membranes, resulting in infection.

1.2.2.3 Fecal–Oral Transmission

Fecal–oral transmission occurs when bacteria or viruses found in the stool enter the human respiratory tract and digestive tract and thus infect people. Whether there is a fecal–oral transmission route for 2019-nCoV is to be determined. It is also believed that the virus in feces may be transmitted by aerosol formed by droplets containing the virus, which also requires further investigation.

1.2.2.4 Aerosol Transmission

Aerosol transmission refers to when the respiratory droplets lose water in the air, and the leftover proteins and pathogens form nuclei or dust that float far away in the form of aerosols, causing long-distance transmissions, and the range of transmission can vary from tens of meters to hundreds of meters.

1.2.2.5 Mother-to-Child Transmission

At present, a case has been reported in which the mother was a confirmed COVID-19 patient, and the throat swab for viral nucleic acid detection showed positive for the 30-hour-old infant, suggesting that 2019-nCoV may cause neonatal infection through mother-to-child transmission, and there is vertical mother-to-child transmission; however, preliminary evidence suggests that infection in the third trimester of pregnancy does not cause vertical transmission.

Other studies suggest that the urinary system might also be a potential route for COVID-19 infection. It has been proven through scientific experiments that the virus will not spread through skin penetration.

1.2.3 Susceptible Groups

As it is a new infectious disease, the mass population generally has no resistance. In terms of age, the ability to resist the virus is no different for people of all age groups, and everyone is susceptible under suitable conditions. The probability of infection increases among the elderly and people with underlying diseases. Children and pregnant and lying-in women are vulnerable to 2019-nCoV infection.

1.2.4 Mortality Rate

On the whole, COVID-19 spreads faster than SARS, with high risk and low mortality rate, but its mortality rate of severe patients is higher than that of SARS and MERS.

1.3 PATHOGENESIS

COVID-19 is a systemic multiorgan injury disease, with the lung as the main target organ. Its pathophysiological mechanisms involve inflammation, fever, hypoxia, water, electrolytes, acid–base balance disorder, shock, and other basic pathological processes. Excessive activation of immune cells, excessive oxidative stress caused by cytokine storm, and hypoxemia may be the common pathophysiological basis for COVID-19 to cause acute respiratory distress syndrome (ARDS), septic shock, and multiple organ failure leading to death.

1.3.1 Excessive Inflammatory Response and Cytokine Storm

ACE2 is the binding receptor of 2019-nCoV, and the specific mutation of base T at the 501st site of the genome of 2019-nCoV enhances its ability to bind to human ACE2. ACE2 is widely expressed in various tissues of the human body, and it is most abundant in alveolar epithelium, small intestinal epithelium, and vascular endothelial cells. However, most COVID-19 patients are characterized by pulmonary manifestations with a few having diarrhea, suggesting that the lungs are the main target organ of 2019-nCoV.

After entering the cell, the virus can induce the release of cytokines, such as monocyte chemoattractant protein 1 (MCP-1), granulocyte-macrophage colony-stimulating factor (GM-CSF), and macrophage colony-stimulating factor (M-CSF), which can be activated by binding to the corresponding receptors on the macrophage surface. Activated macrophages can recruit a large number of mononuclear phagocytes on the one hand, and initiate a specific immune response on the other hand, and at the same time produce and release a large number of interleukin-1β (IL-1β), tumor necrosis factor-α (TNF-α), interleukin-6 (IL-6), MCP-1 and other inflammatory factors, causing tissue damage. MCP-1 can also promote the synthesis of angiotensin II (Ang), further aggravating the inflammatory response. It is speculated that after infection, 2019-nCoV activates immune cells, releases TNFα, IL-1, interferon, chemokines, etc.; mediates a large number of immune cells to gather and infiltrate lung tissues; and activates intracellular signal transduction pathways to initiate inflammatory cascade. The joint reaction releases a large number of cytokines and continuously activates more inflammatory cells, forming a vicious cycle, which eventually leads to a cytokine storm. The combination of coronavirus and ACE2 leads to the decrease in the available amount of ACE2, and the conversion of Ang II to Ang (1-7) is inhibited. The Ang II produced through ACE2 increases continuously, which leads to the accumulation of Ang II, thereby aggravating the inflammatory response.

1.3.2 Oxidative Stress (Peroxidation Damage)

Under physiological conditions, the body's reactive oxygen species (ROS) are in a low level of dynamic equilibrium under the regulation of oxidation and anti-oxidant systems. Pathological factors, such as viral infection, may cause excessive production of ROS or insufficient removal. Excessive ROS can cause lipid oxidation, protein damage, and DNA breakage, leading to and aggravating tissue damage. Inflammatory cells and inflammatory mediators are the main factors that initiate and maintain the early inflammatory response and play a key role in the occurrence and development of ARDS. Inflammatory cytokines are released by inflammatory cells, leading to the accumulation and activation of large numbers of neutrophils in lungs and the release of oxygen free radicals through "respiratory burst", which can lead to tissue and cell damage. After virus infection, the glycolysis pathway of host cells is significantly enhanced, which not only provides energy for the survival and replication of the virus but also mediates the production of large amounts of ROS. The overactivation of immune cells caused by viral infection and the maintenance of persistent inflammatory phenotype depend on immune cells regulating the production of cytokines and ROS through metabolic transformation.

1.3.3 Hypoxemia

The main mechanisms of hypoxemia in COVID-19 patients are as follows: firstly, inflammation damages alveolar epithelial cells and pulmonary capillary endothelial cells and increases alveolar-capillary membrane permeability, causing pulmonary interstitial and alveolar edema and affecting oxygen diffusion. Secondly, the decrease of pulmonary surfactant and the increase of alveolar surface tension result in alveolar collapse due to the decreased number of alveoli that effectively participate in gas exchange and imbalanced ventilation/blood flow ratio. Serious hypoxemia is a pathological feature of ARDS and is an important factor that causes and aggravates the functional damage of various organs in the whole body. Not only does hypoxia directly cause extensive tissue and cell damage, it also causes or aggravates inflammatory response, oxidative stress, and other damaging pathophysiological processes, which may be an important mechanism for the occurrence and development of COVID-19. Hypoxia can increase the expression of adhesion molecules, such as intercellular adhesion molecules of pulmonary vascular endothelial cells-1 (ICAM 1), vascular cell adhesion molecule-1 (VACM-1), and E-selection. It can also promote the adhesion of leukocytes to pulmonary vascular endothelium, cause the inflammatory cell infiltration in lung tissue and the increased secretion of a large number of inflammatory cytokines activated by alveolar macrophages, and enhance TLR4 signaling pathway triggered by LPS, amplifying the inflammatory response. Hypoxia can also cause oxidative stress damage to various tissues and cells.

1.4 PATHOLOGY

The main pathological characteristics of COVID-19 summarized as follows are based on the limited current histopathological observations of autopsy and needle biopsies.

1.4.1 Lungs

The lungs demonstrated different degrees of consolidation. The formation of serous fluid, fibrinous exudate, and transparent membrane was found in alveolar cavity. The exuding cells were mainly monocytes and macrophages, and polynuclear giant cells were easily seen. Type II alveolar epithelial cells proliferated significantly, and some cells fell off. Inclusion bodies could be seen in Type II alveolar epithelial cells and macrophages. The blood vessels of alveolar septum were congested and edematous, with infiltration of monocytes and lymphocytes and intravascular hyaline thrombosis. For focal hemorrhage and necrosis of lung tissue, hemorrhagic infarction may occur. Partial alveolar exudation and pulmonary interstitial fibrosis also appeared. Part of the epithelium of the bronchial mucosa in the lungs fell off, and mucus and mucus plug could be found in the cavity. A few alveoli were overinflated; the alveolar septum was broken or a cyst had formed. Coronavirus particles could be found in the cytoplasm of bronchial mucosal epithelium and Type II alveolar epithelial cells under electron microscope. Immunohistochemical staining showed that some alveolar epithelium and macrophages were positive for 2019-nCoV antigen, and real-time quantitative polymerase chain reaction (PCR) (reverse transcription [RT-PCR]) was positive for 2019-nCoV nucleic acid.

1.4.2 Spleen, Hilar Lymph Nodes, and Bone Marrow

The size of the spleen was reduced significantly. The number of lymphocytes were significantly reduced, the spleen had focal hemorrhage and necrosis, and macrophage proliferation and phagocytosis were observed. The number of lymph cells in lymph nodes were reduced and necrosis was seen. Immunohistochemical staining revealed that CD4+ and CD8+T cells in the spleen and lymph nodes were reduced. The number of bone marrow trilineage cells decreased.

1.4.3 Heart and Blood Vessels

Degeneration and necrosis could be seen in cardiomyocytes, and a few monocytes, lymphocytes, and/or neutrophils infiltration was seen in the interstitium. Part of the blood vessel endothelium peeled off, and intimal inflammation and thrombosis were formed.

1.4.4 Liver and Gallbladder

The sizes of the liver and gallbladder were enlarged, and were dark red in color. Histopathological observations shows hepatocyte degeneration and focal necrosis with neutrophil infiltration; hepatic sinus was congestive, lymphocyte and monocyte infiltration in the portal area were seen, and microthrombus was formed. The gallbladder was highly filled.

1.4.5 Kidney

Protein exudate was seen in the glomerular cavity. The renal tubules were epithelialized and exfoliated, with hyaline cast. The interstitial congestion, microthrombus and focal fibrosis were seen.

1.4.6 Other Organs

Congestion, edema, and degeneration of some neurons were observed in brain tissue. Focal necrosis of adrenal glands were seen. The mucosal epithelium of the esophagus, stomach, and intestine degenerated, necrotized, and fell off to varying degrees.

1.5 CLINICAL MANIFESTATIONS

Based on current clinical data, the clinical symptoms and signs of COVID-19 mainly include the following.

1.5.1 Epidemiological Characteristic

The incubation period of the disease is 1–4 days, mostly 3–7 days.

1.5.2 Main Symptoms

The main manifestations include fever, dry cough, and fatigue. A small number of patients experience nasal congestion, runny nose, sore throat, myalgia, and diarrhea. It is worth noting that, during the course of severe and critically severe cases, patients may have moderate to low fever or even no obvious fever. In some cases of children and newborns, the symptoms may be atypical, manifested as vomiting, diarrhea, and other digestive tract symptoms or only manifested as mental weakness and shortness of breath. Patients with mild cases show the symptoms of only a low fever and mild fatigue, without manifestations of pneumonia. At present, there are a few reports that patients with 2019-nCoV infection may suffer from genitourinary system and nervous system damage, and clinicians should also be vigilant about the relevant conditions.

Typical patients with severe respiratory symptoms develop rapidly into pneumonia after infection. Due to the systemic inflammatory reaction and immune system dysfunction caused by viral infection, various systems of the human body may be damaged to varying degrees. In the course of disease progression, there will be acute myocardial damage, sudden heart rate decline, weakened heart sound, and other manifestations of cardiac impairments, as well as proteinuria, elevated plasma creatinine and urea nitrogen levels, and abnormal renal imaging manifestations. In a small number of patients, the disease progresses rapidly, with dyspnea and/or hypoxemia 1 week after onset, followed by acute respiratory distress syndrome, septic shock, refractory metabolic acidosis, coagulation dysfunction, and multiple organ failure, resulting in a life-threatening condition.

1.5.3 Respiratory System Signs

It is generally believed that the lung signs of COVID-19 are mostly nonspecific. Patients may experience a rapid breathing rate due to hypoxia, and patients with severe respiratory difficulties may even show symptoms of orthopnea. Lung auscultation may cause abnormal breath sounds in the affected lung segments, most of which are reduced sounds or disappeared sounds, but moist rales sounds are rare.

1.5.4 Clinical Outcomes

The progression or outcome of COVID-19 patients varies. Judging from the status of the currently admitted cases, most of the patients have a good prognosis, and a few are in critical condition. The prognosis of the elderly and those with chronic underlying diseases is poor. The clinical course of pregnant and lying-in women with COVID-19 is similar to that of patients of the same age. Symptoms in children are relatively mild. Age > 60 years old, neutrophil/lymphocyte ratio ≥ 3.13, suffering from other underlying diseases (e.g., hypertension, diabetes, cardiovascular disease, respiratory infectious disease, tumor) are high risk factors for severe pneumonia. Timely identification and intensive care management can help reduce the incidence of poor prognosis.

1.6 LABORATORY EXAMINATION AND IMAGING EXAMINATION

1.6.1 Routine Examination

In the early stage of the disease, the total number of leukocytes in the peripheral blood is normal or decreased, and the lymphocyte count is reduced. Some patients may have increased liver enzymes, lactate dehydrogenase (LDH), creatine kinase, and myoglobin; some critically severe patients may have increased troponin. C-reactive protein (CRP) and erythrocyte sedimentation rate are elevated in most patients, and procalcitonin is normal. In severe cases, D-dimer is increased, and peripheral blood lymphocytes are progressively decreased. Inflammatory factors are often increased in severe and critically severe patients. The ratio of neutrophils/lymphocytes ratio is helpful to determine the severity of the disease.

1.6.2 Virological Testing

Common virological testing includes virus nucleic acid detection and serological tests.

1.6.2.1 Virus Nucleic Acid Testing

1.6.2.1.1 Testing Methods
Using RT-PCR and/or Next-Generation Sequencing (NGS) methods, 2019-nCoV nucleic acid can be detected in nasopharyngeal swabs, sputum, and other lower respiratory secretions, blood, feces, and other specimens. It is more accurate to detect lower respiratory tract specimens (sputum or airway extracts). Specimens should be sent for examination as soon as possible after collection.

When collecting samples from the oral, nasopharyngeal swabs, and other parts of the upper respiratory tract, it is recommended to collect nasopharyngeal swabs for virus nucleic acid testing. In order to improve the detection accuracy, it is recommended to collect multiple samples (oropharyngeal swabs, nasopharyngeal swabs, nasal swabs, etc.) from the same patient for combined detection. For suspected patients with digestive tract symptoms, stool or anal swabs can be collected at the same time of testing.

1.6.2.1.2 Reasons for False Negative Results and Countermeasures

The advantage of nucleic acid testing is that it shortens the window period of infection detection and can detect infected persons early. The false negative of nucleic acid testing may be due to poor quality specimens. The possible influencing factors include improper collection, preservation, transportation, and handling of specimens, virus mutation, PCR inhibition, and so on. In addition, as 2019-nCoV is a single-stranded positive-stranded RNA virus with a large molecular weight, it is easy to mutate. Nucleic acid sequence mutations may occur in the process of transmission. If it is located in the primer binding area for nucleic acid amplification, false negative results will occur. It is suggested that multiple nucleic acid regions should be amplified to effectively avoid the influence of nucleic acid variation on the detection results. When the nucleic acid testing result is negative, only the negative result of this testing can be reported. The 2019-nCoV infection cannot be ruled out, and repeated confirmation is required.

1.6.2.2 Serological Test

After the virus infects the body, the immune system defends against the virus and produces the specific antibody. Among them, specific IgM antibody is an early antibody produced after infection, which can indicate acute infection or recent infection. IgG antibody is the main antibody produced by the reimmune response, indicating that the disease has entered the convalescent period or there was a previous infection. Therefore, the combined detection of immunoglobulin IgM and IgG antibodies can not only provide early diagnosis of infectious diseases but also contribute to the evaluation of the infection stage of the body.

The clinical sensitivity of 2019-nCoV-specific IgM antibody and IgG antibody detection is 70.24% and 96.10%, and the clinical specificity is 96.20% and 92.41%, respectively. The total coincidence rate of 2019-nCoV specific antibody detection and nucleic acid detection in diagnosing infection is 88.03%.

Serum specific antibody detection has shown that 2019-nCoV-specific IgM antibodies mostly start to be tested as positive 3–5 days after the onset of the disease, and the titer of IgG antibodies during the convalescent period is 4 times or even higher than that in the acute phase.

2019-nCoV-specific IgM antibody and IgG antibody detection cannot only make up for the inadequacy of nucleic acid testing and improve the diagnosis rate of 2019-nCoV but also avoid the risk of infection during the collection of nasopharyngeal swab specimens. At the same time, it is useful for assessing the immune status of patients, and it is also of great significance for the selection of some high-titer individuals as plasma donors for antibody therapy.

Because any single test has a certain false negative and false positive rate, a reasonable interpretation of the combined detection of nucleic acid and antibodies can better determine the patient's current condition and outcome (see Table 1.1).

1.6.3 Chest Imaging Examination

2019-nCoV mainly infects the lungs through the respiratory tract, so chest imaging manifestations have become an important basis for diagnosis and treatment of COVID-19, and imaging examination has become an important means of case screening, early diagnosis, and efficient evaluation.

1.6.3.1 Chest X-ray

Chest X-rays cannot show the subpleural ground-glass opacity (GGO) at the early stage. With the progression of the disease, it can be manifested as a localized, patchy, increased-density shadow distributed in the lower fields of both lungs. In severe patients, diffuse consolidation shadow of both lungs may occur, with or without a small amount of pleural effusion.

Because it is easy to miss the early GGO in chest X-rays, it is not recommended for screening and early diagnosis of this disease. It can be used for bedside review of severe and critically severe patients.

1.6.3.2 Chest CT Examination

1.6.3.2.1 Advantages and Characteristics

Chest CT examination has certain characteristics in assessing the nature and scope of the lesion, and it is the preferred method of imaging examination for COVID-19.

Although COVID-19 chest CT has certain characteristics, it is impractical to use the CT images as the only criterion to diagnose COVID-19. CT examination allows detection of only relatively specific viral pneumonia in the early stages.

The main signs of chest CT of COVID-19 are single or multiple GGOs and consolidation shadows in both lungs, showing a "paving stone" sign. The pathological changes are mainly distributed around the lung peripheral and subpleural and can also be around the bronchial bundles and blood vessels. There are

TABLE 1.1   INTERPRETATION OF RESULTS OF COVID-19 NUCLEIC ACID TESTING AND SERUM ANTIBODY COMBINED TESTING

Nucleic Acid Testing	IgM	IgG	Clinical Significance
+	–	–	The patient may be in the "window period" of 2019-nCoV infection.
+	+	–	The patient may be in the early stage of 2019-nCoV infection.
+	–	+	The patient may be in the mid and late stage of 2019-nCoV infection or have recurrent infection.
+	+	+	The patient is in the active stage of infection, but the body has developed a certain degree of immunity to 2019-nCoV.
–	+	–	The patient is most likely to be in the acute stage of 2019-nCoV infection; the nucleic acid testing result is in doubt; the patient has other diseases that affect the outcome.
–	–	+	The patient may have been previously infected with 2019-nCoV but has recovered, or the virus has been cleared from the body.
–	weak+	–	The patient is initially infected with 2019-nCoV with an extremely low load and is at an early stage; IgM false positive caused by other reasons.
–	+	+	The patient has recently been infected with 2019-nCoV and is in the recovery phase; the nucleic acid testing result is a false negative, and the patient is in the active stage of infection.

signs of air bronchogram and thickening of interlobular septa in some areas, with very few or a few pleural effusions or lymphadenopathy.

1.6.3.2.2 Stages of Chest CT Manifestations

According to the scope and type of lung lesions, the chest CT manifestations of COVID-19 can be divided into early stage, progression stage, severe stage, and absorption stage.

1) Early stage: The lesions are mostly confined to subpleural or interlobular fissures, with uneven density, and single or multiple patchy, localized GGOs, with or without interlobular septal thickening, with air bronchogram.

2) Progression stage: The distribution area of the lesions increases, and the scope expands to multiple lobes in both lungs, usually in 4–5

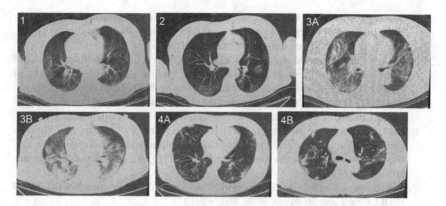

Figure 1.1   CT manifestations of COVID-19. 1. Lung CT manifestations of the early stage of COVID-19: GGO lesions in the right middle lobe lateral segment. 2. CT manifestations of the progression stage of COVID-19: Multiple large GGO lesions in the middle lobe of both lungs, some accompanied by consolidation. 3. CT manifestations of COVID-19 in severe/critical stage: A. Diffuse distribution of consolidated lesions in both lungs. B. Multiple consolidation lesions in both lungs, showing "white lung". 4. CT manifestations during the prognosis of COVID-19: A. The two lungs are absorbed earlier before pathological changes, B. A small amount of residual fibrous stripes, especially in the right lung.

    lobes. The density of the lesions increases and merges into large pieces, showing asymmetric distribution, with visible thickening of bronchial vascular bundles.

3) Severe stage: Both lungs show diffuse lesions, which progress rapidly and become dominant with solidification, combined with GGOs, a small number of "white lungs", and a small amount of pleural effusion.

4) Absorption stage: The scope of lung lesions is reduced, the density decreases, the consolidation foci gradually disappear, and the exudate is absorbed or organized (see Figure 1.1).

BIBLIOGRAPHY

1. General Office of the National Health Commission, Office of the State Administration of Traditional Chinese Medicine. *COVID-19 Diagnosis and Treatment Plan (Trial Version 7) [EB/OL]*. China. 2020.
2. Li Shixue, Shan Ying. A review of the research progress of COVID-19 (Medical Edition) [J/OL]. *Journal of Shandong University*, 58(3): 19–25.

3. Su Shi, Li Xiaocheng, Hao Hua, Wang Xiaoyan, Zhang Mingming, Geng Hui, Ma Mao. Research progress of COVID-19 (SARS-CoV-2) (Medical Edition) [J/OL]. *Journal of Xi'an Jiaotong University*, 2020, 41(04): 479–482+496.
4. Chinese Preventive Medicine Association COVID-19 Prevention and Control Expert Group. The latest understanding of the epidemiological characteristics of COVID-19 [J/OL]. *Chinese Journal of Viral Diseases*, 2020, 10(02): 86–92.
5. Gao Yuqi. Treatment strategies based on the pathophysiological mechanism of COVID-19 [J/OL]. *Chinese Journal of Pathophysiology*, 2020, 36(03): 568–572.
6. Liu Qian, Wang Rongshuai, Qu Guoqiang, Wang Yunyun, Liu Pan, Zhu Yingzhi, Fei Geng, Ren Liang, Zhou Yiwu, Liu Liang. General observation report on systemic anatomy of cadavers died from COVID-19 [J]. *Journal of Forensic Medicine*, 2020, 36(1): 19–21.
7. Fang Sangao, Wei Jianguo. Progress in clinical pathological research of COVID-19 [J/OL]. *Chongqing Medicine*, 2020, 49(17): 7–12.
8. Ning Yating, Hou Xin, Lu Minya, Wu Xian, Li Yongzhe. Application of COVID-19 serum specific antibody detection technology [J/OL]. *Xiehe Medical Journal*, 2020, 11(06): 649–653.
9. Ma Qiong, Shi Xiudong, Lu Yang, Shi Yuxin. Research progress in clinical and imaging studies of COVID-19 [J]. *Chinese Journal of Clinical Medicine*, 2020, 27(1): 23–26.
10. Shi Heshui, Han Xiaoyu, Fan Yanqing, Liang Bo, Yang Fan, Han Ping, Zheng Chuansheng. Clinical features and imaging manifestations of COVID-19 infection[J/OL]. *Journal of Clinical Radiology*, 2020, 39(1): 8–11.
11. Li Zhenhao, Gao Xiaoling, Yang Xiaojuan, Xu Hui. COVID-19 nucleic acid detection and analysis [J/OL]. *Laboratory Medicine and Clinic*, 2020, 17(10): 1313–1315.
12. Chinese Medical Association Laboratory Medicine Branch. Expert consensus on nucleic acid detection of COVID-19 (English edition) [J]. *Chinese Medical Journal*, 2020(13),968–973.
13. Wang Kai, Kang Siru, Tian Ronghua, Wang Yan, Zhang Xiaozhou, Li Hongmei. Analysis of chest CT imaging features of COVID-19 [J]. *Chinese Journal of Clinical Medicine*, 2020, 27(1): 27–31.
14. Radiology Branch of Chinese Medical Association. Radiological diagnosis of COVID-19: Expert recommendations of Chinese medical association radiology branch (1st Edition) [J/OL]. *Chinese Journal of Radiology*, 2020, 54(4): 279–285.
15. Bernheim Adam, Mei Xueyan, Huang Mingqian, Yang Yang, Fayad Zahi, Zhang Ning, Diao Kaiyue, Lin Bin, Zhu Xiqi, Li Kunwei, Li Shaolin, Shan Hong, Jacobi Adam. Chest CT Findings in Coronavirus Disease-19 (COVID-19): Relationship to Duration of Infection. [J]. *Radiology*, 2020, 295: 200463.
16. Liang Qi. Imaging examination, diagnosis and nosocomial infection prevention and control of COVID-19: Hunan province radiology expert consensus (Medical Edition) [J/OL]. *Journal of Central South University*, 2020, 45(03): 221–228.
17. Li Hongjun. Guidelines for imaging-assisted diagnosis of COVID-19 [J/OL]. *Chinese Medical Imaging Technology*, 2020, 36(03): 321–331.

Chapter 2

Diagnosis and Treatment of COVID-19

2.1 CLINICAL DIAGNOSTIC CRITERIA

2.1.1 Diagnostic Criteria

According to the *Diagnosis and Treatment Protocol for COVID-19 (7th Trial Edition)*, jointly released by the National Health Commission (NHC) and the National Administration of Traditional Chinese Medicine, and the *Diagnosis and Treatment of COVID-19 Infection Suitable for Military Medics Supporting Hubei (1st Trial Edition)*, the diagnostic criteria for COVID-19 are divided into two categories: "suspected case" and "confirmed case".

2.1.1.1 Suspected Cases

The following sections contain a comprehensive analysis of the epidemiological history and clinical manifestations of COVID-19.

2.1.1.1.1 Epidemiological History

1) Travel to or reside in Wuhan and surrounding areas or other communities with documented COVID-19 positive cases within 14 days before the onset of illness.
2) History of contact with COVID-19-infected persons (positive for nucleic acid testing) within 14 days before the onset of illness.
3) History of contact with patients presenting fever or respiratory symptoms, who traveled to or resided in Wuhan and surrounding areas or in other communities with documented COVID-19 positive cases within 14 days before the onset of illness.
4) Cluster onset (two or more cases of fever and/or respiratory symptoms within 2 weeks in small areas such as homes, offices, school classes, etc.).

2.1.1.1.2 Clinical Manifestations

1) Presenting with fever and/or respiratory symptoms.
2) With imaging features of COVID-19 mentioned in Chapter 1 (Figure 1.1).
3) In the early stage of the disease, the total number of leukocytes was normal or decreased, and the lymphocyte count was normal or decreased.

A case that meets any one of the epidemiological history criteria and any two of the clinical manifestations can be identified as a suspected case. If there is no clear epidemiological history, the patient can be identified as a suspected case as long as three of the clinical manifestations are met.

2.1.1.2 Confirmed Cases

Suspected cases with one of the following etiology or serological evidences can be identified as confirmed cases.

1) Real-time reverse transcription polymerase chain reaction (RT-PCR detection is positive for COVID-19 nucleic acid.
2) The viral gene identified by gene sequencing is highly homologous with known COVID-19.
3) The COVID-19-specific IgM and IgG antibodies test positive. The titer of COVID-19-specific IgG antibody is 4 times higher in the convalescent period than that in the acute phase.

Instructions:

1) Suspected cases can be classified into two categories: one is with any one of the epidemiological histories and conforming to any two of the clinical manifestations (fever and/or respiratory symptoms; the above-described imaging features of pneumonia (Figure 1.1); normal or decreased total number of leukocytes and decreased lymphocyte count in the early stage of disease).
2) Confirmed cases need a positive result of etiological evidence (real-time RT-PCR detection is positive for COVID-19 nucleic acid; or viral genome sequencing, highly homologous with known COVID-19).
3) It should be noted that it is difficult to distinguish the types based on imaging features alone. Although a chest CT of COVID-19-infected patient has certain characteristics, it is impractical to differentiate COVID-19 from other types of viral pneumonia by image changes alone. CT examination can help to detect a relatively specific viral pneumonia in the early stage.
4) Serological antibody test: The COVID-19-specific IgM antibody usually begins to be positive at 3–5 days after onset, and the titer of IgG

antibody in the convalescent period is 4 times or higher than that in the acute stage.

Not only can the detection of the COVID-19-specific IgM and IgG antibodies make up for the lack of nucleic acid detection, but it can also increase the diagnosis rate of COVID-19 and avoid infection risk as well when collecting nasopharyngeal swab specimens. Meanwhile, it is of great significance to assess patients' immune status and select some high-potency individuals as plasma donors for antibody therapy.

5) Pulmonary signs of COVID-19 are generally considered to be nonspecific. Patients may experience rapid breathing rate due to hypoxia, and patients with severe respiratory difficulties may even show symptoms of orthopnea. Lung auscultation may involve abnormal breath sounds in the affected lung segments, most of which are reduced sounds or disappeared sounds, but moist rales sounds are rare.

6) With the continuous development of the global pandemic, imported cases keep growing gradually. In the epidemiological investigation, travel history to other countries can also be used as an important reference.

2.1.2 Clinical Classification

2.1.2.1 Mild

The clinical symptoms are mild, and there was no sign of pneumonia on chest imaging.

2.1.2.2 Moderate

These patients may have fever and respiratory symptoms. Signs of pneumonia can be found in the imaging.

2.1.2.3 Severe Cases

Adults who meet one of the following criteria:

1) Shortness of breath, RR $\geq$ 30 times/min.
2) Oxygen saturation $\leq$ 93% at rest.
3) Alveolar oxygen partial pressure/fraction of inspired oxygen (PaO_2/FiO_2) $\leq$ 300 mmHg (1 mmHg = 0.133 kPa).

At high altitudes (above 1,000 meters), PaO_2/FiO_2 should be corrected according to the following formula: PaO_2/FiO_2 × [Atmospheric Pressure (mmHg)/760].

Patients whose pulmonary imaging showed significant progression of lesions > 50% within 24–48 hours should be treated as a severe case.

Children who meet one of the following criteria:

1) Shortness of breath (< 2 months of age, RR ≥ 60 times/min; 2–12 months of age, RR ≥ 50 times/min; 1–5 years old, RR ≥ 40 times/min; > 5 years old, RR ≥ 60 times/min), excluding the effects of fever and crying.
2) In the resting state, the oxygen saturation is ≤ 92%.
3) Assisted breathing (groaning, wing flaps, tri-retraction sign), cyanosis, intermittent apnea.
4) Lethargy and convulsions.
5) Refuse to eat or have feeding difficulties, with signs of dehydration.

2.1.2.4 Critically Severe

Patients who meet one of the following criteria:

1) Respiratory failure, requiring mechanical ventilation.
2) Shock.
3) Multiple organ failure, requiring ICU monitoring and treatment.

Instructions:

1) Severe patients may develop dyspnea and/or hypoxemia one week after onset. More severe cases may rapidly progress to acute respiratory distress syndrome, septic shock, refractory metabolic acidosis, coagulation dysfunction, multiple organ failure, and so on.
2) Special groups: some children and neonates may have atypical symptoms; the clinical course of pregnant women with COVID-19 is similar to that of patients of the same age; the elderly, and those with chronic underlying diseases and extreme obesity are more likely to develop severe disease. It is worth noting that during the course of severe and critically severe cases, patients may have medium to low fever, or even no obvious fever.

2.1.3 Warning Signals

The differences in clinical manifestations and prognosis make it particularly important to distinguish the severity of patients' conditions accurately. For patients undergoing treatment or rehabilitation training in general isolation ward, once abnormalities of the following warning signals occur, the following can be an important reference for patients to be transferred to ICU for treatment (children, due to their particularity, have different early-warning signals from adults; the clinical warning signals of pregnant and lying-in women are the same as those of the same age group).

2.1.3.1 Adults

1) Progressive decline in the number of peripheral lymphocytes.
2) Progressive increase in the levels of peripheral inflammatory bio-markers, such as Interleukin-6 (IL-6) and C-reactive protein (CRP).
3) Progressive increase in lactic acid concentration.
4) Pulmonary lesions progress rapidly in a short time.

2.1.3.2 Children

1) Increased respiration rate;
2) Poor mental responsiveness and drowsiness.
3) Progressive increase in lactic concentration.
4) Imaging showed bilateral or multilobar infiltration and pleural effusion; or pulmonary lesions progress rapidly in a short time.
5) Infants under 3 months of age, children with underlying diseases (congenital heart disease, bronchopulmonary dysplasia, respiratory deformity, abnormal hemoglobin, severe malnutrition, etc.), or children with immunodeficiency or weak immune system (long-term use of immunosuppressants).

2.1.4 Auxiliary Examination

2.1.4.1 Laboratory Examination
2.1.4.1.1 Routine Examination

In the early stage of the disease, the total count of peripheral leukocytes could be normal or decreased, and the lymphocytes are decreased. In some patients, liver transaminases, lactate dehydrogenase (LDH), creatine kinase, and myoglobin were elevated. In some critically severe patients, troponins were also increased. In most patients, CRP and erythrocyte sedimentation rate (ESR) were increased, while procalcitonin generally remained in a normal range. Notably, D-dimer was significantly increased in severe patients, and peripheral lymphocytes were progressively decreased (Note: The guidelines of the NHC suggest that inflammatory biomarkers are often elevated in severe and critically severe patients. The *Diagnosis and Treatment of Novel Coronavirus Pneumonia Infection Suitable for Military Medics Supporting Hubei* recommended that the neutrophil-lymphocyte ratio [NLR] should be focused, as this ratio is helpful in determining disease severity. Inflammatory factors are not emphasized.)

2.1.4.1.2 Etiological and Serological Examination

1) Etiological examination: COVID-19 nucleic acids can be detected in nasopharyngeal swabs, sputum and other lower respiratory tract

secretions, blood, and feces by using RT-PCR and next-generation sequencing technology (NGS). It is more accurate to detect the lower respiratory tract specimen (sputum or airway extract). Once collected, specimen examination should be performed as soon as possible.

2) Serological examination: the COVID-19-specific IgM antibody starts to be tested as positive after 3–5 days from onset. In comparison, the titer of COVID-19-specific IgG antibody is 4 times higher in the convalescent period than that in the acute phase.

2.1.4.2 Chest Imaging

At the early stage of the disease, multiple small patchy shadows and interstitial changes appear, which are more obvious in the periphery of the lung. Then it develops into multiple ground-glass opacities (GGOs) and infiltration shadows. In severe cases, pulmonary consolidation may occur. Pleural effusion is rare.

2.1.5 Differential Diagnosis

2.1.5.1 Upper Respiratory Disease

The clinical manifestations of patients with COVID-19 infection lack specificity. Atypical manifestations such as cough, nasal congestion, runny nose, and pharyngitis are easy to be confused with a lot of upper respiratory illnesses, such as the common cold, flu, even rhinitis, pharyngitis, etc.

2.1.5.2 Other Viral and Mycoplasma Pneumonia

COVID-19 needs to be distinguished from other known viral pneumonia or mycoplasma pneumoniae infections, such as influenza virus adenovirus and respiratory syncytial virus. For suspected cases, techniques such as rapid antigen detection and multiplex PCR nucleic acid detection should be taken to detect common respiratory pathogens.

2.1.5.3 Non-Infectious Disease

It should also be distinguished from non-infectious diseases, such as vasculitis, dermatomyositis, and organizing pneumonia.

2.1.6 Reporting and Exclusion System

2.1.6.1 Reporting System

Based on the above diagnostic criteria, it is crucial to isolate the suspected person immediately in a solitary cell for further monitoring and treatment when a COVID-19 case is suspected. If COVID-19 infection is still suspected after consultation by medical experts and/or physicians, a case report should be submitted online within 2 hours. In addition, specimens should be collected for

COVID-19 nucleic acid test. Meanwhile, the suspected person should be transferred to a predesignated hospital immediately and safely. For people who have had close contact with confirmed COVID-19 cases, COVID-19 nucleic acid test should be performed, even if their common respiratory pathogen detection test has shown positive.

2.1.6.2 Exclusion Criteria

If the samples were negative for two consecutive nucleic acid tests (with at least 24 hours' interval between each test), and if COVID-19 specific IgM and IgG antibodies remain negative after 7 days from onset, the suspected diagnosis of COVID-19 can be ruled out (Note: Specific IgM antibody usually tests positive 3–5 days after onset. The accuracy of exclusion criteria can be improved if serum-specific antibody test results show negative 7 days after onset; however, about a 2-week "window period" may occur in a small number of patients. For this particular circumstance, it is recommended to appropriately postpone the detection time of serum antibody for highly suspected patients and make a collective decision through expert consultation, if necessary.)

2.2 CLINICAL TREATMENT

According to the clinical classification of patients, the corresponding clinical treatment plan is formulated. Mild and moderate patients generally have a good prognosis, and strict isolation management and close observation are needed to detect potentially severe/critically severe patients in time. For severe and critically severe patients, it is necessary to concentrate superior medical resources and carry out a comprehensive treatment in the form of multidisciplinary expert consultation (infection department, respiratory department, critical care department, rehabilitation department, etc.), so as to improve the cure rate and reduce the mortality rate as far as possible.

2.2.1 Treatment Place Determination According to the Patient's Condition

1) Suspected and confirmed cases should be isolated and treated in a designated hospital with effective isolation and protection conditions. Suspected cases should be isolated in a single ward; post-discharge convalescent patients can be treated in a designated COVID-19 rehabilitation medical facility.
2) Critically severe cases should be admitted to ICU as soon as possible; rehabilitation work is suggested to be carried out as soon as possible in qualified hospitals.

2.2.2 General Treatment

1) Rest in bed with supportive treatment to ensure sufficient calorie supply. The water and electrolyte balance should be observed to maintain internal environment stability. Vital signs and oxygen saturation should be closely monitored.

2) Monitor the blood routine, urine routine, CRP, biochemical indicators (liver enzyme, myocardial enzyme, renal function, etc.), coagulation function, arterial blood gas analysis, chest imaging according to the condition. If possible, a cytokine test should be performed.

3) Effective oxygen therapy measures should be given in time, including nasal cannula, mask oxygen, and high-flow nasal cannula oxygen therapy. Hydrogen-oxygen inhalation (H_2/O_2: 66.6%/33.3%) treatment can be considered for use.

4) Antiviral therapy: Suggested prescription: α-interferon (5 million U or equivalent for adult, add 2 mL of sterile water, 2 times daily inhalation), lopinavir/ritonavir (200 mg/50 mg/capsule, 2 capsules each time for adults, twice a day, the course of treatment should not exceed 10 days). Ribavirin (it is recommended to combine with interferon or lopinavir/ritonavir, 500 mg each time for adults, 2cc3 times intravenous infusions per day, the course of treatment should not exceed 10 days), chloroquine phosphate (for adults aged between 18 and 65 who weigh over 50 kg, 500 mg each time, twice daily for 7 days; for those who weigh less than 50 kg, 500 mg each time, twice daily for day 1 and day 2, once daily for day 3–day 7), arbidol (200 mg each time, three times a day for adults, the course of treatment should not exceed 10 days).

Instructions:

a)   It is not recommended to use three or more antiviral drugs at the same time. The use of related drugs should be stopped when intolerable side effects occur. Treatment of maternal patients should consider the number of weeks of pregnancy. If possible, choose drugs that will have less impact on the fetus, and consider whether to terminate pregnancy prior to treatment, and keep the patients informed.

b)   Attention should be paid to the adverse reactions and contraindications of the above drugs (for example, arbidol may have digestive reactions such as diarrhea, lopinavir/ritonavir may even have a risk of fatal pancreatitis, chloroquine is contraindicated in patients with heart disease) and interactions with other drugs. Minor tolerable adverse reactions should be closely observed, and the drugs should be stopped immediately once intolerable adverse reactions occur. The efficacy of the drugs in clinical application should also be further evaluated.

5) Antibacterial drug treatment: Inappropriate use of antibacterial drugs should be avoided, especially the broad-spectrum antibacterial drugs. However, in the case of severe/critically severe patients with confirmed bacterial infection, drugs should be used after weighing the pros and cons.

2.2.3 Treatment of Severe and Critically Severe Cases

2.2.3.1 Principles of Treatment

In addition to symptomatic treatments, it is important to actively prevent complications, treat underlying diseases, prevent secondary infections, and provide organ function support.

2.2.3.2 Respiratory Support

1) Oxygen therapy: Severe patients should receive nasal cannula or ventilator to inhale oxygen and assess in time whether respiratory distress and/or hypoxemia is relieved.

2) High-flow nasal cannula oxygen therapy or noninvasive mechanical ventilation: When patients with respiratory distress and/or hypoxemia cannot be relieved after receiving standard oxygen therapy, high-flow nasal cannula oxygen therapy or noninvasive ventilation can be considered. If the condition does not improve or worsens within a short time (1–2 hours), tracheal intubation and invasive mechanical ventilation should be performed in time.

3) Invasive mechanical ventilation: Use lung protective ventilation strategy, that is, small tidal volume (6–8 mL/kg ideal body weight) and low level of airway plateau pressure ($\leq$ 30 cm H_2O) for mechanical ventilation to reduce ventilator-related lung injury. When the airway plateau pressure is $\leq$ 35 cm H_2O, high positive end-expiratory pressure (PEEP) can be appropriately used. Keep the airway warm and humid, avoid prolonged sedation, awaken patients early, and perform pulmonary rehabilitation treatment. For those patients who encounter problems with man-machine synchronization, sedation and muscle relaxants should be used in time. According to the airway secretions, closed sputum suction should be considered, and bronchoscopy should be performed if necessary.

4) Salvage treatment: For patients with severe acute respiratory distress syndrome (ARDS), it is recommended to perform lung expansion. Prone ventilation should be performed for more than 12 hours per day. When the patient is in the prone position, mechanical ventilation is not effective; if possible, extracorporeal membrane pulmonary

oxygenation (ECMO) should be performed as soon as possible. Related indications:

a)   When $FiO_2 > 90\%$, the oxygenation index is less than 80 mmHg, which lasts more than 3–4 hours.

b)   When the airway plateau pressure ≥ 35 cmH_2O. For patients with simple respiratory failure the VV-ECMO mode is preferred; if circulatory support is needed, then VA-ECMO mode should be used. When the underlying disease is under control and cardiopulmonary function shows signs of recovery, a weaning test should be considered.

2.2.3.3 Circulation Support

Based on adequate fluid resuscitation, improvement of microcirculation and use of vasoactive drugs may be considered. Changes in patients' blood pressure, heart rate, and urine output, as well as lactic acid and alkali residuals in arterial blood gas analysis, should be closely monitored. Noninvasive or invasive hemodynamic monitoring, such as Doppler echocardiography, echocardiography, invasive blood pressure, or pulse index continuous cardiac output (PiCCO) monitoring is necessary. In the process of treatment, attention should be paid to the liquid balance to avoid excess and deficiency.

When the patient's heart rate suddenly increases over 20% of the baseline value or the blood pressure has dropped by more than 20% of the baseline value, accompanying symptoms, such as poor skin perfusion and decreased urine output, may indicate patients have septic shock, gastrointestinal bleeding, or severe heart failure.

2.2.3.4 Renal Failure and Renal Replacement Therapy

When renal insufficiency occurs in critically severe patients, the causes of renal function insufficiency, such as hypoperfusion and drugs, should be analyzed. The treatment of patients with renal failure should pay attention to fluid balance, acid-base balance, and electrolyte balance. For nutrition support treatment, attention should be paid to nitrogen balance, and calories and minerals should be supplemented. Continuous Renal Replacement Therapy (CRRT) can be considered in severe patients. The indications include:

1) Hyperkalemia.
2) Acidosis; Pulmonary edema or excessive water load.
3) Fluid management when multiple organ dysfunction occurs.

2.2.3.5 Recovered Patients' Plasma Therapy

This therapy is suitable for severe and critically severe patients with rapid disease progression.

Instructions:

Recruitment requirements for plasma donors:

1) People who have recovered from COVID-19 infection.
2) No fewer than 3 weeks from the first symptom.
3) Meet the latest COVID-19 protocol standards for isolation and discharge.
4) Are between the ages of 18–55.
5) Weigh at least 50 kg for male donors and 45 kg for female donors.
6) No history of menstrual blood borne diseases.
7) People who are considered eligible after being evaluated by clinicians for comprehensive treatment.

    For detailed dosage, please refer to the *Convalescent Plasma Treatment Plan for COVID-19 Patients* (*2nd Trial Edition*).

Special testing of donor plasma:

1) The single test result of COVID-19 nucleic acid blood sample should be negative.
2) The qualitative test of COVID-19 serum/plasma IgG antibody is reactive, and, after 160 times dilution, the test is still positive, as required by the reagent instructions. Or the qualitative test of COVID-19 serum/plasma IgG antibody is reactive, and, after 320 times dilution, the test is still positive, as required by the reagent instructions.
3) If possible, a virus neutralization test can be carried out to determine the antibody titers.
4) Plasma donors with a history of pregnancy or blood transfusion should be screened for HNA and HLA antibodies.
5) Depending on the epidemiological characteristics of the area in which the plasma donor is located, additional tests may be added as appropriate.

2.2.3.6 Blood Purification Treatment

The blood purification system includes plasma exchange, adsorption, perfusion, blood/plasma filtration, etc., which can remove inflammatory factors and block the "cytokine storm", thereby reducing the damage to the body caused by the inflammatory response. It can be used for treatment of early and midstage cytokine storms in severe and critically severe patients.

2.2.3.7 Immunotherapy

For patients with extensive lung lesions and severe patients with elevated IL-6 levels, tocilizumab treatment can be considered. The starting dose is 4–8 mg/kg, the recommended dose is 400 mg. Dilute it in a 100 mL 0.9% Normal Saline (NS), and inject it into the patient for more than 1 hour. If the first administration is ineffective, it can be given again after 12 hours (the dose is the same as before), with a cumulative administration of no more than two times, and a single maximum dose of no more than 800 mg. Pay attention to allergic reactions. Patients with active infections such as tuberculosis are forbidden to use this drug.

2.2.3.8 Other Treatment Measures

For patients with progressive deterioration of oxygenation indicators, rapid imaging progress, and excessive activation of inflammatory response, the use of glucocorticoids in the short term (3–5 days) should be considered. The dosage of methylprednisolone should not exceed 1–2 mg/kg/day. It should be noted that large doses of glucocorticoids will delay the removal of coronavirus due to immunosuppressive effects. Intestinal microecological regulators can be used to maintain intestinal microecological balance and prevent secondary bacterial infections. For severe and critically severe children, intravenous gamma globulin should be considered.

Pregnant women with severe or critically severe COVID-19 should consider pregnancy termination, and cesarean delivery is preferred.

2.2.3.9 Rehabilitation Treatment

Rehabilitation treatment should follow the following principles:

1) Individualization: Treatment should be carried out according to the different stages, complications, and underlying diseases of COVID-19 and systemic conditions as well.
2) Integration: Treatment should target not only respiratory function but also cardiac function, nerve function, digestive function, kidney function, systemic physical function, psychological function, and environmental factors.
3) Strict observation: Pay attention to different rehabilitation methods, especially the reaction during and after activities and exercises.
4) Gradual progress: All treatment must be carried out without affecting clinical care and comprehensive assessment and with safety. For severe and critically severe patients, special attention should be paid to a comprehensive assessment of their state of consciousness, respiratory, cardiovascular, and musculoskeletal systems.

2.2.3.10 Psychotherapy

Psychological counseling should be strengthened in patients with anxiety and phobia. Rehabilitation professionals, when discovering psychological problems in patients, can adopt professional techniques for rehabilitation or clinical psychological knowledge acquired through formal training to play an assisting role in psychological intervention, rather than replacing the role of psychological professionals. Once a patient is found to have signs of deteriorating mental health, rehabilitation professionals should report to the competent medical team immediately and cooperate with the team to guide the patient to receive help from mental health professionals. Through proper assessment, patients with severe mental illness can receive help from psychologists/psychiatrists in time.

Psychological issues that rehabilitation professionals can help with:

1) Emotional problems: It is recommended to accept the assessment of psychological professionals. In the absence of professional psychological resources, self-rating scales such as PHQ-9 and GAD-7 can be used to quickly assess or screen the type and degree of psychological disorders existing in patients. These scales mainly use rehabilitation treatment techniques, such as the pleasure effect of occupational therapy and sports and leisure activities, as well as distraction skills, to regulate emotions and relieve stress. The "retelling of the traumatic event" technique should be used with caution to avoid causing repeated trauma to patients.

2) Cognitive problems: Use cognitive behavioral therapy and other methods, such as explaining medical knowledge, scientific exercise, and the need for comprehensive rehabilitation measures of COVID-19 through science programs or mental health hotlines; correct the patient's confused or distorted beliefs to facilitate their transition to the psychological endurance phase in conjunction with rehabilitation program.

3) Interpersonal problems: Cooperate with professional teams to provide positive guidance to patients, helping them to recognize their ability to reinvent themselves and their social identity, reduce their feelings of humiliation and discrimination, and return to the society and work.

4) Sleep problems: Maintain a regular routine and get enough sleep. Relaxation training such as meditation, hypnosis, music therapy, yoga, qigong, tai chi chuan (a kind of traditional Chinese shadow boxing), and other exercises can relieve negative emotions, which help the body to maintain balance and stability.

2.2.4 Treatment and Prevention of Complications

2.2.4.1 Prevention of Ventilator-Associated Pneumonia

Recommendations:

1) Goal-directed sedation and analgesia, as mild as possible.
2) Endotracheal intubation should be preferred.
3) Lift bed head 30°–45°.
4) Adopt closed suction device.
5) Replace ventilator tube and humidification device immediately in case of contamination.

2.2.4.2 Prevention of Deep Vein Thrombosis

Recommendations:

1) If there is no contraindication, the first choice is LMWH 4000 U, subcutaneous injection, once a day.
2) For patients with anticoagulant contraindications, mechanical prevention can be used, such as intermittent pneumatic compression (IPC), graduated compression stockings (GCS), and so on.
3) For patients with severe renal insufficiency, ordinary heparin 5000 U can be selected and injected subcutaneously twice a day.
4) Early mobilization.

For details, please refer to the *First Edition of Recommendations for Prevention and Treatment of COVID-19 Related Venous Thromboembolism (Trial)* formulated by the Respiratory Society of Chinese Medical Association, Respiratory Physicians Society of Chinese Medical Doctor Association, and the National Collaborating Group on Prevention and Treatment of Pulmonary Embolism and Pulmonary Vascular Disease.

2.2.4.3 Prevention of Catheter-Related Bloodstream Infection

Recommendations:

1) Take maximal sterile barrier precautions during arteriovenous catheterization.
2) Emphasize hand hygiene.
3) Assess daily whether the catheter can be removed.

2.2.4.4 Prevention of Stress Ulcers

Recommendations:

1) Early enteral nutrition.
2) H_2 receptor antagonists or proton pump inhibitors are used in patients with a high risk of gastrointestinal bleeding.

2.2.4.5 Prevention of ICU-Related Complications

Recommendations: Implement comprehensive management of ICU patients as far as possible, pay attention to sedation and analgesia, humanistic care, and early activity and exercise and prevent short and long-term complications such as ICU-related myasthenia, delirium, and post-ICU syndrome.

2.2.5 Traditional Chinese Medicine Treatment

In traditional Chinese medicine (TCM), COVID-19 falls under the category of "pestilences". The disease is divided into medical observation and clinical treatment period (confirmed cases) according to the plan of the NHC, and the clinical treatment period is divided into mild cases, moderate cases, severe cases, critically severe cases, and convalescent period, and so on. For specific prescriptions, please refer to the contents of "TCM Treatment" in Section 1, Chapter 6.

2.2.5.1 Medication Observation

Clinical manifestations: fatigue with gastrointestinal discomfort or fatigue with fever.

2.2.5.2 Clinical Treatment (Confirmed Cases)

2.2.5.2.1 Mild Cases

1) Cold dampness stagnating in the lung.
2) Damp heat accumulating in the lung.

2.2.5.2.2 Moderate Cases

1) Damp toxin stagnating in the lung.
2) Cold damp obstructing the lung.

2.2.5.2.3 Severe Cases

1) Pandemic toxin blocking the lung.
2) Flaring heat in both qi and ying phases.

2.2.5.2.4 Critically Severe Cases

1) Internal blocking causing external collapse.

2.2.5.2.5 Convalescent Period

1) Qi deficiency of the lung and spleen.
2) Deficiency of qi and yin.

2.2.6 Criteria and Precautions after Being Discharged from the Hospital

2.2.6.1 Discharge Criteria

1) The body temperature returns to normal for more than 3 days.
2) Significant improvement in respiratory symptoms.
3) Pulmonary imaging shows a marked improvement in acute exudative lesions.
4) Sputum, nasopharyngeal swabs, and other respiratory specimens appear negative for two consecutive nucleic acid tests (at least a 24-hour interval between each test).

Patients who meet all the above conditions can be discharged.

2.2.6.2 Precautions after Being Discharged from the Hospital

1) The hospital should keep contact with the local medical and health institutions, tracing where the patients live, sharing the medical records, and sending the discharged patients' information to the residential committee and the basic medical and health institutions in a timely manner.
2) After the patient is discharged from the hospital, it is recommended that the patient continue isolation management and health monitoring for 14 days, wear a mask, live in a well-ventilated single room, reduce close contact with family members, wash hands frequently, and avoid going out.
3) It is recommended to follow up and return to the hospital in the second and fourth week after discharge.

2.2.6.3 Re-Positive Nucleic Acid Conversion after Being Discharged from the Hospital

2.2.6.3.1 Analysis of Re-Positive Nucleic Acid Conversion

Re-positive nucleic acid conversion means that the nucleic acid test for COVID-19 patients who have been discharged changes from negative to positive. There are several explanations for this, including:

1) False negatives due to sampling and test kit.
2) The patients did not fully recover, and the virus still remains in the body.
3) The patients become infected again after recovery. Because COVID-19 is a new disease that humans have never been exposed to in the past, its exact cause requires further observation and research.

2.2.6.3.2 Management Measures

1) For symptomatic patients, the emergency center, also known as "120", should be notified by the receiving medical institution, from which the patient shall be transferred to designated hospitals for treatment. The patient should be discharged when the discharge criteria are met again. Two weeks of isolation and rehabilitation observation are required after discharge.

2) For asymptomatic patients, they should be transferred to the relevant centralized isolation location. After 2 weeks' centralized isolation and rehabilitation observation, patients who meet the quarantine-exit criteria may be released from quarantine.

3) Patients with re-positive nucleic acid tests have been included in the report of confirmed cases according to the national requirements at the first diagnosis, so they will not be repeatedly reported as new confirmed cases at the time of rediagnosis.

2.2.6.3.3 Treatment Measures for Patients with "Re-Positive" Nucleic Acid Tests

1) After transferring symptomatic patients to designated hospitals, specific treatment should be given according to patients' specific conditions and laboratory tests. It is generally not recommended to continue the use of antiviral drugs for patients who have reached the maximum treatment course.

2) For asymptomatic patients, it is recommended to manage them according to convalescent period and improve the detection of COVID-19 antibody IgG and IgM to assess the overall condition of patients.

2.2.6.3.4 The Infectivity of Patients with Re-Positive Nucleic Acid Tests

Presently, there is a big difference in the reinfection ratio among all reported data. The sputum, feces, and other specimens of the patients with reinfection were cultivated in P3 laboratory, but no live virus has been successfully cultivated. There have also been no reported cases from people who had close contact with re-positive patients. Related problems need to be observed and studied further.

BIBLIOGRAPHY

1. Military Front Expert Group. Diagnosis and treatment of novel coronavirus pneumonia infection suitable for military medics supporting Hubei (1st trial edition) [J/OL]. *Chinese Journal of Tuberculosis and Respiratory Diseases,* 43. [2020-02-25].http://rs.yiigle.com/yufa-biao/1182686.htm.doi:10.3760/cma.j.cn112147-20200224-00172.

2. General Office of National Health Commission, National Administration of Traditional Chinese Medicine Office. *Diagnosis and Treatment Protocol for Novel Coronavirus Pneumonia (7th Trial Edition) [EB/OL]*. [2020-03-03].

3. National Health Commission, National Administration of Traditional Chinese Medicine. Diagnosis and treatment plan for severe and critically severe COVID-19 cases (2nd trial edition) [EB/OL]. *National Health Commission Office Medical Letter*, 127. [2020-02-19].

4. Chinese Thoracic Society. Guidelines for diagnosis and treatment of community acquired pneumonia of Chinese adults (2016 edition) [J]. *Chinese Journal of Tuberculosis and Respiratory Diseases*, 39(4): 253–279. [2016]. doi:10.3760/cma.j.issn.10010939.2016.04.005.

5. Zhao Jianping, Hu Yi, Du Ronghui, Cheng Zhenshun, Jin Yang, Zhou Min, Zhang Jing, Qu Jieming, Cao Bin. Suggestions for application of glucocorticoid therapy for COVID-19 patients [J/OL]. *Chinese Journal of Tuberculosis and Respiratory Diseases*, 2020(03): 183–184. doi:10.3760/cma.j.issn.1001-0939.2020.0007.

6. Chinese Association of Rehabilitation Medicine, Respiratory Rehabilitation Committee of Chinese Association of Rehabilitation Medicine, Cardiopulmonary Rehabilitation Group of Chinese Society of Physical Medicine and Rehabilitation. Recommendations for respiratory rehabilitation of COVID-19 patients (2nd Edition) [J/OL]. *Chinese Journal of Tuberculosis and Respiratory Diseases*, 43 [2020-03-03]. http://rs.yiigle.com/yufabiao//1183323.htm. doi:10.3160/cma.j.cn112147-20200228-00206.

7. National Health Commission Office. Notice on printing and distributing the rehabilitation plan (trial) for discharged COVID-19 patients [EB/OL]. *National Health Commission Office Medical Letter*, 189. [2020-03-04].

8. Liu Qian, Wang Rongshuai, Qu Guoqiang, Wang Yunyun, Liu Pan, Zhu Yingzhi, Fei Geng, Ren Liang, Zhou Yiwu. A general observation report on systematic anatomy of dead bodies of COVID-19 patients [J]. *Journal of Forensic Medicine*, 36(1): 19–21. [2020].

9. Li Hui, Li Yongyin, Zhang Zhigao, Lu Zhen, Wang Yi, Lin Guanfeng. Establishment and clinical performance evaluation of COVID-19 antibody colloidal gold detection method [J/OL]. *Chinese Journal of Infectious Diseases*, 38. [2020-03-03]. http://rs.yiigle.com/yufabiao/1183332.htm. doi:10.3760/cma.j.cn311365-20200221-00101.

10. Chen Huagen, Liu Xiaohua, Xu Ying. Laboratory detection of common respiratory pathogens [J]. *Laboratory Medicine and Clinic*, 11(20): 2920–2921. [2014]. doi:10.3969/j.issn.1672-9455.2014.20.055.

11. Chaolin Huang, Yeming Wang, Xingwang Li. Clinical features of patients infected with 2019 novel coronavirus in Wuhan, China [J]. *Lancet*, 395(10223): 497–506. [2020]. doi: 10.1016/ S0140-6736(20)30183-5.

12. Dawei Wang, Bo Hu, Chang Hu. Clinical characteristics of 138 hospitalized patients with 2019 COVID-19 in Wuhan, China [J]. *JAMA*, 323(11): 1061–1069. [2020]. doi:10.1001/jama.2020.1585.

13. World Health Organization. *Statement on the Second Meeting of the International Health Regulations (2005) Emergency Committee Regarding the Outbreak of Novel Coronavirus (COVID-19) [EB/OL]*. [2020-1-30]. https://www.who.Int/news–room/

detail/30-01-2020-statement-on-the-second-meeting-of-the-international-heal th-regulations-(2005)-emergency-committee-regarding-the-outbreak-of-novel-c oronavirus–(COVID-19).

14. N Chen, M Zhou, X Dong, J Qu, F Gong, Y Han, Y Qiu, J Wang, Y Liu, Y Wei, J Xia, T Yu, X Zhang, L Zhang. Epidemiological and clinical characteristics of 99 cases of 2019 novel coronavirus pneumonia in Wuhan, China: A descriptive study. *Lancet*, 395(10223): 507–513. [2020].

15. World Health Organization. *Clinical management of severe acute respiratory infection when novel coronavirus (nCoV) infection is suspected [EB/OL]*. [2020-1-28]. https://www.who.Int/publications-detail/clinical-management-of-severe-acute-respiratory-infection-when-novel-coronavirus-(ncov)-infection-is-suspe cted.09601200Information Classification: General00Information Classification: General

Chapter 3

Dysfunctions of COVID-19

3.1 RESPIRATORY DYSFUNCTION

Respiratory dysfunction in COVID-19 patients is closely related to the severity of the disease after onset. According to the clinical classification criteria in the *Pneumonia Diagnosis and Treatment Protocol for COVID-19 Infection (6th Trial Edition)* issued by the National Health Commission (NHC), except patients with mild clinical symptoms and no manifestations of pneumonia in imaging, normal, severe, and critically severe patients all have respiratory dysfunction to varying degrees. Understanding the pathophysiological mechanisms of respiratory dysfunction in COVID-19 patients determines the timing of rehabilitation intervention. According to existing studies and literature reports, patients with COVID-19 have been found to often suffer from the following respiratory dysfunctions.

3.1.1 Dyspnea

Dyspnea is one of the more common dysfunctions in COVID-19 patients. From the patient's subjective point of view, dyspnea is laborious breath, suffocation, and discomfort. Symptoms of dyspnea are often seen clinically as a sign of the severity of the disease, but it has been observed that, in some COVID-19 patients, the improvement in dyspnea is disproportionate to the recovery from the disease. A few patients in nucleic acid testing twice had negative results, indicating oxygen saturation of 98% or more, but there were still obvious symptoms. This suggests that the symptoms of dyspnea may also be related to psychosocial factors, and it is necessary to carry out professional psychological intervention for COVID-19 patients during the convalescent period.

3.1.1.1 Definition of Dyspnea

The American Thoracic Society has defined dyspnea as "a symptom characterized by a subjective sense of labored breathing, which differs significantly in intensity". This sense of labored breathing can result from the interaction of multidisciplinary factors, including physiological, psychosocial, social, and environmental factors, which may induce secondary physiological and behavioral responses. So, dyspnea is typically characterized by labored breathing, which is different from shortness of breath, polypnea, hyperpnea, and hyperventilation. It is a subjective feeling of the patient and is closely correlated with the life quality of the patient.

3.1.1.2 Mechanisms That Cause Dyspnea

Dyspnea, as a subjective feeling, is caused by different stimuli (such as exercise, hypoxemia, acidosis, anxiety, etc.). They activate the cerebral sensory cortex and limbic lobe of the brain. Then sensory signals are sent to the center, and the brain processes signals and finally leads to dyspnea. During this process, other regulatory systems in the body are also involved in the regulation of respiration.

3.1.1.3 Pathophysiology of Dyspnea

The pathophysiological mechanism of dyspnea was first introduced by Campbell and Howell in 1960 with the theory of "length-tension inappropriateness". The core of this theory is to propose that dyspnea is caused by the separation or mismatch among the central respiratory dynamic activation and the afferent information of the airway, lung, and chest wall receptors. On the one hand, feedback from peripheral receptors enables the brain to assess the effectiveness of dynamic instructions in reaching the respiratory muscles as well as the adequacy of flow and volume instructions. When the respiratory pressure, airflow, or movement of the lungs or chest wall changes, the center fails to issue appropriate dynamic instructions, thereby increasing the intensity of dyspnea. On the other hand, the mismatch between the central respiratory movement instructions and the mechanical response of the respiratory system will also lead to the feeling of dyspnea. When patients have an abnormal mechanical load of the respiratory system, such as resistance load, elastic load, abnormal respiratory muscle, etc., it will cause the separation of outgoing and incoming information during respiratory movement. Some researchers have found that inadequate neural activity and ventilation can cause intense dyspnea.

1) Increased ventilation instruction: There was a close correlation between ventilation level and dyspnea intensity. COVID-19 patients in the state of calm often experience labored breathing and discomfort. At this time, increased ventilation is usually due to dyspnea caused by excessive physiological activity level. For example, in order to compensate for the invalid cavity enlargement caused by lung consolidation, the patient needs to increase ventilation. This increase in respiratory

dynamic instruction can produce dyspnea symptoms. In addition, malnutrition and hypoxemia can also impair respiratory function and peripheral muscle function, leading to limited exercise endurance and dyspnea. It was found that the intensity of dyspnea was different with different ventilation levels, and supplementation of oxygen could relieve exercise-related dyspnea.

2) Abnormal respiratory muscles: Respiratory muscle weakness leads to a mismatch between central power output and completion of ventilation. This mismatch may explain the reason for dyspnea in patients with neuromuscular disease. It is the weakness of muscle tissue that led to reduced ventilation. Respiratory muscle weakness in COVID-19 patients often results from fatigue, muscle soreness, hypokalemia, anemia, bed rest, and immobilization. Recovery can be achieved within a short period of time through symptomatic treatment and rehabilitation intervention after vital signs are stable.

3) Abnormal ventilation resistance: Increased elastic resistance due to airway constriction and lung consolidation can lead to dyspnea. CT findings of COVID-19 patients were dominated by subpleural ground-glass opacity (GGO). Lesions were mainly distributed under the pleura, often accompanied by localized thickening of the adjacent pleura. Bilateral lung involvement is more common, mainly in the lower lobe of the lung. The formation of GGO suggests that the virus causes inflammatory exudation and edema dominated by pulmonary interstitium, in which thickened interlobular septa and interlobular septal line shadow superimposed on the GGO background form typical paving-stone-like changes. In the lesion, air bronchogram and halo were also seen. During the progression of the disease, the exudation in the pulmonary interstitium gradually increased, and on the basis of GGO, lung consolidation is often associated. In some patients, the formation of fibrous stripes can be seen during the convalescent period. According to the above imaging conclusions, moderate, severe. and critically severe COVID-19 patients all experienced increased ventilation resistance throughout the course of the disease. This increase in ventilation resistance adds to the peripheral elastic load, and when the external ventilation load increases, the intensity of dyspnea grows. The increasing intensity of dyspnea during the external ventilation load is consistent with the peak air pressure associated with respiratory muscle contraction, inspiratory cycle, and respiratory rate.

4) Abnormal respiratory patterns: Dyspnea is usually caused by a lesion involving the lung parenchyma. The most common abnormal respiratory pattern in lung parenchyma lesions is rapid shallow breathing.

Pursed lip breathing can reduce dyspnea in chronic obstructive pulmonary disease (COPD) patients, as this technique can reduce respiratory rate, restore the normal breathing patterns in respiratory muscle, prolong expiratory time, and increase tidal volume. For COVID-19 patients, pulmonary function tests should be performed first. Patients with obstructive ventilatory impairment found after the test can refer to the respiratory training methods for COPD patients, and patients with restrictive ventilatory impairment can increase lung ventilation through deep breathing exercises combined with thoracic expansion exercise. Patients with negative results for reverse transcription polymerase chain reaction (RT-PCR) assays will be more benefited from airway clearance techniques (ACT), which can promote the removal of exudation within the lesion and the removal of small-airway mucus plugs. As COVID-19 is an acute respiratory infectious disease, priority should be given to how to avoid aerosol spread, reduce the risk of virus transmission, and reduce occupational exposure of health care workers when adopting ACT.

5) Abnormal blood gas: Abnormal blood gas is the worst consequence of most cardiopulmonary diseases, and because of compensation of kidneys, the correlation between abnormal blood gas and dyspnea changes significantly under different conditions. Based on the medullary chemoreceptor, it is dependent on changes of hydrogen ion concentration and can lead to dyspnea when acidosis occurs.

3.1.2 Hypoxemia

Hypoxia is a major pathophysiological change in the progression of respiratory disease to respiratory dysfunction and is one of the common dysfunctions in COVID-19 patients, except in mild cases.

The main generation mechanisms of hypoxemia in COVID-19 patients are discussed below.

3.1.2.1 Hypoventilation

Hypoventilation can be caused by decreased respiratory power, increased dead space, decreased chest wall and lung compliance, and increased airway resistance. When respiratory muscle power is weakened, the chest expands feebly and the alveoli do not fill normally, resulting in decreased ventilation. The increase of dead space volume is seen in rapid shallow breathing, which leads to the increase of anatomic ineffective air cavity and the decrease of effective air exchange capacity in alveoli. Bronchiectasis increases the airway volume, which also gives rise to the enlargement of the anatomic cavity, leading to hypoventilation.

A decrease in chest wall compliance and lung compliance leads to alveolar filling, which gives rise to poor ventilation. The compliance of the chest wall is related to its activity. When extensive pleural adhesion, pleural effusion, pneumothorax, severe thoracic deformity and other conditions occur, the expansion of the thorax will be limited, and the compliance of the chest wall will be reduced. Alveolar surfactant can reduce the surface tension and play an important role in maintaining alveolar filling and preventing alveolar collapse. A large amount of inflammatory substances exuded from the lesions of COVID-19 patients. In pulmonary edema, alveolar surfactant is diluted, which damages the stability of the alveoli, leading to atelectasis, and ultimately leads to inadequate ventilation.

The increase in airway resistance is mainly because of the decrease in airway diameter, which is caused by the edema of airway mucosa and increased secretions.

3.1.2.2 Diffusion Impairment

The physical division between gas and blood or the reduced transport time of red blood cells through pulmonary capillaries will lead to the diffusion impairment. The main factors affecting the diffusion function are diffusion distance and diffusion area. When the diffusion distance increases or the diffusion area decreases, the diffusion capacity of carbon dioxide is much faster than that of oxygen, so the diffusion impairment generally only affects oxygenation. In COVID-19 patients, the diffusion impairment alone is rarely seen, and it is often accompanied by decreased ventilation and disordered ventilation/blood flow.

3.1.2.3 Local Ventilation/Blood Flow Disorder

Ventilation/blood flow disorder is the most common cause of hypoxemia. It is often seen in diseases that can cause poor ventilation of multiple pulmonary units at the same time, such as airway obstruction, atelectasis, lung consolidation, and pulmonary edema. Rapidly advancing GGO can be seen on lung computed tomography (CT) scans in COVID-19 patients in the exacerbation phase, suggesting a high probability of severe ventilation/blood flow disorder.

3.1.2.4 Increase of Dead Space

Rapid shallow breathing can increase ventilation of the anatomic dead space. This rapid shallow breathing is extremely common in severe and critically severe COVID-19 patients.

3.1.2.5 Decreased Oxygen-Carrying Capacity

When hemoglobin's oxygen-carrying capacity is reduced, persistent hypoxemia can occur even when arterial partial oxygen pressure is normal. In the acute phase of COVID-19, patients often have fever, fatigue, and poor appetite, and are in a negative nitrogen balance with insufficient iron intake. Elderly patients often have iron-deficiency anemia, which affects the oxygen-carrying capacity of the blood to a certain extent, and then causes the reflexivity heart rate to increase.

3.1.3 Acute Respiratory Distress Syndrome and Respiratory Failure

According to current clinical data, complications in COVID-19 patients include acute respiratory distress syndrome (ARDS), ribonucleic acidemia, acute heart injury, and secondary infection. The clinical characteristics of severe patients include older age (median age: 66 years), more underlying diseases, the time from onset to dyspnea is 5 days, while the time for ARDS is 8 days. Most patients need oxygen therapy, and a few patients need invasive ventilation and even extracorporeal membrane oxygenation (ECMO). Laboratory tests suggest that critically severe patients often have higher leukocyte and neutrophil counts, as well as higher D-dimer, creatine kinase, and creatine levels, with significant lymphopenia. This suggests that severe patients develop an overactivation of immune cells and a cytokine storm in the immune response targeting the virus.

Mechanisms of respiratory failure usually include:

1) Ventilation dysfunction: Inflammation in the airway, bronchial wall edema, increased secretion, and thickened mucosal and other factors together lead to narrow lumen, increased airway resistance, blocked airflow, and reduced ventilation.
2) Air exchange dysfunction: Bronchiolar inflammation, the formation of small-airway mucus plugs, lung consolidation, interstitial fibrosis, and other pathological changes can lead to ventilation-perfusion ratio imbalance, increased ventilation of dead space, increased functional shunt, and decreased diffusion area, thus causing ventilation dysfunction.

For COVID-19 patients, damage to multiple organs and respiratory failure caused by a cytokine storm must be taken into account. The pathological changes of viral pneumonia include pulmonary interstitial and parenchymal involvement. Biopsy of the COVID-19 victim revealed that histopathological changes were very similar to the viral pneumonia caused by severe acute respiratory syndrome coronavirus (SARS-CoV) and Middle East respiratory syndrome coronavirus (MERS-CoV). It is worth noting that the current autopsy found that COVID-19 is different from atypical pneumonia caused by the SARS virus. The COVID-19 patients who died in the early stage showed obvious lung damage. Patchy shadows were found by visual observation, with gray-white lesions and dark red bleeding. The texture was tough, and the lung has lost its inherent sponge texture, which is consistent with the distribution of lung imaging changes of patients. Pulmonary fibrosis and consolidation were not as serious as those caused to SARS, but the exudative reaction was more obvious than SARS. This also explains why it is difficult to correct hypoxemia in critically severe patients who rely solely on ventilators to increase inspiratory pressure.

3.2 PHYSICAL DYSFUNCTION

The inevitable long-term bed rest and inactivity of COVID-19 patients during the course of the disease is a major cause of physical dysfunction. Its symptoms are malaise, easy fatigue, muscle soreness, and palpitate and some patients have amyotrophy and decrease of muscle strength. At the same time, in addition to the psychological stress and trauma brought by the disease, there are also physical symptoms closely related to psychological factors, such as insomnia, fatigue, palpitation, chest tightness, dysphagia, urinary frequency, and so on. These physical symptoms may involve nervous, circulatory, digestive, respiratory, urogenital, endocrine, motor, and other systems. Therefore, in the assessment of patients' physical dysfunction, the whole psychological and physiological analyses should be carried out, and careful observation should be made to identify whether physiological factors or psychological factors are dominant, which guides the formation of the rehabilitation treatment plan. The more common physical dysfunctions in COVID-19 patients during the convalescent period are discussed below.

3.2.1 Tachycardias

Tachycardia is common in COVID-19 patients in a calm state, and can occur even with moderate physical exertion. With a certain oxygen uptake, the heart rate of COVID-19 patients is higher than the normal level, indicating a lower stroke volume. Because the cardiac output of the general population without special training is similar, tachycardia reflects a decrease in cardiopulmonary function in COVID-19 patients.

3.2.1.1 Cause of Tachycardia

There are 33 known causes of tachycardia. There are six causes associated with the pathophysiological mechanisms of COVID-19, including ARDS, anemia, fever, tachycardia, hypoxemia, and hypovolemia. Hypoproteinemia, caused by nutritional deficiency and infection in COVID-19 patients, can lead to a decrease in effective circulating blood volume, often accompanied by mild anemia, resulting in a significantly faster heart rate at rest than before the onset of the disease. To meet the increase of peripheral muscle oxygen consumption, it is necessary to further increase cardiac output to meet the needs of oxygenation when carrying out daily activities with low metabolic equivalent. During low-power exercises, such as baduan jin exercise (baduanjin qigong) and tai chi chuan, it can be observed that patients' heart rates often quickly exceed the standard rate predicted by age.

3.2.1.2 Heart Rate and Oxygen Uptake

Oxygen uptake reflects the body's ability to absorb and consume oxygen, which is determined by the level of oxygen demand in cells and the maximum amount of oxygen transport. Oxygen uptake can be calculated by oxygen uptake into the bloodstream and tissues. Maximal oxygen uptake (VO2max) is the most important index to reflect aerobic capacity and exercise potential. Factors affecting oxygen uptake include oxygen-carrying capacity of blood, cardiac function, peripheral blood flow redistribution, tissue uptake, etc. The relationship between heart rate and oxygen uptake is usually nonlinear in low power motion but becomes nearly linear when the power gradually increases to the maximum. When an age-predicted heart rate is reached during exercise, it usually reflects that the patient has made the most effort and is close to reaching VO2max. The difference between the heart rate predicted by age and the maximum heart rate during exercise is the heart rate reserve. For COVID-19 patients, after correction of hypoxemia, anemia, and hypoproteinemia, tachycardia in calm state and low metabolic equivalent during exercise exceed the predicted value, both of which reflect the patient's reduced exercise ability.

3.2.2 Decreased Exercise Ability and Tolerance

Exercise ability refers to the ability the human body shows when exercising, which can be divided into general exercise ability and athletic ability. The former mainly refers to the basic abilities of walking, running, jumping, throwing, climbing, and scrambling that people have in daily life, labor, and general sports, while the latter refers to the athletic ability to complete a certain athletic competition. Exercise tolerance refers to the ability of the human body to carry out muscle activities for a long time, also known as antifatigue ability. Tolerance quality reflects the comprehensive condition of muscular endurance, cardiopulmonary endurance, and whole-body endurance. It is closely related to the improvement of the function of muscle tissue, cardiopulmonary system, and other basic system functions of the body. Patients with COVID-19 have a decrease in both exercise ability and tolerance.

3.2.2.1 Fatigue

Fatigue is one of the most common symptoms in clinical practice, which belongs to nonspecific fatigue. Its symptoms are perceived exertion and limb weakness. Under the physiological state, fatigue can be relieved after rest or eating, and pathological fatigue cannot be relieved. According to the severity of fatigue, it is divided into three degrees clinically: mild fatigue is manifested as listlessness and constant tiredness or weakness. Patients with mild fatigue can perform manual labor, and the symptoms of fatigue can be relieved after rest, yet they cannot return to the normal state. Moderate fatigue is manifested as mental fatigue and physical weakness. Patients can perform their daily life and work, but they feel very tired after light physical work, and cannot return to normal state after a long rest. Severe fatigue is manifested as extreme mental exhaustion, inability to carry out normal activities, feeling of tiredness, and reluctance to speak even when resting.

Fatigue is one of the first symptoms in COVID-19 patients. It has been reported that fatigue is also one of the most common symptoms after fever, cough, and expectoration. In severe and critically severe patients, the severity of fatigue was significantly higher than that of normal patients. Symptoms of fatigue can last until the nucleic acid turns negative; however, even after the nucleic acid turns negative for a period of time, there will still be symptoms of exhaustion, which is the root cause for the decline in exercise ability and exercise tolerance of COVID-19 patients.

3.2.2.2 Immobilization Syndrome

Immobilization syndrome refers to a series of pathophysiological reactions caused by limb motor dysfunction or function loss due to diseases or trauma, or prolonged bed rest and immobilization after fracture. The specific manifestations are as follows:

1) Nervous system: Skin and limb sensory abnormalities, decreased sensitivity to pain, decreased motor function, and emotional instability.
2) Circulatory system: Increased heart rate and orthostatic hypotension.
3) Exercise system: Declined muscle strength and endurance, muscle atrophy, osteoporosis, etc.
4) Digestive system: Loss of appetite or anorexia and constipation.
5) Respiratory system: Decreased vital capacity, decreased respiratory ability, weak cough, etc.
6) Endocrine and urinary system: Polyuria and sometimes kidney stones occur due to heavy urinary calcium.
7) Others: Some patients will suffer from skin nutrition problems and ulcers.

COVID-19 patients have to stay in bed during the acute phase of disease progression. The severity of the disease is directly proportional to the time spent in bed, and respiratory muscle weakness and muscular atrophy caused by immobilization are also directly proportional to the severity of the disease. It is not difficult to see, from the influence of immobilization on the functions of various systems and organs of the whole body, that immobilization further aggravates the decline of exercise capacity and endurance.

3.3 PSYCHOLOGICAL AND SOCIAL DYSFUNCTION

With the development of medicine, the change of disease category and the improvement of people's health needs, the outlook on health and the medical model of modern people has changed, and the medical model has changed from biological model to biological-psychological-social medical model. This means that the objects of medical research are patients rather than diseases. When studying the psychological and social dysfunction of COVID-19 patients, researchers should know more clearly that COVID-19 is not only a disease but also a collective crisis. In terms of the psychological and social dysfunction of COVID-19 patients, attention should be paid to two levels of psychological reactions to stress: first, the adverse emotional reactions brought by the disease itself to patients, often manifested as anxiety, depression, fear, etc.; second, post-traumatic stress disorder (PTSD) will also cause psychological and social dysfunction of patients.

3.3.1 Post-Traumatic Stress Disorder (PTSD)

PTSD is a stress-related disorder that can develop after a person is exposed to a traumatic event, such as a natural disaster, traffic accident, or sudden death of a loved one. It is also a kind of stress disorder with serious clinical symptoms, poor prognosis, and possible brain damage among trauma and stress-related disorders. Trauma-exposed individuals usually experience a typical psychological reaction process of "shock-denial-invasion-constant correction-end". However, when the traumatic event exceeds the limit of the patient's psychological endurance, or the psychological reaction is too strong, physiological and mental pathological changes will occur and eventually develop into PTSD. The U.S. Research Center announced that PTSD would be the fourth most common mental disease since the September 11 attacks. Hubei Province, especially Wuhan City, is the region with the largest number of confirmed COVID-19 cases and deaths. In the early stage of disease transmission, the sharp increase in the number of patients greatly exceeded the load capacity of local medical resources, resulting in serious medical runs and great psychological blows to patients, their families, and frontline medical staff. These groups are the high-risk groups to suffer from PTSD. From the epidemiology of PTSD, women are more likely to suffer from the disease than men. People with a low education level, harsh environments in childhood, and introverted personalities are also considered high-risk groups that need special attention.

3.3.1.1 Clinical Symptoms of PTSD

1. Traumatic re-experience: Trauma re-experience is the most common and specific symptom of PTSD, including flashback; under the condition of clear consciousness, sudden memories or scenes of traumatic events are constantly appearing in the brain; nightmares related to traumatic events continue to occur in sleep; the time, place and people related to traumatic events stir up the patients' feelings and serious mental pain or physiological reaction to stress occur.

   Increased alertness: It is one of the typical symptoms of PTSD, often manifested as excessive alertness, panic attack, inattention, irritability and anxiety. Physical symptoms may include palpitations, hidrosis, headache, general malaise, etc.

2. Avoidance or emotional paralysis: Avoidance can be manifested as conscious or unconscious continuous avoidance of scenes or events related to trauma occurrence. Emotional paralysis refers to emotional anesthesia, such as slow response to the stimulation of the surrounding environment; loss of interest in previous hobbies; gradually keeping away from social and interpersonal relationships; lack of vision for the future. Patients suffering from emotional paralysis often give people a superficial impression of being indifferent and dull, but they are always alert.

3. Depression: Depression is a fairly common simultaneous phenomenon of PTSD. Patients find it difficult to be interested in things, alienate or isolate the outside world, have no thinking and longing for the future, have decreased memory, and find it difficult to think and concentrate.

4. Sleep disorders: Sleep disorders in patients with PTSD mainly include difficulty in sleeping, nightmares and being easily awakened. For patients with COVID-19, there are many causes of sleep disorders, which need to be carefully screened.

   Sleep disorders in patients with PTSD mainly include difficulty in sleeping, nightmares and being easily awakened. For patients with COVID-19, there are many causes of sleep disorders, which need to be carefully screened.

3.3.1.2 Prognosis and Influence of PTSD

It is normal for patients to feel depressed and unstable for a period of time after traumatic events; however, if the emotional reaction is too intense or the stress reaction persists and has an impact on daily life, it is necessary to be alert of having PTSD, and they should go to the psychology and psychiatric department as soon as possible. Because the pathogenesis of PTSD is not completely clear, the main treatment methods are empirical therapies, including drug therapy, physical therapy, and psychotherapy. PTSD is characterized by persistent and recurrent onset and is a stress-related disorder with the most serious clinical symptoms and the worst prognosis. Patients' social, work, and study functions are impaired, which often leads to their loss of labor ability, accompanied by substance abuse, depression, anxiety-related disorders, and other mental disorders, with a very high suicide rate. Timely and effective treatment is very important for PTSD patients.

3.3.2 Adjustment Disorder

Adjustment disorder is mainly characterized by emotional disorder, which manifests itself in various forms, such as depression and anxiety, as well as maladjusted conduct disorder, which is related to age. Emotional symptoms are more common in adults. Stress, depression, and related physical symptoms can appear but may not necessarily meet the diagnostic criteria of anxiety disorder or depression disorder.

The mental stress events causing adjustment disorder are weak in intensity, and most of them are common events in daily life. The milder condition of adjustment disorder is closely related to personality and individual coping style, and there is a lack of research on the pathological mechanism of this disorder. There is also a lack of epidemiological reports on the incidence rate in adjustment disorder. It has been reported in foreign countries that patients with adjustment disorder account for 5%–20% of psychiatric outpatient clinics.

Adjustment disorder usually occurs within 1–3 months after stressful events happen in life, with various clinical manifestations, including depression, anxiety or worry, feeling unable to cope with the present life or planning for the future, insomnia, stress-related physical dysfunction (headache, abdominal discomfort, chest tightness, and palpitation), and impaired social function or work. The course of the disease is generally not more than 6 months. If the stressors persist, the course of the disease may be prolonged, and the prognosis is good regardless of the course of the disease, especially in adult patients.

3.3.3 Bereavement and Mourning Reaction

Bereavement and mourning reaction refers to the state of depression, sadness, or grief caused by the patient's reaction to the stressful life event of the death of a relative, which is also called grief reaction. Bereavement and mourning reaction or grief reaction does not belong to affective disorder, but to adjustment disorder. According to DSM-IV, the exclusion criteria for major depression is not diagnosed if the depressive symptoms persist for less than 2 months after the loss of a loved one. However, in DSM-IV, this exclusion criterion has been removed, and it can be seen that the bereavement and mourning reaction is not easily distinguished from major depression. In fact, mourning and depression do not conflict each other. Bereavement and mourning reaction is often involved in the onset of depression.

Wuhan is the city with the largest number of deaths during the pandemic, and because of the family clustering onset of COVID-19, many members of a family may be infected or even die. After the pandemic is totally controlled, medical professionals should be alert to the impact of the bereavement and mourning reaction.

3.3.4 Sleep Disorder

Sleep disorder refers to the abnormal amount of sleep and abnormal behavior during sleep and is also the manifestation of normal rhythmic alternating disorder of sleep and awakening. It can be caused by a variety of factors and is often related to physical diseases, including sleep disorders and abnormal sleep. Sleep is closely related to human health. A survey shows that many people suffer from sleep disorders or sleep-related diseases, and the proportion of adults suffering from sleep disorders is as high as 30%. Sleep is an extremely important physiological function to maintain human life and is essential to the human body. The incidence of sleep disorder in COVID-19 patients is much higher than 30%, which should be addressed.

Sleep disorders in COVID-19 patients are mainly manifested by abnormal sleep volume, including sleep difficulties and early awakening. Frequent cough and dyspnea affect people's sleep; on the other hand, anxiety leads to difficulty in falling asleep. Considering that there are both physiological and psychological reasons for the sleep disorders in patients with COVID-19, drug treatment is suggested and behavioral treatment should be adopted for intervention at the same time, so as to improve the sleep disorder of patients to the maximum extent and provide favorable conditions for the rehabilitation of other physical dysfunctions.

3.3.5 Activities of Daily Living Dysfunction

Activities of daily living (ADL) refers to a series of basic activities necessary for people to take care of their own clothing, food, housing, transportation, and personal hygiene, allowing them to live independently in the community in daily living. ADL reflects the most basic abilities of people's activities in families (or medical institutions) and communities. It is divided into basic activities of daily living (BADL), i.e., eating, grooming, washing, bathing, toileting, and dressing, and instrumental activities of daily living (IADL), such as turning over, sitting up from the bed, moving, walking, driving wheelchairs, and going up and down the stairs. COVID-19 patients generally have a decline in ADL score during the course of the disease, and the degree of decline is positively correlated with the severity of the disease. In the early course of the disease, the patient's functional activity is decreased due to fever, fatigue, and myalgia. As the disease progresses, patients' ability to take care of themselves can be affected. Severe patients are often unable to eat and use a bedpan in bed with assistance from others. Patients in convalescent period still have functional problems, such as inability to take a bath independently, prolonged washing time, short of breath when dressing, etc. At present, it is observed that some severe patients still have a decline in functional activity after discharge, which is the result of a decline in cardiopulmonary function, exercise capacity, and endurance.

3.3.6 Social Engagement Dysfunction

In 2001, the World Health Organization (WHO) put forward the theoretical framework in the *International Classification of Functioning, Disability, and Health* (ICF), which provides an update and more comprehensive understanding of health evaluation. The ICF framework points out that disability is an inclusive term that includes disability, limited activities, and social participation dysfunction, and reflects the health status in terms of functionality at the body organ or structure level and the individual and social levels. Among them, social participation dysfunction refers to the restriction of individuals' participation in daily living, which is a comprehensive manifestation of the impact of personal health status on normal individual and social functions. Compared with physical disability, social participation belongs to a higher level of needs and has a more significant impact on the quality of life. Studies have shown that the function of social participation is affected by multiple factors, at the individual level, such as demography, socioeconomic and physical conditions, and at the environmental level, such as place of residence.

As a highly contagious acute respiratory infectious disease, COVID-19 will not only bring long-term psychological pressure to patients but also have a certain impact on the social group where the patients are located and the social environment in the concentrated outbreak areas. As the pandemic has been gradually controlled and the order of production and living has been gradually restored, the social participation inability of COVID-19 patients should be considered by all sectors of society. On the basis of identifying the bad psychological state of the patients and improving their physical dysfunction through systematic rehabilitation, and with the evaluation and assistance of the psychological professionals, we should actively deal with various psychological problems, build a healthy and positive social environment, avoid negative social phenomena such as phobias, discrimination, exclusion, and isolation and help the cured patients who once suffered from COVID-19 to smoothly return to normal social life.

BIBLIOGRAPHY

1. Shen Meng, Siyuan Chen. *Lung rehabilitation [M]*. Beijing: People's Health Publishing House. [2007].
2. National Health Commission. Diagnosis and treatment plan for COVID-19 (6th trial edition) [J]. *Chinese Journal of Virus*, 10(2): 88–92. [2020].
3. Chen Wang, Guoen Fang, Yuxiao Xie. Guidelines for respiratory rehabilitation of COVID-19 patients (1st edition) [J]. *Chinese Journal of Reparative and Reconstructive Surgery*, 34(3): 275–279. [2019].
4. Kebin Cheng, Ming Wei, Hong Shen, Wu Chaoming, Chen Dechang, Xiong Weining, Zhou Xin, Zhang Dinyu, Zheng Junhua. Analysis of clinical characteristics of 463 patients during rehabilitation from common and severe COVID-19 [J/OL]. *Shanghai Medical Journal*, 43(04): 224–232 [2020-03-27]. http://kns.cnki.net/kcms/detail/31.1366.r.20200312.1254.004.html.
5. Huang CL, Wang YM, Li XW. Clinical features of patients infected with 2019 novel coronavirus in Wuhan, China [J]. *Lancet*. 395(10223): 497–506. [2020]. doi: 10.10 16/S0140-6736(20)30183–5org/10.1101/2020.02.08.20021212.
6. Hui DSC, Zumla A. Severe acute respiratory syndrome historical, epidemiologic, and clinical features [J]. *Infectious Disease Clinics of North America*, 33(4): 869–889. [2019].
7. Chen N, Zhou M, Dong X, Qu J, Gong F, Han Y, Zhang L. Epidemiological and clinical characteristics of 99 cases of 2019 novel coronavirus pneumonia in Wuhan, China: a descriptive study[J]. *Lancet*, 395(10223): 507–513. [2020].
8. Wang DW, Hu B, Hu C, et al. Clinical characteristics of 138 hospitalized patients with COVID-19 in Wuhan, China[J]. *JAMA*, 323(11): 1061–1069. [2020].
9. Zare Mehrjardi M, Kahkouee S, Pourabdollah M. Radio – pathological correlation of organizing pneumonia (OP): A pictorial review [J]. *British Journal of Radiology*, 90(1071): 20160723. [2017].
10. Xu Z, Shi L, Wang Y, et al. Pathological findings of COVID-19 associated with acute respiratory distress syndrome [J]. *Lancet Respiratory Medicine*, 8(4): 420-422, [2020]. doi: 10. 1016/S2213-2600(20)30076-X

11. Xi Liu, Rongshuai Wang, Guoqiang Qu, et al. A general observation report on systematic anatomy of dead bodies of COVID-19 patients [J]. *Journal of Forensic Medicine*, 36(1): 19–21. [2020].

12. Shengyu Zhou, Chunting Wang, Wei Zhang, et al. Clinical features and therapeutic effects of 537 patients with COVID-19 in Shandong Province [J/OL]. *Journal of Shandong University (Health Sciences)*, 58(3): 44–51, [2020-03-27]. http://kns.cnki.net/kcms/detail/37.1390.r.20200310.1047.002.html.

13. Stroebe M, Schut H, Finkenauer C. The traumatization of grief? A conceptual framework for understanding the trauma – bereavement interface [J]. *Journal of Psychiatry and Related Sciences*, 38(3): 185–201. [2001].

14. Katz CL, Pellegrino L, Pandya A, et al. Research on psychiatric out-come and interventions subsequent to disasters: A review of the literature [J]. *Psychiatry Research*, 110(3): 201–217. [2002].

15. Breslau N, Davis GC, Peterson EL, et al. Psychiatric sequence of posttraumatic stress disorder in women [J]. *Archives of General Psychiatry*, 54(1): 81–87. [1997].

16. He Yue, Zhang Hongtao, Psychological effect and rehabilitation of PTSD patients [J]. *Chinese Journal of Clinical Rehabilitation*, 7(16): 2346–2347. [2003].

17. Yang Rui, Li Yajie, Psychological effect and nursing of trauma patients [J]. *Chinese Nursing Research*, 4(18): 577–579. [2004].

18. Jiang Kaida, Zhou Dongfeng, Li Lingjiang, et al. *Advanced Course in Psychiatry[M]*. Beijing: People's Military Medical Press. [2009].

19. World Health Organization. *International Classification of Functioning, Disability and Health (ICF) [M]*. Gevena: World Health Organization. [2001].

20. Svestkova O. International classification of functioning, disability and health of world health organization (ICF) [J]. *Prague Medical Report*, 109(4): 268–274. [2008].

21. Curvers N, Pavlova M, Hajema KJ, et al. Social participation among older adults (55+): Results of a survey in the region of South Limburg in the Netherlands [J]. *Health & Social Care in the Community*, 26(1): e85–93. [2018].

22. Broer T, Nieboer AP, Strating MM, et al. Constructing the social: An evaluation study of the outcomes and processes of a 'social participation' improvement project [J]. *Journal of Psychiatric and Mental Health Nursing*, 18(4): 323–332. [2011].

23. Woodruff Prescott G, van den Berge Maarten, Boucher Richard C et al. American thoracic society/national heart, lung, and blood institute asthma-chronic obstructive pulmonary disease overlap workshop report.[J]. *American Journal of Respiratory and Critical Care Medicine*, 2017, 196: 375–381.

24. Campbell EJ, Howell JB. The sensation of breathlessness. *British Medical Bulletin[J]*, 1963, 19: 36–40. doi: 10.1093/oxfordjournals.bmb.a070002

Chapter 4

Assessment for Rehabilitation of COVID-19

Despite effective treatment, COVID-19 patients still often suffer from respiratory, physical, psychological, and social dysfunction to varying degrees. Therefore, it is urged that patients should receive rehabilitation intervention for their comprehensive recovery as well as quality of life. Rehabilitation training for COVID-19 patients requires professional rehabilitation physicians to formulate exercise prescriptions based on patients' specific conditions. The formulation of exercise prescription depends on systematic assessment for rehabilitation, which should run through the whole process of rehabilitation treatment. The system of rehabilitation assessment for COVID-19 patients mainly includes assessments for respiratory function, physical function, and psychosocial function.

4.1 ASSESSMENT FOR RESPIRATORY FUNCTION

Examination of lung function is required to diagnose many respiratory diseases. The examination results can determine the degree and type of lung damage caused by the disease, helping clinicians make accurate diagnoses and develop scientific treatment plans.

Generally speaking, an examination of the respiratory function includes a pulmonary ventilation test, a respiratory mechanism test, and a small-airway test. This examination is used not only in rehabilitation but also in occupational evaluation.

Two important factors must be taken into account when conducting the above tests:

1) Mental factors: Respiration is more directly affected by mental factors; therefore, the examination of respiratory function requires active doctor–patient cooperation, the degree of which has a significant impact on the

results. Therefore, this examination must be repeated several times to find out a relatively constant value, with generally ±20% as its normal range.

2) Respiratory system state factors: Respiratory function changes more obviously in different respiratory system states. For example, the results of examinations are usually significantly different in the case of respiratory tract inflammation and after the elimination of respiratory tract inflammation. In fact, this difference should be regarded not as an improvement in respiratory function, but as the elimination of inflammation's effect on respiratory function. For that reason, attention must be paid to the consistency of the basic conditions in the predynamic and postdynamic examinations.

4.1.1 Assessment of Respiratory Function

Clinical assessment of respiratory function includes subjective symptoms and objective examinations.

4.1.1.1 Subjective Symptoms

Generally speaking, subjective symptoms are divided into six levels based on the presence of shortness of breath and panting symptoms in daily life.

- Level 0: Patients can act normally even if they have respiratory dysfunction. They have a normal life like ordinary people without shortness of breath or panting.
- Level 1: Unlike ordinary people, patients may experience shortness of breath during manual labor.
- Level 2: Patients can walk at a normal speed without shortness of breath, but they will show symptoms of shortness of breath when walking fast, climbing stairs, or climbing uphill, while other healthy peers of the same age will not show shortness of breath.
- Level 3: Patients will show shortness of breath when walking fewer than 100 slow steps.
- Level 4: Patients will show shortness of breath during slight movements, such as speaking or dressing.
- Level 5: Patients will still show shortness of breath even in a quiet state. They are unable to lie on their backs.

4.1.1.2 Objective Examination

4.1.1.2.1 Lung Volume

Lung volume includes tidal volume, inspiratory reverse volume, inspiratory capacity, vital capacity, residual volume, functional residual capacity, and total lung capacity, among which vital capacity is the most commonly used.

Vital capacity of healthy adults varies greatly depending on genders, ages, body types, and exercises. Generally, males have higher vital capacity than females. Tall and obese people have higher vital capacity than short and slim people. Exercise can improve vital capacity. And adults' lung capacity decreases with age. The specific inspection methods of vital capacity are as follows.

1) Routine spirometry: After deep inhalation, the patient should blow the air into the lung measuring cylinder with force at the inlet of the measuring cylinder, which can be repeated several times to take the highest value. It is more significant to observe the change of vital capacity than to pay attention to the absolute value of vital capacity clinically.

2) Multiple spirometry: Patients should perform the spirometry every 30 seconds three to five times in a row. Normally, vital capacity remains basically unchanged (with an error value of ± 2%) or is slightly increased. A decrease in the measured vital capacity often indicates poor lung function or respiratory muscle fatigue.

4.1.1.2.2 Pulmonary Ventilation Volume
Common clinical indexes are maximum ventilatory volume (MVV), forced vital capacity (FVC), or forced expiratory volume (FEV).

1) Maximum ventilatory volume: First, measure the maximum fast and deep breathing within 5 seconds, then record it on the kymograph for subsequent measurement and calculation. But that is not suitable for people with body deficiency, serious heart or lung diseases, or patients with recent hemoptysis symptoms. This method is also not recommended for people with asthma. Its standard values may vary widely from measured values. For instance, even healthy people's MVV may be 30% more or less than the standard values; therefore, only when there is a significant change will MVV become valuable. It is affected by less thoracic movement caused by ankylosing spondylitis, senile emphysema, senile kyphosis, or dysfunction and unbalanced respiratory muscles caused by emphysema.

2) Forced vital capacity: This is used to measure airway obstruction as well as strength and coordination of respiratory muscles. The value of vital capacity in the first second is often taken and expressed as a percentage of the total volume. Healthy people can exhale 83% of their lung capacity in one second, 94% in two seconds and 96% in three seconds. A drop in exhalation in the first second indicates airway obstruction, most commonly in loss of elasticity of lung tissue, bronchospasm, or stenosis.

4.1.1.2.3 Respiratory Gas Analysis

Respiratory gas analysis is a noninvasive method for measuring gas metabolism. When patients develop heart or lung disease, oxygen intake volume and related indexes will change significantly. The measurement can be carried out by a specific pulmonary function instrument to measure the oxygen consumption in the resting state, after quantitative activities and in the convalescent period, respectively, or to measure the maximum oxygen consumption with maximal exercise capacity or the oxygen consumption per minute during one specific activity. Heart rate should be recorded at the same time during the measurement. Pulmonary ventilation per minute should be recorded. Then, oxygen uptake, oxygen equivalence, carbon dioxide equivalence, oxygen pulse, and respiratory quotient, etc., can be calculated according to the measured indexes, the oxygen difference between exhaled air and atmosphere, and carbon dioxide difference.

4.1.1.2.4 Others

Other respiratory function measures include U-tube test (Valsalva), breath-holding test, fire-blowing test, bottle-blowing test, etc. These methods are relatively cursory but simple to carry out, so they can be used to compare observations between patients' pretreatment and post-treatment state.

4.1.2 Measurement of Respiratory Muscle Function

The basic function of respiratory muscles is to provide power for pulmonary ventilation through regular, nonstop contractile and diastolic movements. In pathological conditions, respiratory muscle fatigue and function decline will cause pulmonary ventilation disorders and respiratory failure, even affecting normal life. The main clinical manifestations of respiratory muscle fatigue include:

1) Dyspnea.
2) Changes in breathing patterns, such as rapid shallow breathing, or prolonged exhalation, wheezing, etc.
3) Decrease in diaphragm motion amplitude.
4) Recovery of respiratory muscle function after rest.
5) Changes in lung function; lung capacity and pulmonary ventilation functions, such as vital capacity, tidal volume, maximum ventilatory volume, etc., can be reduced to different degrees when respiratory muscle fatigue occurs.

Measurement of respiratory muscle function mainly includes measurement of respiratory muscle strength, measurement of respiratory muscle endurance, and measurement of respiratory muscle fatigue.

4.1.2.1 Measurement of Respiratory Muscle Strength

The strength of respiratory muscles can be indirectly determined by measuring changes in respiratory system pressure. The measurement indexes include maximum inspiratory and expiratory pressure, transdiaphragmatic pressure and maximum transdiaphragmatic pressure, and pressure induced by exogenous stimulus.

4.1.2.2 Measurement of Respiratory Muscle Endurance

Measurement of respiratory muscle endurance includes diaphragmatic muscle tension time index, diaphragmatic muscle tolerance time, and diaphragmatic muscle function and motion monitoring during exercise.

4.1.2.3 Measurement of Respiratory Muscle Fatigue

When the respiratory muscle is overloaded, with the passage of time, the whole neuromuscle-respiratory chain in the muscle will undergo various changes, resulting in respiratory muscle fatigue. The direct measures include maximum isometric systolic pressure or force drop, failure to reach the predetermined inspiratory pressure or drop, and electrical stimulation of phrenic nerve to induce a decrease in twitch transdiaphragmatic pressure (TwPdi), etc.

4.1.3 Small Airway Function Examination

Generally speaking, small airway refers to the airway with less than 2 mm diameter during inhalation, below Level 17 of the bronchial tree, including the entire bronchioles and terminal bronchus. The purpose of the small-airway function examination is to detect early-stage airway lesions that are clinically asymptomatic and cannot be detected by routine lung function tests. The main contents of the examination include maximum expiratory flow-volume curve (MEFV), closed capacity (CC), isovolumetric volume (VisoV), maximum midexpiratory flow velocity (MMEF), dynamic compliance, and resistance measurement.

4.1.4 Common Assessment of Respiratory Function

4.1.4.1 Dyspnea Scale

Common dyspnea scale includes the Borg scale, the modified Medical Research Council (mMRC) scale, etc.

   1) Borg scale: Rated from Level 0 to Level 10, corresponding to mild to severe, to assess the degree of dyspnea or fatigue caused by patients' actions from rest to vigorous exercise.

2) mMRC scale: Rated from Level 0 to Level 4, corresponding to mild to severe, to assess dyspnea caused by patients' actions of walking or walking upstairs.

4.1.4.2 Body-Weight Assessment of Cardiopulmonary Function

1) 6-minute walking test (6MWT): Measures the distance an individual is able to walk over a total of 6 minutes on a flat surface. It is divided into 1–4 grades from low to high, which can reflect the maximum exercise ability of lower limbs and indirectly reflect the patient's oxygen uptake ability and body force.
2) 2-minute step test: Count the number of times that patients' unilateral knee can reach the specified height (usually the height of the midpoint of the line between bone and anterior upper iliac spine) within 2 minutes.
3) Step test: Patients step on and off the stair with their left and right legs alternately to test their cardiopulmonary fitness level.

4.1.4.3 Cardiopulmonary Exercise Test (CPET)

The cardiopulmonary exercise test determines the exercise ability of subjects by the method of respiratory metabolism, including the stress response of the respiratory system, cardiovascular system, blood system, neurophysiology, and skeletal muscle system to the same exercise. And it can make real-time measurements of oxygen intake, carbon dioxide output, pulmonary ventilation, heart rate, blood pressure, electrocardiogram, and other indexes during subjects' rest, exercise, and convalescent period. Combined with patients' symptoms during exercise, comprehensive and objective assessments of patients' exercise response, cardiopulmonary functional reserve, and degree of functional impairment can be gained. CPET is an objective, quantitative, and noninvasive method that can reflect cardiopulmonary metabolism and overall function at the same time. It is also a noninvasive examination method widely used to assess human respiratory and circulatory function that is regarded as the "gold standard" for cardiopulmonary function assessment.

4.2 ASSESSMENT OF PHYSICAL FUNCTION

4.2.1 Body-Weight Assessment of Muscle Strength

4.2.1.1 30-Second Chair Standing Test

This test measures the number of times a subject can stand in 30 seconds. It is used to evaluate the function of lower limbs and is significantly correlated with the strength of laps.

4.2.1.2 30-Second Arm Curl Test

This test is a measure of upper body strength by counting the number of arm curls a subject can complete in 30 seconds to assess the patient's power.

4.2.2 Assessment of Flexibility

4.2.2.1 Sit-and-Reach Test

This is a precise and reliable modification of the standard seated forward flexion test and is a safe and generally acceptable method for assessing the flexibility of lower limbs and lower back.

4.2.2.2 Improved Twist Test

This test is used to measure the flexibility of trunk rotation, which is important for assessing core muscle mass.

4.2.2.3 Back-Scratch Test

As one of the flexibility tests, the shoulder flexibility test is most closely related to the subject's daily activities and physical tasks. The back-scratch test is a very simple test that assesses the shoulder flexibility by the distance the subjects can reach with both hands.

4.2.3 Assessment of Balance

4.2.3.1 One-Leg Standing Balance Test

This test is not only a method to test postural stability but also a clinical training method to help patients prevent accidental falls. It can be divided into two types, standing on one leg with eyes open and standing on one leg with eyes closed. Obviously, the latter is more difficult than the former.

4.2.3.2 Functional Reach Test

This test is used to assess the balance of the elderly.

4.2.3.3 Timed Up and Go Test

Also known as the timed up and go test (TUG), it is one of the most common and reliable ways to test muscle strength and fitness.

4.2.4 Assessment of Pain

4.2.4.1 Single-Dimensional Assessment

Visual Analogue Scale (VAS), for example, is simple and easy to operate, but it has slightly lower accuracy.

4.2.4.2 Multi-Dimensional Assessment

The McGill Pain Questionnaire (MPQ), for example, can accurately assess the intensity and nature of patients' pain with patients' physiological sensation, emotional factors, cognitive ability, and other factors taken into account; however, its results are also susceptible to patients' education background and emotional factors.

4.3 ASSESSMENT FOR PSYCHOSOCIAL FUNCTION

4.3.1 Assessment of Psychological Function

The mental and psychological state of COVID-19 patients is often associated with their symptoms; therefore, psychological intervention is an important means of rehabilitation. Necessary evaluation provides the basis for psychological intervention.

4.3.1.1 Evaluation of Mental and Psychological State

Generally speaking, there are mainly four aspects to evaluate the patient's mental and psychological state clinically:

1) Emotional aspect, including depression, worry, anger, guilt, embarrassment, and repression of intense emotions.
2) Cognitive aspect, including mild impairment, impaired problem-solving ability, and impaired attention.
3) Social aspect, including the decrease of social activities, the change of family role, and the decrease of independence.
4) Behavior aspect, including activities of daily living (ADL) impairment, smoking, malnutrition, reduced capacity of exercise, disobedience to medical treatment, etc.

4.3.1.2 Commonly Used Psychological Assessment Scales

1) Nine-item Patient Health Questionnaire (PHQ-9): This questionnaire is used for screening and assessing depressive symptoms and can be divided into two parts. The first part consists of nine items, namely, nine depressive symptoms. In the second part, there is one item, in which patients' responses are given a score of 0–3 (0 means not at all, and 3 means every day. The lowest total score is 0. The highest total score is 27). According to the scores, patients' degree of depression can be classified as mild depression, moderate depression, or severe depression. The specific assessment criteria are as follows: 6–9 is classified is mild depression, 10–14 is moderate depression, 15–19 is severe depression, and 20–27 is extremely severe depression.

2) Seven-Item Generalized Anxiety Disorder (GAD-7): Used for assessing the severity of anxiety symptoms. Consisting of 7 items, GAD-7 is a self-rating scale with four levels, for which patients are given a score of 0–3 (0 means not at all, and 3 means almost every day. The score ranges from 0 to 21). According to the score, a patient's degree of anxiety can be classified as mild anxiety, moderate anxiety, or severe anxiety. Specific evaluation criteria are as follows: 6–9 is mild anxiety, 10–14 is moderate anxiety, and 15–21 is severe anxiety.

3) PTSD Checklist (PCL): Used to assess whether the patient has symptoms of PTSD.

4) Assessment of sleep disorders: The Pittsburgh Sleep Quality Index (PSDI) is used to assess the sleep quality of patients with organic or inorganic sleep disorders in the past month. It is one of the most widely used sleep quality assessment scales. The Athens Insomnia Scale (AIS) is a self-rating scale of insomnia severity based on the 10th revision of the International Statistical Classification of Diseases and Related Health Problems (ICD-10) insomnia diagnostic criteria.

4.3.2 Assessment of ADL

ADL refers to the ability of individuals to carry out necessary activities every day in order to meet the needs of daily life. The main purpose of ADL evaluation is to understand the degree to which ADL is affected by dyspnea. The commonly used evaluation method is the Barthel index, which includes 10 items. ADL can be divided into different levels according to the need for help and the degree of help. The higher the score, the stronger the independence.

4.3.3 Health-Related Quality of Life (HQRL) Scale

The assessment indexes of health-related quality of life scale, HRQL scale, are the most important symptoms of a disease, and can also cover many aspects such as the patient's mental state, social state, daily life and entertainment activities, etc. The HRQL scale can be used to evaluate the overall quality of life of patients. It can also assess specific quality of life associated with a specific disease. Therefore, HRQL can be divided into HRQL overall scale and disease-specific scale. The latter one is more susceptible to small changes, so it is often used to observe the effect of clinical treatment trials. The advantage of the former one is that it is applicable to different health states and different diseases to assess the overall quality of life status of patients.

4.3.4 World Health Organization Quality of Life–BREF (WHOQOL-BREF)

This scale contains the following four evaluations regarding the patients, e.g., the feeling of certain things being experienced in the past 2 weeks; the ability to do certain things in the past 2 weeks; the level of satisfaction about various aspects of life over the past 2 weeks; and the frequency of such feeling or experiences in the past 2 weeks. The scores of these four aspects are then calculated. The higher the scores in each aspect, the better the quality of life.

BIBLIOGRAPHY

1. Meng Shen, Chen Siyuan. *Pulmonary rehabilitation [M]*. Beijing: People's Medical Publishing House. [2007].
2. Xiaolin Huang, Tiebin Yan. *Rehabilitation medicine [M]*. Beijing: People's Medical Publishing House. [2018].
3. Wu Liang, Guo Qi, Hu Ling, Huang Lifeng, Wang Minghang, Yu Pengming, Yuan Ying. Consensus of technical experts on rehabilitation treatment of serious respiratory diseases in China [J]. *Chinese Journal of Geriatric Care*, 16 (5): 3–11. [2016].
4. Pan Huaping, Ge Weixing. Research progress of cardiopulmonary rehabilitation for severe diseases [J]. *Chinese Journal of Rehabilitation*, 28 (6): 61–66. [2018].
5. Chronic Obstructive Pulmonary Disease Group, Respiratory Society, Chinese Medical Association. Guidelines for the diagnosis and treatment of chronic obstructive pulmonary disease. (revised in 2013) [J]. *Chinese Journal of the Frontiers of Medical Science*, 6 (2): 67–80. [2014].
6. Li Jiansheng, Wang Minghang, Li Suyun. Progress in the evaluation of dyspnea in patients with chronic obstructive pulmonary disease [J]. *Journal of Henan University of Chinese Medicine*, 22 (2): 79–82. [2017].
7. Andrew L. Ries. Impact of chronic obstructive pulmonary disease on quality of life: The role of dyspnea [J]. *Am J Med*, 119 (10A): 12–20. [2006].
8. Chen Wei, Fan Qiuji. Application situation and prospect of cardiopulmonary exercise test in cardiopulmonary rehabilitation [J]. *Practical Journal of Cardiac Cerebral Pneumal and Vascular Disease*, 27 (11): 1–5. [2019].
9. Ali Teymoori, Ruben Real, Anastasia Gorbunova, E.F. Haghish, Nada Andelic, Lindsay Wilson, Thomas Asendorf, David Menon, Nicole von Steinbüchel. Measurement invariance of assessments of depression (PHQ-9) and anxiety (GAD-7) across sex, strata and linguistic backgrounds in a European-wide sample of patients after Traumatic Brain Injury [J]. *Journal of Affective Disorders*, 262: 278–285. [2020]. doi:10.1016/j.jad.2019.10.035.
10. Duan Ying, Sun Shuchen. Commonly used assessment scale for sleep disorders [J]. *World Journal of Sleep Medicine*, 3 (4): 201–203. [2016].

Chapter 5

Modern Rehabilitation Techniques for COVID-19

COVID-19 can cause respiratory damage, resulting in lung function damage, respiratory muscle involvement, deterioration of lung function, and dyspnea. There are some breathing recovery measures, such as training of breathing pattern, training of breathing muscles, and breathing exercises. Airway clearance techniques (ACTs) are ideal for respiratory rehabilitation especially for severe and critically severe patients who have difficulties in sputum excretion as a result of long-term bed rest that resulted in a decrease in respiratory muscle strength, deteriorating function of tracheal cilia, and adhesion of secretions to bronchial wall.

The progress of this disease may lead to systemic hypoxia, inducing systemic inflammation and aggravating respiratory system injury. At the same time, compensatory rapid deep breathing will occur under the condition of hypoxia and respiratory muscle weakness, leading to a significant increase in transpulmonary pressure, resulting in ventilator-induced lung injury and shearing injury. In addition to directly causing lung tissue injury, the cytokine storm triggered by it will further aggravate the inflammatory response. Then, abnormally elevated cytokines and overactivated immune cells are activated and recruited in the lung, causing diffuse damage to pulmonary capillary endothelial cells and alveolar epithelial cells, large exudate airway obstruction, deterioration of lung function increases sharply, finally leading to acute respiratory distress syndrome (ARDS) and respiratory cycle failure. For COVID-19 patients with respiratory muscle weakness and lung tissue injury, respiratory rehabilitation methods, such as respiratory pattern training, respiratory muscle training (RMT), and respiratory body exercise, can be adopted in clinical rehabilitation.

After discharge, patients may have shortness of breath after activities, which hinders their ability to perform daily tasks. According to the existing evidence of severe acute respiratory syndrome (SARS) patients discharged from the hospital, some patients still have general weakness, shortness of breath and other symptoms, and their exercise ability is limited due to respiratory muscle weakness and surrounding muscle weakness. Lung function is characterized by restrictive ventilatory dysfunction, impaired diffuse function, and is associated with pulmonary fibrosis changes demonstrated by chest computed tomography (CT) examination, which may persist. Aerobic training is one of the most effective rehabilitation treatment methods for respiratory diseases. Long-term regular aerobic training can effectively improve the exercise tolerance of patients with chronic respiratory diseases by improving the function of skeletal muscles and cardiopulmonary adaptability, thus achieving the goal of improving shortness of breath after activities.

Modern rehabilitation techniques for COVID-19 mainly include respiratory rehabilitation techniques, physical rehabilitation techniques and psychosocial rehabilitation techniques. Rehabilitation practitioners should work with teams as much as possible to improve respiratory symptoms and dysfunction in COVID-19 patients, reduce complications, relieve anxiety and depression, reduce disability, and maximize the ability to perform daily tasks and improve the quality of life of patients.

5.1 RESPIRATORY REHABILITATION THERAPY TECHNIQUES

Patients with COVID-19 are at risk for respiratory dysfunction at all stages of the disease, as well as limited ability to participate in daily activities and society due to the effects of the disease itself and isolation restrictions. Techniques such as body position management, airway clearance, breathing training, chest physical therapy and breathing exercises in respiratory rehabilitation can effectively help patients relieve respiratory symptoms, improve function, and improve quality of life.

5.1.1 Intervention Activities in the Early Stage

Rehabilitation intervention in the early stage plays an important role in patients' prognosis, quality of life, and the return of normal life.

5.1.1.1 Respiratory Control Techniques

The breathing control (BC) technique is a breathing method that relaxes the shoulder and neck, assisting inspiratory muscles in a comfortable and relaxed position. And they require patients to slowly inhale through the nose, slowly exhale through the mouth, and expand the lower chest, which can reduce the work intensiveness of breathing and relieve dyspnea.

5.1.1.2 Energy-Saving Techniques

Energy-saving techniques require avoiding unnecessary energy consumption or reducing strenuous activities. Actions are planned in stages before those techniques, and actions with light and moderate energy consumption are completed alternately. They require the patients to control the activity speed and complete the activity slowly and rhythmically; grasp the rhythm of breathing (i.e., pay attention to interval rest when strongly exhaling or inhaling); notice the possible effects of the environment on energy, such as high temperature, low temperature, tension; and incorporate breath control techniques during the activity to save energy.

5.1.2 Posture Management

Posture management is the use of body position to optimize the oxygen transport, reflecting that oxygen transport pathway has multiple, straight links. Therefore, these effects can be preferentially produced on oxygen transport. Therapeutic position placement can effectively increase lung volume, improve pulmonary ventilation and blood flow ratio, optimize respiratory mechanics, and promote airway secretion clearance. Dynamic monitoring should be performed during posture management to avoid compression atelectasis. Severe and critically severe COVID-19 patients are in a supine position for a long time, and this nonphysiological position limits oxygen transport. Common therapeutic positions include the prone position and the upright position. The correct physiological position of the upright position is combined with actions, such as walking, cycling, or sitting, in accordance with the requirements of daily activities. To meet the energy requirements of these activities, oxygen transport function needs to be maximized, and ventilatory perfusion is more consistent without additional motor stimulation. Apart from reducing closure capacity, the upright position can maximize lung volume and lung capacity. Prone position enhances arterial oxygenation and reduces respiratory work in patients with cardiovascular and pulmonary dysfunction, no matter with or without mechanical ventilation. The prone position moves the unfixed structures in the chest and abdomen, allowing the heart and great vessels to move forward, and the liver, spleen, and kidneys can move forward and toward caudal.

Prone position can increase arterial blood oxygen partial pressure, tidal volume, and dynamic lung compliance. Prone position is used to guide the treatment of patients with ARDS. But complications from lying prone for long periods of time, especially skin problems, are common. Therefore, close monitoring of the skin at the osseous processes is essential. To prevent or treat these complications, an intermittent prone position is recommended.

5.1.2.1 For Patients with ARDS

For patients with ARDS, prone position for more than 12 hours is clinically used to improve ventilation and blood flow ratio, reduce pulmonary edema, increase functional residual capacity, and reduce the probability of intubation. A large number of reports have confirmed that sheer prone position or prone position combined with artificial mechanical ventilation can effectively improve blood oxygen and ventilation in COVID-19 patients with acute respiratory distress.

5.1.2.2 For Patients with Sedation or Consciousness Disorders

For patients with sedation or consciousness disorders, a standing bed or bed with its head position raised can be used to assist the patient with the therapeutic position placement when physiological conditions permit. Doctors can gradually increase the simulated antigravity position until the patients can maintain an upright position.

Patients can start from adaptation training of 30°–45° headboard elevation for body position, and gradually transit to 60° position. While raising the head position of the bed, doctors can raise the knee joint position up to 10°–15° or add a small pillow underneath the knee to put the lower limbs and abdomen in a relaxed position, then gradually transition to the bedside sitting position. It should be noted that the tray table can be provided to help the patient maintain a comfortable sitting position (forward-leaning position in which the forearm is supported on the table and the elbow flexed 80°–110°). When the patient's feet cannot touch the ground, the footstool and other support assistance should be provided, with the assistance of therapist and nurse beside the patients. This can be done under the supervision of a therapist or with patients sitting in a protected therapeutic chair. Finally, patients can transition to a standing position next to the bed.

To prevent the tube from shifting during all body position changes, the selection and duration of body position should be based on the premise that the patient can tolerate and feel comfortable and relaxed.

5.1.3 ACT

ACT uses physical or mechanical means to act on the airflow to help sputum discharge in the trachea and bronchus or induce coughing to make sputum discharge. Airway clearance is designed to minimize airway obstruction, infection, and mucous congestion resulting in pulmonary inflammation, as well as damaging effects on the airway and lung parenchyma.

When patients have airway secretion retention, they can be instructed to perform spontaneous sputum excretion techniques, including usage of effective cough, active cycle of breathing techniques (ACBTs) and oscillating positive expiratory pressure (OPEP) equipment. Patients should strictly pay attention to the protection and isolation of sputum during voluntary sputum discharge. When patients are coughing or forcefully exhaling, doctors should use the isolation bag to cover the mouth and nose to avoid virus transmission.

5.1.3.1 Effective Cough

An effective cough is divided into four stages. The first step is to breathe in enough air to provide the necessary gas for a vigorous cough. Generally speaking, the cough should be fully aspirated, with the inhalation volume reaching at least 60% of the person's lung capacity. The second stage involves closing the glottis (vocal cords) and preparing the abdominal and intercostal muscles. The third stage is the active contraction of these muscles. The fourth and final stage is when the glottis is opened, and the air is forcefully exhaled. Usually, patients can cough three to six times during one deep exhalation. Problems in one or more of those four steps will affect the results of an effective cough.

Doctors should pay attention to cough intensity to avoid excessive oxygen consumption caused by continuous coughing, patients should be asked to inhale deeply. After reaching the necessary inspiratory capacity, let patients hold the breath briefly to close the glottis to maintain intrapulmonary pressure. Intrathoracic and abdominal pressure are further increased before coughing. Finally, patients suddenly open the glottis, release plosive airstream with their lips relaxed.

5.1.3.2 ACBTs

ACBTs can effectively remove bronchial secretions and improve lung function without aggravating hypoxemia and airflow obstruction. The technique consists of three stages of ventilation, according to the patient's condition and selection. Those three stages will occur in circulation of BC, thoracic expansion exercises (TEE), and forced expiration technique (FET).

1) BC: A rest interval between two active parts, encouraging the patients to relax the upper chest and shoulders, and to perform tidal breathing at their own breathing rate and amplitude, using diaphragmatic breathing patterns whenever possible. To prevent airway spasm, respiratory control should be performed between the two active parts. COVID-19 patients increase abdominal pressure by contracting the lower chest and abdomen, forcing more air from the alveolar through the respiratory tract. By paying attention to the shoulder and upper chest to stay relaxed, COVID-19 patients can reduce the participation of auxiliary respiratory muscles, strengthen the coordination of diaphragmatic and abdominal activities during breathing exercises, and reduce the work intensiveness of respiratory muscles.

2) TEE: Let the patients take a deep inhalation, usually holding the breath for 3 seconds at the end of inhalation, and then make passive exhalation. The final breath holding allows the airflow to pass through the ventilation bypass system to the rear of the secretions, thereby moving the secretions from the small airway to the atmospheric channel. At the same time, the interalveolar interdependence cannot only make adjacent alveoli dilate but also loosen secretions. Respiratory control is generally performed after three thoracic dilations. The therapist's hand may also be placed on the area of chest wall to stimulate the expansion of the chest by proprioception.

3) FET: Consists of one to two forced exhalations. Low lung volume breathing can make the peripheral secretions move outward. When the secretions move to a larger bronchus, deep inhalation and exhalation may cause the secretions to be discharged or gently coughed out after moving to a larger bronchus. Expiratory flow is a rapid but not maximum exhalation that removes more peripheral secretions from the lower lung volume position. As the secretions reach the larger, more proximal upper airway, the exudative flow or cough at the higher lung volume position clears these secretions. At the same time, breathing can stabilize the collapsed wall of the branch air tube and increase the expiratory flow. For COVID-19 patients, using breathing techniques instead of coughing for sputum drainage can reduce the work intensiveness of respiratory muscles and promote sputum drainage.

Specific clinical applications are shown in Figure 5.1.

Start here: Start from here. BC: Breathing control. TEE: Thoracic expansion exercises.

FET: Forced expiration technique. Huff: Blow out loudly.

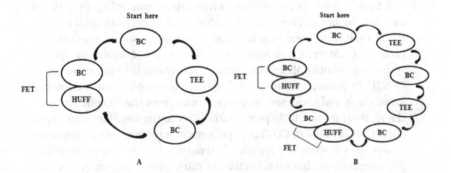

Figure 5.1 Active cycle of breathing techniques.

5.1.3.3 OPEP

The OPEP device combines positive expiratory pressure with endobronchial vibration therapy. The vibrations will produce an effect similar to percussive ventilation in the lungs, loosening secretions from the tracheal walls. Positive expiratory pressure keeps the airway open during exhalation, while airflow passes through the ventilation bypass system, making it easier for patients to expel airway secretions, improve lung function, and prevent lung complications. Acapella and Flutter are commonly applied to clinical situations.

5.1.3.4 High-Frequency Chest Wall Oscillation (HFCWO)

The high-frequency chest wall oscillation (HFCWO) device can effectively reduce the viscosity of the secretion so that the secretion can be discharged from the peripheral airway to the central airway. In addition, it can also prevent atelectasis and control pneumonia.

5.1.3.5 Postural Drainage Techniques

When secretions are retained in patients, corresponding pulmonary segment position drainage can be performed according to imaging. Postural drainage maximizes the effect of gravity on different drainage segments by placing the patient in a specific position. The target lung segments drain vertically into the main bronchi to help the bronchial secretions flow out of the airway. Each lobe needs to be at a higher position for drainage. Combined with gravity and pressure, secretions can move from the periphery to a larger, more central airway. When secretions are retained in patients, gravity can be taken advantage of to promote the excretion of secretions accumulated in each lung segment. Different lesions were treated with different drainage positions, and the drainage frequency was determined by the amount of secretions (Figure 5.2). The effects are better when these techniques are combined with other sputum removal techniques. For those with less secretion, drainage is performed once in the morning and once in the afternoon. For those with more secretion, drainage is performed three to four times a day. Each session targets only one part. If there are several parts to deal with, the total time should not exceed 30–45 minutes to avoid patient fatigue.

5.1.3.6 Other Chest Physical Therapy Techniques

Other chest physical therapy techniques, such as tapping, vibration, and shaking, also help the patients to expel sputum and clear airway secretions.

Physiotherapists should consider carefully when selecting ACTs. There is evidence that tapping, vibration, shaking, postural drainage, and coughing cause pain and discomfort and may cause hypoxemia and arrhythmias.

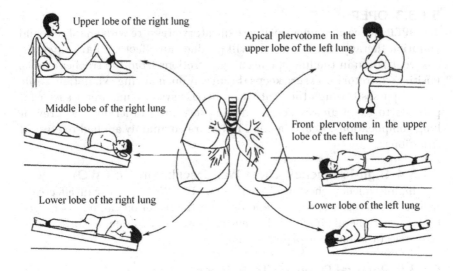

Figure 5.2   Diagram of different postural drainaging.

It is generally recommended that airway clearance be performed 1 hour after the patients have eaten, especially when it comes to patients with position changes and cough symptoms. It is better to use a combination of ACTs and sophisticated devices. The usage of airway clearance should be combined with atomization and humidification. In atomization treatment, bronchodilators can be used to make the small airway open better. Phlegm-reducing drugs can reduce the viscosity of secretions. Humidification treatment can reduce the consistency of secretions, thus improving the expelling of secretions.

5.1.4 Breathing Training

COVID-19 patients often get dyspnea, and many critically severe patients who are discharged from hospitals still have symptoms, such as wheezing and dyspnea. For that reason, interventional respiratory training is necessary to help patients improve ventilation and respiratory patterns. Ventilatory strategies and respiratory control techniques can help maximize symptom relief and activity potential. Respiratory training is mainly to teach patients to relax the neck as well as chest auxiliary breathing muscles, to use normal breathing mode more, and to increase the effectiveness of breathing. This treatment regimen focuses on energy savings, relaxation of assisted breathing muscles, and the combination of activity and BC.

5.1.4.1 Respiratory Pattern Training

Breathing pattern training includes adjusting breathing rhythm (inhalation: exhalation = 1:2), abdominal breathing training, pursed-lip breathing training, etc.

5.1.4.1.1 Abdominal Breathing Exercises

Abdominal breathing exercises involve inhaling deeply and slowly through the nose as the belly expands and exhaling slowly with abdominal contraction. During the exercise, the abdomen can be slightly pressurized with hands, repeat 10 times, relax for 1 minute, and then continue. This exercise should be done 10 times for 1 group, 3 groups/time, 2–3 times a day. During training, patients should relax the neck, shoulders, and back of the chest. Abdominal breathing training can increase the tidal expiratory volume, reduce ineffective dead cavity, increase alveolar ventilation volume, improve gas distribution, reduce oxygen consumption of respiratory function, relieve dyspnea, and shortness of breath symptoms. At the same time, it is important to have a high degree of synchronization between the diaphragm, abdominal, and other assisted breathing muscles. Competing output signals from multiple driving centers lead to disordered breathing rhythm and synchronization between the assisted respiratory muscles and the diaphragm, which can cause dyspnea. Therefore, ineffective respiration is related to the dysfunction of the respiratory muscles. The guidance of abdominal breathing training for COVID-19 patients can correct abnormal chest wall actions, reduce the work of auxiliary inspiratory muscles, reduce the subjective feeling of dyspnea, improve the ventilatory function by coordinating diaphragmatic and abdominal muscle activity during respiratory movement, and improve the effectiveness of ventilation function. In addition, it can also improve tidal volume and oxygenation.

5.1.4.1.2 Pursed-Lip Breathing Training

This training requires patients to sit up with their hands on their knees. The tip of the tongue slightly touches the palate. Let them inhale slowly and count for 3 seconds silently. Then let them purse their lips like whistling, slowly exhaling, and silently count 6–9 seconds. Then let them breathe out as far as possible to maintain two to three times of the breathing-in time. And let them repeat 10 times and then relax 1 minute, 10 times for 1 group, 3 groups/time, and 2–3 times a day. The slow exhaling process of breathing air through narrowly opened mouth can keep the airway open for a long time, in order to increase the release of residual gas in the ventilation and lungs and extend the exhale process, thereby reducing the respiratory rate and work of breathing and lung volume at the end of the process. Additionally, it can also let COVID-19 patients be less affected by the extension of the respiratory cycle, increase the residual gas discharge and fresh gas suction, and improve their breathing pattern, relieve their shortness of breath and other symptoms after activities.

5.1.4.1.3 Breathing Rhythm Adjusting Training

Shortness of breath commonly occurs among COVID-19 patients. When the respiratory rate is accelerated, the respiratory amplitude is necessarily shallow, and the tidal volume is reduced. The anatomic invalid cavity remains unchanged, while the alveolar ventilation capacity is small, affecting the exchange of air and pulmonary capillary blood fluid gas. The ability of the respiratory muscle pump is critical to the flow of air through the respiratory system up to the level of gas exchange. Damage to the respiratory pump can affect ventilation, gas exchange, and tissue respiration. Respiratory muscles promote ventilation. Respiratory muscle weakness may occur in diseases with increased respiratory muscle load or decreased respiratory muscle energy. Changes in breathing patterns may help relieve respiratory muscle fatigue. A slow and deep breathing pattern can guarantee an efficient breathing process. Rapid shallow breathing can reduce respiratory muscle fatigue. Although this rhythm reduces the effectiveness of gas exchange, lower tidal volume and faster breathing rates can help reduce respiratory muscle fatigue; therefore, it is important to adjust the breathing rate in the breathing pattern training. The reasonable timing of inhalation and exhalation plays a key role in adjusting the breathing rate.

1) From panting breathing to deep breathing: An important chief complaint of COVID-19 patients is chest tightness and shortness of breath. Deep breathing training can help patients improve oxygen transport and relieve shortness of breath caused by movements or actions.

   When shortness of breath occurs, first try to do the training in a comfortable position, such as reclining at 60° (with a pillow under the knee to maintain knee joint flexion between 10°–15°) sitting up with body slightly leaning forward or standing against a wall. Then start by breathing calmly from 30 seconds to 1 minute. Attention should be paid to adjusting breathing based on the original respiratory rhythm, and excessive slowdown and deepening are not required in case of fatigue and discomfort.

2) Deep and slow breathing: When inhaling, try to mobilize the diaphragm to participate actively and breathe as deeply and slowly as possible to avoid the reduction of ventilation efficiency caused by panting breathing. This breathing mode has less work intensiveness than chest breathing, and it is better used to measure tidal volume and ventilator-perfusion ratio. It can be used to adjust breathing during shortness of breath. The key is to reduce the participation of the auxiliary breathing muscle as much as possible. Doctors can guide the patients to carry out the tense auxiliary breathing muscle and chest drawing when necessary.

5.1.4.2 Relaxation Training

Relaxation training refers to the relaxation of the neck and chest auxiliary breathing muscles to encourage normal breathing mode, effectively reducing the work intensiveness of breathing.

For those with stable vital signs, their thoracic compliance can be improved by thorax draft, thus improving respiratory function. Thorax draft can be completed autonomously. When the chest is tight and the effect of voluntary drawing is not ideal, the patients can complete with the assistance of the therapist. When the patients have auxiliary inspiratory muscle tension, the palpation of auxiliary inspiratory muscle can be used to confirm the muscle tension. Then the muscle energy technology can be used to improve the shortened muscle. Auxiliary inspiratory palpation is to experience the tension of the abdominal muscles and tendons of the corresponding muscles, including the superior trapezius, levator scapulae, sternocleidomastoid, pectoralis major, and pectoralis minor. When doing the limb drafting, the patients should be in the inspiratory phase with the posture of bending forward and abducting the upper limb to avoid breathing resistance.

5.1.4.3 Local Dilation Breathing Training

Imaging examination can determine the presence of specific lobe collapse or inflammation. If combined with postural drainage, it can determine more targeted specific lobe expansion. With the enlarged lung parenchyma in an upward position, the patients or assistants can place their hands on the projection side of the body surface of the lung tissue, maintaining the patient's lung volume through deep inspiration.

During breathing training, pay attention to monitoring vital signs strictly. If patients show obvious fatigue (when Rating of Perceived Exertion [RPE] is 11–13), shortness of breath ($SPO_2 \leq 90\%$ or falls by more than 4%, showing obvious phenomena of significant shortness of breath, dyspnea, chest tightness), pain, etc., suspend the treatment in time and adjust the training intensity to guarantee their basic health condition try not to hold breath during the process of training.

5.1.5 RMT

RMT is generally carried out not only by means of respiratory training apparatus but also by means of simple instruments, such as balloons and whistles. In the course of RMT with the help of specific training equipment, the required pressure of RMT is given and adjusted to give the exercise load of respiratory muscle, so as to achieve the purpose of RMT, and conform to the principles of overload, pertinence, and reversibility of RMT. Under a certain intensity load, for a specific respiratory muscle or muscle group, it is necessary to make gradual exercise to achieve the desired optimal functional state. Patients in this training process are required to produce enough negative pressure in the respiratory movement to overcome exercise load and stimulated by load series of adaptive change. Regular breathing muscle training can improve the cell oxidase activity, enhance strength and endurance, guarantee effective cough and sputum expelling, and help improve breathing difficulties. During RMT, COVID-19 patients can overcome respiratory load and increase tidal volume and alveolar ventilation volume to improve blood gas exchange rate and respiratory function. Respiratory muscle dysfunction is more common in severe patients, often due to early biological retraining, mechanical ventilation, and other operations. Studies have shown that the pace of diaphragmatic muscles atrophy is 8 times faster than skeletal muscles during early biological retraining. Mechanical ventilation can also induce accelerated diaphragmatic atrophy. As the strength of the breathing muscles decreases, the body's need to inhale and exhale increases. It increases the work intensiveness of breathing and exacerbates symptoms such as dyspnea and decreased mobility. Therefore, the training of respiratory muscles should not be neglected in the rehabilitation of discharged patients.

For some patients with acquired weakness in the intensive care unit (ICU), inspiratory muscle training (IMT) should be performed. This requires patients to use breathing training devices with an initial load of 30% of the maximum inspiratory pressure, inhaling five times in each group with an interval of not less than 6 seconds. Six groups should be performed for each training, with a 1-minute rest between groups. The frequency is once a day. During the training, if patients show obvious fatigue, polypnea, shortness of breath, wheezing, chest tightness, pain, etc., the treatment should be suspended in time, and the training intensity should be adjusted.

5.1.6 Breathing Exercises

Breathing exercises are suitable for patients with mild symptoms. Different from aerobic training, they do not require certain intensity and emphasize the rhythm and depth of breathing to help patients breathe better, relieve their breathing difficulties, and enhance their comfort. Breathing exercises can be divided into three positions: semisupine position, sitting position, and upright position. Breathing exercises in different positions can be selected according to the patient's condition. It is recommended to try to do eight breath exercises each time, with four sets of eight beats per breath. The rhythm of breathing is based on the movements of the body. Generally speaking, patients inhale when the chest is open, exhale when the breath is relaxed, and try not to hold the breath.

Breathing exercises can be performed in either a sitting or standing position depending on the patient's condition.

The principles of breathing exercises include:

1) Strictly follow the three steps of warm-up, movement, and relaxation.
2) The movement should be in accordance with the frequency of breath, as far as possible to avoid breath closure and movement in the breath resistance, namely, stretching when inhaling or relaxing when exhaling.
3) Patients should perform as slowly and thoroughly as possible with the participation of multijoint motions and avoid the rapid repetition of small joint motions. Suspend training at any time if patients feel unwell.

5.1.7 Respiratory Intervention Techniques

Patients who have suffered from COVID-19 to a certain severe degree (refractory respiratory failure or multiorgan failure) may need to receive extracorporeal membrane oxygenation (ECMO) intervention, and then carry out rehabilitation training (early motion and respiratory training), which can improve the prognosis.

A comprehensive respiratory function assessment should be performed prior to respiratory training, including ECMO setting, ventilation mode, flow curve and compliance, arterial blood gas, oxygen saturation, auscultation, observation and palpation of chest wall motion and chatter, and re-examination of chest radiograph or CT scan.

5.1.7.1 Patient's Position
The patient's position is recommended to be determined in consultation with the physician and specialist nurse. Be mindful of the cannula position, the risk of ventilator-perfusion mismatch, and the stability of the patient's condition.

5.1.7.2 Sputum Suction
Closed suction is recommended. Be mindful of airway bleeding and lung collapse, and monitor platelet levels and Activated Clotting Time/Activated Partial Thromboplastin Time (ACT/APTT) ratio.

5.1.7.3 Mechanical/Artificial Dilated Ventilation
Patients with high positive end-expiratory pressure (PEEP) are advised to use mechanical or end-expiratory positive valves in the artificial extension ventilation circuit before treatment. The maximum peak stress should be agreed upon by the multidisciplinary treatment team. As far as lung compliance is concerned, this intervention may not be appropriate for "super" protective pulmonary ventilation (e.g., barotrauma) and may not be appropriate for ECMO

flow insufficiency or instability. Artificial dilatation ventilation barometer pressure should refer to the specific established pressure. Artificial dilatation ventilation should be avoided with PEEP > 10 cm H_2O. At this time, mechanical dilatation ventilation is recommended.

5.1.7.4 Precautions in Manual Treatment

It is recommended to begin with gentle manipulation. Considering the position of the cannula within the vessel, this intervention may not be appropriate when ECMO flow is insufficient/unstable.

5.1.7.5 Precautions for HFCWO

It is recommended to consult ECMO specialists and specialist nurse. It is also necessary to take arrhythmias, clotting, cannula locations, and wound positions into consideration.

5.1.7.6 Precautions for ACBTs

If the cardiovascular system has adverse reactions, modification to the treatment regimen is recommended. It is necessary to take the effects of the increase in intrathoracic pressure during treatment into consideration.

During respiratory therapy, doctors and patients should comply with the requirements of personal protection because aerosol particles will be produced.

5.1.8 Principles of Techniques Implementation

1) According to regulations, COVID-19 discharged patients are required to undergo clinical observation for 2 weeks. All personnel who come into contact with patients for respiratory rehabilitation assessment and treatment must pass the local nosocomial infection control training and assessment before they can return to work.

2) The objective of respiratory rehabilitation is to restore the physical and mental functions of patients as soon as possible and to improve their mobility in order to help the patient return to society and work.

3) The timing of rehabilitation intervention should be based on the confirmation of stable vital signs, no signs of underlying diseases, and exclusion of relevant contraindications.

4) The time of suspension of rehabilitation may refer to the results of vital signs monitoring and should be combined with the patient's chief complaint. If the patient does not adapt to the interruption at any time, corresponding measures should be taken.

5) Treatment is not given until assessment is done. Assessment and monitoring should be carried out throughout the respiratory rehabilitation treatment.

6) No matter what type of rehabilitation intervention is adopted, the principle of individuation should be followed. Teamwork is needed to develop a detailed individualized rehabilitation plan, especially for severe cases, elderly patients, and patients with a variety of underlying diseases.

5.2 REHABILITATION TREATMENT TECHNIQUES FOR PHYSICAL FUNCTION

COVID-19 not only will directly impair the cardiopulmonary, neurological, and renal functions of patients, but also cause patients to lie in bed for a long period of time. Due to their lack of activity or motion, there are complications that can lead to physical dysfunction. Body dysfunction of COVID-19 patients is usually characterized by general fatigue, easy fatigue, and muscle soreness, some of which may be accompanied by muscle atrophy and decreased muscle strength. Physical function can be assessed by using the Borg conscious fatigue scale and freehand muscle strength test. In addition, there is a wide range of rehabilitation techniques that can improve physical function. For of COVID-19 patients' main problems, such as decreased muscle strength and reduced exercise tolerance, the rehabilitation treatment technology that can be adopted is mainly exercise therapy, including aerobic exercise, strength training, and balance training. On the premise of safety protection, the cardiopulmonary function, psychological state, physical ability, and other aspects of patients in different stages of the disease should be thoroughly assessed step by step according to their conditions. With usage of these techniques, safe, scientific, reasonable, and feasible exercise prescription should be given to patients for intervention.

5.2.1 Aerobic Exercise

Aerobic exercise refers to the physical exercise that the human body undertakes in the circumstance of oxygen supply adequately. That is, in athletic process, the amount of oxygen that the human body inhales and the amount required are equal, achieving balance on physiology. In addition to the participation of oxygen, aerobic exercise also requires the participation of major muscle groups throughout the body, which can strengthen the heart and lung functions, making the cardiovascular system more effective and rapid oxygen transmission to every part of the body. Aerobic training, combined with respiratory control and postural changes, can increase alveolar ventilation, improve mucosal ciliary oscillation and gas exchange capacity, improve body function, and reduce fatigue. In the meantime, it is acceptable to combine other appropriate measures (e.g. oxygen therapy and/or aerosolization). During aerobic training in the acute phase, patients should be prevented from overwork and improper exercise intensity, which may lead to oxygen demand exceeding their oxygen supply capacity. An excessive increase in oxygen demand may even worsen the patient's gas exchange impairment.

The exercise prescription is formulated according to the principles of FITT (frequency, intensity, time, and type).

1) **F** (frequency): The general frequency of aerobic exercise is 3 to 5 times a week, but it can be adjusted according to different types and periods of COVID-19 patients.

2) **I** (intensity): According to the cardiopulmonary function of patients, the intensity can be adjusted from the very low intensity (heart rate during exercise < 57% HRmax, or increase in heart rate < 30% HRr, or RPE < 9/20) to the low intensity (heart rate during exercise < 57%– 63% HRmax, or increase in heart rate < 30%–39% HRr, or RPE < 9/20–11/20) then to moderate intensity (heart rate during exercise < 64%–76% HRmax, or increase in heart rate < 40%–59% HRr, or RPE < 12/20–14/20).

3) **T** (time): The aerobic exercise time is generally 10–30 minutes once. The first 3 minutes are the warm-up stage, and the last 5 minutes are the finishing stage, which reflects 30%–40% of the intensity during the exercise. According to the situation of COVID-19 patients, the time can be slightly extended with the intensity reduced (if intermittent exercise is adopted, the accumulated exercise time can be calculated).

4) **T** (type): There are various types of aerobic exercises, such as continuous or intermittent standing time, indoor/outdoor walking, indoor/outdoor treadmill, tai chi chuan, and other traditional Chinese exercises.

For example, for patients with mild symptoms, the recommendations are as follows. *Exercise intensity*: Borg dyspnea score ≤ 3 (out of 10 points), with no fatigue phenomenon on the second day. *Exercise frequency*: twice a day. *Exercise time*: 15–45 minutes each time, starting 1 hour after meals. *Exercise types*: respiratory rehabilitation exercises, tai chi chuan, or square dancing, etc.

Activities recommended for ordinary patients during hospitalization are as follows. *Exercise intensity*: the intensity between resting (1.0 METs) and mild physical activity (< 3.0 METs) is recommended. *Exercise frequency*: twice a day, starting 1 hour after meals. *Exercise time*: activity time is determined according to the patient's physical condition, maintaining 15–45 minutes each time. For patients who are prone to fatigue or are weak, they can perform interval training. *Exercise types*: respiratory rehabilitation exercise, walking on the spot, tai chi chuan, and exercises to prevent thrombosis.

For severe and critically severe patients, the recommended activities are as follows (pay attention to preventing the tubes connecting patients from disconnecting during the whole activity process, and monitor vital signs throughout the whole activity process). *Exercise intensity*: patients with poor physical strength can reduce the intensity of exertion. With time or activity range maintained, they are just required to complete the movement. *Exercise frequency*: once or twice a day. *Exercise time*: the total training time should not exceed 30 minutes each time to avoid the aggravation of fatigue. *Exercise types*: first, regularly turning over and moving on the bed, siting up from the bed, transferring from the bed to the chair, sitting on the chair, standing up and walking on the spot, carrying out these exercises step by step in this order. Second, active/passive range of motion training. Third, for patients with sedation or cognitive impairment or biological constraints, passive lower limbs function bicycle ergometer, passive range of motion (PROM), and stretch and neuromuscular electrical stimulation (Table 5.1) are recommended.

Here are two forms of exercises. The first one is walking on the spot with low intensity. Note that patients should not bow their heads or hold their breath in the process of walking on the spot and try to keep breathing evenly. The patients can adjust the intensity of movement by step frequency and height of leg lifting. The second one is the exercise of feet shifting on the step, suitable for patients in good physical condition. The patients can prepare a wooden box with a suitable height and large surface. This exercise requires patients to put Foot A on the box and Foot B under the box and then put Foot B on the box and Foot A under the box. Repeat those feet-shifting processes several times. During this exercise, patients should not lower their heads or hold their breath, so as to keep even breathing. The patients can adjust the exercise intensity by the frequency of lifting the leg and the height of the wooden box. Patients with balance disorders should cautiously choose this form of exercise to prevent falls.

5.2.2 Strength Training

Antiresistance training method is recommended for strength training. The training frequency of each target muscle group is two to three times a week, and its load is 8–12 RM (repeating 8–12 reps at most for each set). Patients should perform one to three groups each time. At the beginning, patients can perform body-weight strength training, then gradually transition to carrying light weights. Take body-weight training as an example to illustrate different muscle groups.

TABLE 5.1   ACTIVITIES RECOMMENDED FOR DIFFERENT TYPES OF PATIENTS DURING HOSPITALIZATION

	Exercise Intensity	Exercise Frequency	Exercise Duration	Exercise Types
Mild	Borg dyspnea score ≤ 3 (out of 10 scores), with no fatigue on the second day.	2 times/day, start at 1 hour after meals.	15–45 minutes each time.	Respiratory rehabilitation exercises, tai chi chuan or square dancing, etc.
Ordinary	Between resting (1.0 METs) and mild physical activity (< 3.0 METs).	2 times/day, start 1 hour after meals.	Activity duration is determined according to the patient's physical condition, maintaining 15–45 minutes each time. For patients who are prone to fatigue or weak, they can perform interval training.	Respiratory rehabilitation exercise, walking on the spot, tai chi chuan, and exercises to prevent thrombosis.
Severe/ Critically Severe	Patients with poor physical strength can reduce the intensity of exertion. With time or activity range maintained, they are just required to complete the movement.	1–2 times a day.	The total training time should not exceed 30 minutes each time to avoid the aggravation of fatigue.	First, regularly turning over and moving on the bed, siting up from the bed, transferring from the bed to the chair, sitting on the chair, standing up, and walking on the spot, carrying out these exercises step by step in this order. Second, active/passive range of motion training. Third, for patients with sedation or cognitive impairment or biological constraints, passive lower limbs function bicycle ergometer, passive range of motion and stretch and neuromuscular electrical stimulation.

5.2.2.1 Upper Limbs Strength Training

1) Elbow flexors: Patients can choose standing, sitting, semirecumbent, or recumbent po sition for training. Take standing position as an example.

Place the upper limbs on either side of the torso. Keep the torso upright and keep eyesight straight forward with hands relaxed. Keep upper arms close to the chest. Bend the elbows when exhaling and return to the original position during inhaling. Do not hold the breath during exercise. Patients can select the appropriate weight load during exercise. A set consists of 8–12 reps. Three to four sets are required and should be performed on both sides in turn.

2) Elbow extensors: Patients can choose standing, sitting, semirecumbent, or recumbent positions for training. Take the sitting position and the recumbent position for examples.

In the sitting position, ask the patients to bend one shoulder forward to the maximum degree, keeping the torso upright, looking at the front, hanging the forearm naturally behind the head, bringing the upper arm close to the ear. Then extend the elbow when exhaling and return to the original position when inhaling. Do not hold breath during exercise. Patients can select the appropriate weight load during exercise. A set consists of 8–12 reps. Three to four sets are required and should be performed on both sides in turn.

Patients who cannot perform the above exercises while sitting can do these exercises while lying down, where their legs can flex so that the lumbar vertebra is attached to the bed surface and the shoulders of both upper limbs can be bent forward to the maximum degree with one forearm naturally under the bed edge. Extend the elbow when exhaling and return to the original position when inhaling. Do not hold breath during exercise. Patients can select the appropriate weight load during exercise. A set consists of 8–12 reps. Three to four sets are required and should be performed on both sides in turn.

3) Shoulder anterior flexors: Patients can choose standing, sitting, semi-recumbent, or recumbent positions for training. Take the sitting and recumbent positions as examples.

In the sitting position, place upper limbs on both sides of torso, and keep torso upright, looking at the front with hands relaxed. Then bend one shoulder joint forward. Bend shoulder joints forward when exhaling and return to the original position when inhaling. Do not hold breath during exercise. Patients can select the appropriate weight load during exercise. A set consists of 8–12 reps. Three to four sets are required and should be performed on both sides in turn.

Patients who cannot perform the above exercises while sitting can do these exercises while lying, where the legs are flexing so that the lumbar spine is close to the bed surface. Bend one side of the upper limbs forward. Bend shoulders forward when exhaling and return to the original position when inhaling. Do not hold breath during exercise. Patients can select the appropriate weight load during exercise. A set consists of 8–12 reps. Three to four sets are required and should be performed on both sides in turn.

4) Shoulder abductors: Patients can choose standing, sitting, semire-cumbent, or recumbent positions for training. Take the sitting and recumbent positions as examples.

In the sitting position, ask the patient to lay upper limbs on the sides of body, keeping the torso upright, looking at the front, keeping hands relaxed. Then stretch the upper limbs with elbow joints slightly flexed. Stretch shoulders out when exhaling and return to the original position when inhaling. Do not hold breath during exercise. Patients can select the appropriate weight load during exercise. A set consists of 8–12 reps. Three to four sets are required and should be performed on both sides in turn.

Patients who cannot perform the above exercises while sitting can do these exercises while lying, where the legs are flexed so that the lumbar vertebra is close to the bed surface. Patients should stretch their upper limbs with elbow joints slightly flexed. Stretch shoulders out when exhaling and return to the original position when inhaling. In the supine position, the upper limbs can be slightly lifted from the bed. Do not hold breath during exercise. Patients can select the appropriate weight load during exercise. A set consists of 8–12 reps. Three to four sets are required and should be performed on both sides in turn.

5) Shoulder posterior extensors: Patients can choose standing, sitting, semirecumbent, or recumbent positions for training.

In the standing position, ask patients to place both upper limbs on both sides of the torso, keeping the torso upright, eyesight on the front, and hands relaxed. Stretch one upper limb backward with elbow joints slightly bent. Stretch shoulders out when exhaling and return to the original position when inhaling. In the supine position, the upper limbs can be slightly lifted from the bed. Do not hold breath during exercise. Patients can select the appropriate weight load during exercise. A set consists of 8–12 reps. Three to four sets are required and should be performed on both sides in turn.

In the semirecumbent and recumbent positions, the legs are flexed so that the lumbar spine is attached to the bed surface. Keep the elbows flexed on both sides and the upper arm attached to the bed surface. When exhaling, try to exert efforts on the upper arm to approach the bottom of the bed as far as possible. At the same time, the upper back can be lifted slightly from the bed surface. When inhaling, return to the original position.

5.2.2.2 Core Strength Training

1) Abdominal muscles: Patients can choose the supine position for training.

First perform hip and knee flexion at 90° and bring legs together so that calves are parallel to the floor and thighs are perpendicular to the floor. When exhaling, move thighs closer to the abdomen and, when inhaling, return to the original position. Do not hold breath during exercise. Patients can select the appropriate weight load during exercise. A set consists of 8–12 reps. Three to four sets are required.

If patients have difficulty completing those exercises, the patient can put the leg on the starting position with the others' help to bring the thigh close to the abdomen, and then let the patient slowly put it down. Do not hold breath during exercise. Patients can select the appropriate weight load during exercise. A set consists of 8–12 reps. Three to four sets are required.

2) Posterior chain such as lower back, buttocks, etc.: Patients can choose the supine position for training.

First, place feet flat on the surface of the bed. Feet should be hip-width apart. Then place upper limbs on either side of torso. When exhaling, the buttocks should be squeezed and the hip should be lifted to the maximum extent. When inhaling, return to the original position. Do not hold breath during exercise. Patients can select the appropriate weight load during exercise. A set consists of 8–12 reps. Three to four sets are required.

If patients have difficulty completing those exercises, they can lift their hips with external help, and then let the patient slowly put the hip down. Do not hold breath during exercise. Patients can select the appropriate weight load during exercise. A set consists of 8–12 reps. Three to four sets are required.

5.2.2.3 Lower Limbs Strength Training

1) Hip flexors: Patients can choose standing, sitting, semirecumbent, or recumbent positions for training. Take the sitting position and the recumbent position as examples.

In the sitting position, patients can choose a slightly higher and stable chair under the sitting position, make sure the feet are flat on the ground, and lift the thighs alternately on both sides. Do not hold breath during exercise. Patients can select the appropriate weight load during exercise. A set consists of 8–12 reps. Three to four sets are required.

Patients who cannot perform the above exercises while sitting can do these exercises in the recumbent position, with the legs flat on the bed. Then perform hip and knee flexion alternatively. When exhaling, raise the hip and knees and, when inhaling, put them down. Do not hold breath during exercise. A set consists of 8–12 reps. Three to four sets are required.

2) Knee extensors: Patients can choose standing, sitting, semirecumbent, or recumbent position for training.

In the standing position, place a stool behind the patient. Keep body upright, feet shoulder-width apart, toes facing forward, hands crossed on the opposite shoulder. Inhale and sit with hips back, touch the stool gently. Exhale and stretch knees. The knee cannot extend beyond toe position, so the knee must always be in a straight line with the toes. Do not hold breath during exercise. Patients can select the appropriate weight load during exercise. A set consists of 8–12 reps. Three to four sets are required.

In the sitting position, patients should stand, with feet on the ground, hands beside the body. When exhaling, stretch knees and **make shank parallel to the floor**, and slowly lower them when **inhaling**. Do not hold breath during exercise. Patients can select the appropriate weight load during exercise. A set consists of 8–12 reps. Three to four sets are required.

Patients who cannot perform the above exercises while sitting can do these exercises in the recumbent position by placing a cushion under the knees so that there is an angle of 90° between the lap the lower legs. Stretch knees out when exhaling and drop them when inhaling. Do not hold breath during exercise. Patients can select the appropriate weight load during exercise. A set consists of 8–12 reps. Three to four sets are required.

3) Knee flexors: Patients can choose standing, semirecumbent, or recumbent position for training.

In the standing position, ask patients to remain upright with hands on the table for stability. Take a deep breath with one knee bent when exhaling, stretch heels as close to hips as possible, and return to the original position when inhaling. Do not hold breath during exercise. Patients can select the appropriate weight load during exercise. A set consists of 8–12 reps. Three to four sets are required.

Patients who cannot perform the above exercises while sitting can do these exercises in the recumbent position. Slide the heels back as close to the hips as possible. Then extend the knee on one side when exhaling and put it back when inhaling. Do not hold breath during exercise. Patients can select the appropriate weight load during exercise. A set consists of 8–12 reps. Three to four sets are required.

4) Ankle plantar and dorsal flexor muscles: Patients can choose standing, sitting, semirecumbent, or recumbent position for training.

In the standing position, keep the body upright with one heel touching the
ground and do dorsal-flexion in maximum degrees. Then transit to the end
part of the forefoot, raise the heel of the foot for plantar flexion in maximum
degrees. And step forward with alternative usage of forepart, middle part,
and back of the entire soles. Keep breathing evenly. If patients cannot perform
these exercises, they can do the heel lift training (i.e., "lifting the heel") in the
standing position. Then lift the feet when exhaling, gradually put down half-
way when inhaling and then continue to lift them. A set consists of 8–12 reps.
Patients can rest after each set. It is recommended to do this exercise two to
three times a week.

In the sitting position, the patients can do the sitting and foot hooking exercise. Keep body upright with feet flat on the floor and knees facing in the same
direction as the toes. Lift up when exhaling and drop back when inhaling. Do
not hold breath during exercise. A set consists of 8–12 reps. Three to four sets
are required.

Patients who cannot perform the above exercises while sitting can do these
exercises in the recumbent position. Ask the patients to straighten their lower
limbs, try their best to hook the feet up when exhaling and keep it for 2–4 seconds. Then return to the original position when inhaling. Next, step on the floor
hard when exhaling and keep it for 2–4 seconds. After that, return to the original position again when inhaling. Hook the feet up when exhaling, and so on.
Do not hold breath during exercise. A set consists of 8–12 reps. Three to four
sets are required.

5.2.3 Balance Training

Maintaining good balance requires multiple conditions: vision, vestibular
function, proprioceptors, tactile input and sensitivity, central nervous system
function, coordination of active and antagonistic muscles, muscle strength
and endurance, flexibility of joints, and soft tissue flexibility. Damage by one
or more factors can affect the maintenance of balance. Among them, the
decrease of muscle strength and endurance will greatly affect the balance
function of patients. Balance requires a certain amount of muscle strength
in the trunk and both upper and lower limbs to adjust the posture. When the
person's balance is disturbed temporarily, the whole body can make timely
corresponding protective responses to maintain the body's balance to prevent fall or injury. But for patients with reduced upper limb muscle strength, if
they cannot adjust body reaction, corresponding protective reactions, such as
upper limbs' protective reaction, the patient's sitting balance will be destroyed.

However, if the muscle strength of the lower limbs is insufficient, the patient's orthostatic balance cannot be maintained, and there is no reaction such as striding and jumping, etc., and the patients are likely to fall and get injured. COVID-19 patients were forced to rest in bed during the acute phase of the disease, and the respiratory muscle weakness and decline of muscle strength and endurance caused by immobilization destroyed the patient's balance ability. The recovery of balance ability is of great importance, especially for middle-aged and elderly patients. Therefore, it is necessary to improve patients' muscle strength and endurance, as well as their core strength. Only by improving the stability of the core area can they move coordinately and effectively. At the same time, it can also effectively prevent them from falling or getting injured during sports.

Patients with balance dysfunction should be involved in balance training under the guidance of rehabilitation therapists, such as unarmed balance training, balance trainers, etc. When the patient can maintain the sitting position but cannot stand, the method of center of gravity transfer under the sitting position can be used for training.

5.2.3.1 For Patients Who Can't Stand

Ask patients to perform balance training in a seated position with a little more space between feet. Ask patients to pick up things from the table alone and put them on the other side from one end. Be sure to have someone nearby to protect them from falling.

5.2.3.2 For Patients Who Can Barely Get Up

Patients stand with feet apart and gradually reduce the distance between the feet. While the patients are able to maintain an upright position, let the patients move the object on the table while standing. Be sure to have someone nearby to protect them from falling.

5.2.3.3 For Patients Who Can Stand on a Flat Surface for a Certain Time

Clinical practice can achieve the purpose of training by destroying the patient's balance temporarily, such as throwing and catching the ball. This type of balance training can also make the process interesting with the interaction between patients and doctors. Be sure to have someone nearby to protect them from falling.

5.2.4 Flexibility Training

Flexibility training involves stretching the major muscle groups of the body to prevent sports injuries and relieve muscle fatigue.

5.2.5 Precautions

5.2.5.1 Pain

Exercise prescriptions should be adjusted appropriately when patients have symptoms of musculoskeletal pain.

5.2.5.2 Fatigue

For discharged patients with mild symptoms, the motion intensity can be gradually increased to moderate intensity under the condition of blood oxygen monitoring. For patients with severe symptoms, a longer period of intensity adjustment is recommended.

5.2.5.3 Panting

Monitoring of blood oxygen and symptoms should be strengthened before and during exercise. In case of shortness of breath, dyspnea, chest tightness, and other symptoms, it is necessary to know the patient's oxygen level. The motions should be terminated if the level is less than 93%.

5.2.5.4 Difficulty in Breathing

1) For bedridden patients, wedge pads or thick quilts at the back so that the trunk and bed can form the angle of 60°. Put a pillow under the knee joints to ensure knee flexion is slightly higher than hips and relax the neck and shoulders to assist breathing muscles. Then ask the patient to prop themselves up with the upper limbs into the lying position. After that, have them inhale slowly through the nose and exhale slowly through the mouth.

2) For nonbedridden patients, find a stable surface to sit down, relax the neck and shoulders to assist breathing muscle relaxation, etc. Then support the whole body with upper limbs. After that, inhale slowly through the nose and exhale slowly through the mouth.

5.3 TREATMENT TECHNIQUES OF PSYCHOSOCIAL FUNCTIONAL REHABILITATION

Treatment techniques of psychosocial function rehabilitation are approaches to treat patients with physical and psychological aspects of dysfunction mainly through selective and purposeful application to daily life, work, study, and leisure activities, and so on. They can prevent loss of living and work ability or disability; improve patients' physical and mental potentials; restore patients' ability to function physically, psychologically, and socially; and improve the quality of life, helping them return home and to society early.

5.3.1 Activities of Daily Living Training

The ability to carry out activities of daily living (ADL) is a basic function necessary to maintain one's daily life. The main purpose of daily activity training is to help patients establish self-rehabilitation consciousness, give full play to their subjective initiative, improve their self-confidence, and further improve patients' physical functions, including joint flexibility, coordination, and balance ability, so that they may return to their families and society.

ADL training is divided into two types: basic activities of daily living training and instrumental activities of daily living training. Different diseases lead to different types of dysfunction. ADL training is required to assess the ability of COVID-19 patients to transfer, modify, go to the toilet, bathe, and other daily activities, followed by targeted training. During training, patients can reduce body energy consumption and manage to complete functional activities accurately with high quality by adopting ergonomic principles, proper posture, correct activity methods and/or assistive techniques, and by combining with patients' functional state.

The main principles in the process of training are as follows.

1) Have sufficient balance between work and rest. Let patients do easy and complicated actions in turn. After they complete one action, let them have proper rest before continuing the following actions, or break the actions in daily life activities down into small sections that can be carried out intermittently according to the patient's own conditions. When patients' strength is regained, let them perform actions consistently.

2) Pay attention to breathing during performing actions. Let patients control their breathing rhythm. The time of exhaling and inhaling once is 4–6 seconds. Inhale before exerting force and exhale when exerting force.

5.3.1.1 Basic Activities of Daily Living (BADL) Training

BADL training mainly includes turning over, sitting up, standing, walking, dressing, putting on shoes, washing face, brushing teeth, bathing, eating, etc.

1) Turning over: Ask patients to bend both knees to 90°, then turn their heads to the side to which they want to turn. Extend hands forward and shake hands. Note that patients do not exert force on abdominal muscles in this process and prevent breath holding. Complete turning over while exhaling. Axial turning can avoid using abdominal force and save energy. Do not hold breath and breathe evenly while turning over.

2) Sitting up: Ask patients to remain in the turning over position. Then let them put their legs under the bed and raise their heads upward. Hold the bed with both hands and complete sitting up while exhalation. They should use the strength of their extremities to lessen the load on core abdominal muscles and make sitting up easier. Do not hold breath and breathe evenly while sitting up.

3) Standing up: When the patients are sitting on the bed with feet shoulder-width apart, ask them to slide their heels backward so that their knees fall in front of the toes, then lean the torso forward until their hips leave the support surface, and exhale and stretch knees to complete standing. Patients can also do this while sitting on a chair. Patients with weak strength or balance problems can use a walker to help them stand. Adjust the walker to the same height as the greater trochanter of the femur, with the upper and lower arms at the angle of 150°. Instruct the patients to hold the armrests at both ends with both hands, and separate the feet as wide as the shoulders, slide the heels backward so that the patient's knees fall in front of the toes, and lean the torso forward until their hips leave the support surface. While exhaling, the upper and lower limbs exert force at the same time to stand up. With a walker, the patient can make good use of their upper limbs to stand. To ensure safety, be sure not to move feet while standing. Keep breathing evenly while standing up, and do not hold breath. During the training, the therapist should pay attention to the patient's condition. If the symptoms do not relieve or worsen during the training, stop immediately and report to the doctor.

4) Walking: Many muscles need to participate in order to maintain balance and stability during walking, which will increase oxygen consumption. Patients can use appropriate walkers to make walking smooth and easy. A suitable walker can help increase the area of the support surface, reducing oxygen consumption with usage of their upper limbs. During walking, the ratio of inhalation and exhalation should be 1:2. Blood oxygen should be maintained within an appropriate range. And respiratory rhythm should be controlled to prevent heart rate increase or blood oxygen decrease caused by disordered inhalation and exhalation ratio.

5) Dressing: For patients with dyspnea who need oxygen inhalation, it is recommended to wear cardigan-type clothes to prevent dyspnea due to oxygen cut-off when putting on pullovers. Note that the position of their hands should not go above the shoulders when dressing. If it is necessary to wear a pullover, the patients should put the clothes on the forearm in advance, arrange the oxygen tubes, remove the oxygen, and quickly put on the clothes once. When the patients have put their head

through the appropriate hole in the item of clothing, patients should put on the oxygen tube first, and arrange the clothes later, so as to shorten oxygen cut-off time.

6) Putting on shoes: Patients with dyspnea should avoid bending down to put on shoes because the contents of the abdominal cavity may limit the movement of the diaphragm. It is recommended that patients should sit on a firm and stable support surface that is slightly higher than the lower leg and use a long shoehorn to put on their shoes.

7) Washing face: Patients with dyspnea should avoid bending down to wash their face because the contents of the abdominal cavity will limit the movement of diaphragm. To reduce oxygen consumption, it is recommended that patients take a sitting position. Patients can put both upper limbs on the table and wipe their faces instead of washing them to avoid oxygen cut-off. Be careful not to hold breath during this process.

8) Brushing teeth: It is recommended to brush teeth in standing position. Keep eyesight straight forward and avoid bowing head, as the contents of the abdominal cavity may limit the movement of the diaphragm and affect breathing. When patients cannot stand, they can brush teeth in the sitting position, holding upper limbs against the sink to reduce oxygen consumption. They can gargle with two cups. One is for receiving water and the other is for spitting water. Use them quickly in turn to reduce breath-holding time.

9) Bathing: Ask the patients to choose a nonslip shower stool, nonslip mat, and a long-handled bath brush to help with bathing. The shower stool enables the patients to take a shower in the sitting position, which can greatly reduce the physical consumption of standing. Nonslip mats can increase safety. The long-handled bath brush can offer easy access to hard-to-reach areas while using a smaller range of activities, reducing oxygen consumption, and saving energy. Patients should wear a special shower cap when washing their hair. When the water flows from top to bottom, it will cover their faces and affect their breathing, and even cause coughing. The shower cap can block the water from entering their eyes, nose, or ears, playing a good protective role to ensure smooth breathing. It should be noted that excessive indoor humidity may cause breathing difficulties. It is recommended to keep good ventilation. If extra oxygen is needed, a long oxygen tube can be passed under the door. For those who can bathe while standing, handrails should be installed to prevent slipping or falling while standing on one leg.

10) Eating: If the patients can sit alone, they can eat in the sitting position. If the patients cannot sit alone, they can eat in the semisitting and

supine position. If the patients cannot eat alone, they can be fed in the supine position at 30° from the surface. While eating, try to ensure that the patients do not eat more than 10 mL once (about half a spoon once), and finish swallowing at the end of inhalation. When swallowing, patients can lower rather than raise head to avoid coughing.

5.3.1.2 Instrumental Activities of Daily Living (IADL)

The training of instrumental activities of daily living (IADL) mainly focuses on the ability of social participation in daily life activities at a higher level, such as household chores, handling personal affairs, purchasing, etc. It is necessary to comprehensively consider the patient's psychological and physical functional ability in completing these activities by simulating the actual scene in the training by creating tasks and obstacles against task completion while under the guidance of the occupational therapist.

5.3.2 Therapeutic Activities

Therapeutic activities refer to carefully selected and targeted activities aimed at helping people with physical, mental, social adaptability, and emotional disorders. These activities enable patients to recover, develop, and maintain an appropriate lifestyle that can reflect their own values, improve their quality of life, and bring satisfaction physically and mentally.

5.3.2.1 Psychological Therapy

1) To enhance the sense of independence and build confidence, activities such as painting, calligraphy, clay sculpture, weaving, origami, mosaic, etc., may be used.
2) To boost the sense of accomplishment and satisfaction, activities such as woodworking, pottery making, painting, calligraphy, weaving, origami, mosaic, and other operations that can produce physical objects may be used.
3) To adjust emotions and divert attention, activities such as playing music, board games, card games, or video games as well as painting, calligraphy, clay sculpture, weaving, origami, mosaic, etc., may be used.
4) To regulate emotions and promote psychological balance, cathartic activities such as woodworking, hammering, paper-cutting, and clay sculpture allow patients to vent out negative emotions and promote psychological balance.
5) To improve cognitive and perceptual functions, activities such as playing music, board games, card games, and electronic games as well

as painting and calligraphy can improve patients' attention, problem-solving, and execution ability (mainly for elderly COVID-19 patients).

5.3.2.2 Occupational Therapy

1) To enhance labor skills, activities such as carpentry, metalworking, typing, handicraft making, gardening, etc., can be used.
2) To improve occupational adaptability, collective activities such as board games, card games, and ball games can enhance the sense of competition and cooperation, promote interpersonal communication, improve the relationship between colleagues, thus improving occupational adaptability.
3) To boost patients' confidence in re-employment, making products through therapeutic activities such as carpentry, pottery, clay modeling, painting, calligraphy, weaving, origami, mosaic, and art crafting may be used.

5.3.2.3 Social Therapy

1) To improve social contact and relationships, activities such as gardening and playing board games, card games, and music may be used.
2) To promote social reintegration, productive, competitive, and recreational activities can help patients adapt to the social environment and return to society sooner.

5.3.3 Main Techniques and Methods for Psychological Rehabilitation of COVID-19 Patients

5.3.3.1 Supportive Therapy

Supportive therapy can help patients express their emotional and cognitive problems, remove doubts, improve their mood, correct bad behaviors, and boost their confidence to overcome the disease, thus promoting the process of physical and mental recovery.

The main methods of supportive therapy are as follows:

1) Guiding and encouraging patients to express their emotions: First, establish a good doctor–patient relationship through conversation, care, and understanding so that patients are willing to express their deep feelings. For patients who are not good at expressing themselves, doctors can guide them or demonstrate ways they can express themselves. If the patient makes emotional reactions, the therapist should show tolerance and understanding and give timely

affirmations and strengthening. Patients' expression of psychological requirements and emotions play an important role in easing emotions.

2) Explanation: This helps patients to ease excessive worries, establish confidence, and strengthen cooperation. It also helps create good psychological conditions for treatment and encourage patients to cooperate with the treatment to the maximum extent. Different explanation methods and techniques should be applied to different patients according to the nature and regularity of the diseases. For some patients, doctors keep their existing psychological problems confidential for the time being, so as to avoid aggravating the psychological burden of patients and make patients feel at ease to receive treatment actively. In addition, doctors can also give some patients a scientific explanation to establish their confidence to overcome the disease.

3) Encouraging and comforting: COVID-19 patients tend to have extreme psychological reactions, such as showing fear, worry, anxiety, depression, pessimism, despair, or even attempting to commit suicide. Especially when the treatment effect is not obvious, patients may have greater emotional fluctuations. Therefore, the treatment personnel should give timely enthusiastic and pertinent encouragement as well as comfort according to patients' psychological problems and characteristics, so that they can cheer them up and boost their confidence.

4) Guaranteeing: Ensure that patients can accept examination and treatment results, so as to boost their confidence in overcoming the disease. However, doctors can only give patients a neutral or limited guarantee under practical conditions, in order to relieve patients' pressure and enhance their confidence. Unrealistic guarantees are forbidden.

5) Improving the environment: This mainly refers to improving the interpersonal environment related to patients. On the one hand, medical staff should help patients eliminate the adverse factors in interpersonal relationship. On the other hand, they should help add some new and beneficial factors. In addition, doctors should seek mental support from patients' family members and relatives and ensure that they are able to communicate effectively.

Supportive therapy is a therapeutic method for COVID-19 patients. It can help patients relieve their depressed emotions or concerns about the rehabilitation of COVID-19. It can also enhance their confidence in pulmonary rehabilitation treatment, improve their interpersonal relationships, and establish a positive and reasonably therapeutic doctor–patient relationship.

5.3.3.2 Cognitive Therapy

Generally speaking, cognition refers to the cognition activity or cognition process, including beliefs and belief systems, thinking, and imagination, etc. Cognitive therapy is the general term of therapies that change patients' poor cognition through cognitive behavior techniques according to the theoretical assumption that the cognitive process affects emotion and behavior. The basic ideas of cognitive therapy are that cognitive processes are mediators of behavior and emotion and that maladaptive behaviors and emotion are associated with maladaptive cognition. The task of the therapist is to work with the patient to identify these maladaptive perceptions and provide learning or training methods to correct these perceptions, keeping the patient's cognition more in line with reality.

5.3.3.2.1 Main Strategies of Cognitive Therapy

1) Education: Introduce basic knowledge about the disease and treatment prognosis to patients. It also includes an introduction about how to cope with social support and emotional impact on the psychological and physical aspects. Provided with relevant skills, patients can form a more objective and correct understanding. This kind of intervention has positive effects on improving patients' coping skills, increasing knowledge about the disease, and improving the obedience to treatment.

2) Cognitive reconstruction: This helps patients change and establish cognition to fight against a variety of incorrect cognition or attitudes, especially negative thinking of failure. This kind of cognitive therapy often requires much more patience because patients' newly established cognition is difficult to be reinforced in a short time, but their old cognition often reappears.

3) Role reversal: This requires patients to put themselves in other people's shoes and consider other's feelings. Some patients, especially those who have conjugal affection or happy families, often want to die early or even refuse to receive any treatment, considering the impact on their work and personal life. The best way to treat those patients is to change their cognition by putting them in other people's shoes, for example, considering how they would feel and act if a beloved family member had a similar disease.

4) Downward comparison: This involves comparing patients to those who are less fortunate than they are in some way. Through comparison,

patients can find their own strengths and believe that they are not the most unfortunate people, even if they are seriously ill. By recognizing that those who are more seriously ill than themselves can be happy and actively cooperate with treatment, patients may wonder why they stay pessimistic. This technique enables patients to evaluate their condition realistically and positively. They can also identify the ways to think about questions so that they can deal with the problems more positively and rationally.

5.3.2.2.2 Methods for Cognitive Therapy

Rational emotive therapy (RET) and Beck's cognitive therapy are the most commonly used methods of cognitive therapy.

RET, one of the cognitive therapies (some scholars call it "cognitive behavioral therapy"), was founded in the 1950s by Ellis and aims to correct patients' unreasonable beliefs, motivate patients to adapt to reasonable beliefs, and change the patient's behavior and cognition in combination with behavior modification techniques. Its theoretical basis is the A-B-C theory for psychological dysfunction, which assumes that psychological disorder is caused not directly by events or life circumstances but by the individuals' interpretation or their own evaluation. A represents activating events that the individuals go through, B represents individuals' beliefs system in their cognitive field, and C represents individuals' emotional and behavioral consequences under the stimulation events. C cannot be caused by A directly, but by B as an intermediary part. Emotions come from thinking, so changing thinking can advance the process of changing mood or behavior. Because it is peoples' misjudgments and interpretations of events that cause problems, people can also change their irrational thinking and self-defeating behavior by accepting rational thinking. RET enables patients to realize their irrational beliefs and their negative emotional consequences. Through modifying the underlying irrational beliefs, patients can finally lead a rational life.

Ellis classified unreasonable beliefs into three kinds, namely, people's irrational beliefs about themselves, about others, and about their surroundings and events. These unreasonable beliefs have three characteristics. First, those beliefs are too absolute. For example, "My illness must be cured, otherwise my life would become worthless!" Second, those beliefs contain over-generalization. For example, if a treatment does not work as it should, the patient would think that there is no possibility of being cured. When a person does something that does not meet their own standard of satisfaction, they think it will lead to terrible or disastrous consequences. For example, if a patient needs a tracheotomy, they may think, "Once the tracheotomy is done, my life will soon be over". To correct patients' irrational beliefs, the therapist can act as an active instructor to persuade and guide patients to rethink their assumptions, reasoning, and views of life that they concluded due to psychological imbalance. Ellis noted that successful therapy involves changing not only the way people deal with problem but also their behavior. For that reason, the therapist can give the patients homework, asking them to do something that contributes to developing a reasonable outlook on life. RET can help patients deal with anxiety, depression, fear, and interpersonal problems from both cognitive and behavioral perspectives.

5.3.4 Behavior Therapy

Behavioral therapy, or conditioned reflex therapy, is a kind of psychological therapy guided by behavioral learning theory. It can eliminate or correct patients' abnormal or bad behaviors with certain therapeutic procedures. Behavioral therapy emphasizes that patients' symptoms, namely abnormal behaviors or physiological functions, are fixed by the individuals' learning process through conditioned reflex in the past. Therefore, special therapeutic procedures can be designed to eliminate or correct abnormal behaviors or physiological functions by means of conditioned reflex.

There are five main approaches of behavior therapy.

1) Systematic desensitization: This method can be used to treat anxiety and fear and other emotional disorders for COVID-19 patients in rehabilitation. The principle of therapy is based on fighting against conditioned reflexes. During the treatment, it is necessary to have a deep understanding of which stimulating situation leads to patients' abnormal behavior (anxiety and fear). Then arrange all anxiety responses in order from the lowest level to the highest level (levels range from 0 to 10, with 0 being completely calm and 10 being extremely anxious). After that, patients are taught a way to fight against anxiety and fear, namely relaxation training, so that patients can feel relaxed and relieve anxiety. Moreover, relaxation training techniques should be gradually and systematically paired with corresponding anxiety response levels from 0 to 10 to form an interactive inhibition situation. In this way, the bad conditions-based anxiety responses can be gradually and systematically eliminated one by one from the mildest to the severest.

2) Aversion therapy: This therapy helps patients combine abnormal behaviors with some disgusting or punitive stimuli to achieve the purpose of abstaining or reducing the occurrence of those abnormal behaviors through aversion conditioning. Disgust stimulation includes painful stimulation, such as pain caused by snapping a rubber band against the skin or pricking skin with the point of a needle.

Clinical aversion treatment can correct some patients' bad behaviors, such as smoking, coercion, etc.

3) Behavior-shaping method: This is a behavioral therapy that creates a certain desired good behavior through positive reinforcement. This method is more effective in correcting patients' passive behavior and improving their attention as well as compliance. During the implementation, patients can be asked to complete a moderate task. In the process of patients completing their homework, timely feedback and positive strengthening on their progress should be given, such as praise, encouragement, reward, etc.

4) Token economy: This requires some kind of rewards. When the patients make the expected good behavior performance, they are rewarded so that the patient's good behavior can be formed and reinforced, and their bad behaviors can be eliminated. Tokens, as positive reinforcements, can be in various symbolic forms, such as scorecards, chips, and bank drafts.

5) Relaxation response training: This is mainly used to treat patients' anxiety, depression, and sleep disorders. Relaxation response training is a kind of self-adjustment training, during which the whole body and then the mind can relax. It can contribute to resistance against the sympathetic nerve tension response caused by psychological stress, helping to eliminate psychological tension and adjust the mental balance. Relaxation response training methods are more commonly used in progressive muscle relaxation. That is to say, the muscles of the whole body should be relaxed systematically in a certain order. Before relaxation, psychological counseling and suggestion must be done to emphasize the mutual relationship between the mind and the body. At the same time, patients should experience the feeling of real relaxation. When experiencing the feeling of relaxation, the patients can first keep both hands tense, then relax them, repeat in this order several times. After that, let the patients compare the difference between relaxation and tension, and then let patients experience the feeling of relaxation again. At first, the therapists will give patients the verbal hints to relax. After several times, the patients can follow therapists' relaxation tape to practice relaxation. Finally, the patients manage to relax themselves without any external hints.

The basic steps of progressive muscle relaxation are as follows.

- Clench fists and then relax. Stretch five fingers and then relax.
- Tighten biceps and then relax. Tighten triceps and then relax.
- Shrug shoulders backward and then relax. Raise shoulders forward and then relax.

- Turn head to the right with shoulders straight and then relax. Turn head to the left with shoulders straight and then relax.
- Bend the neck so that the lower jaw touches the chest and then relax.
- Open mouth as wide as possible and then relax. Clench teeth and then relax.
- Stretch tongue as much as possible and then relax. Roll tongue as much as possible and then relax.
- Press the tongue firmly against the palate and then relax. Press the tongue firmly against the lower jaw and then relax.
- Open eyes and keep eyes wide-open and then relax. Close eyes and then relax.
- Take a breath as deep as possible and then relax.
- Press the shoulder blade against the chair and arch the back and then relax.
- Tighten hip muscles and then relax. Press gluteus against the cushion and then relax.
- Stretch and lift legs for 15–20 cm from the ground and then relax.
- Keep abdomen tight as much as possible and then relax. Stretch abdomen and keep it tight and then relax.
- Straighten legs and bend toes upward and then relax. Flex toes and then relax.
- Bend toes and then relax. Lift toes upward and then relax.

Cognitive behavioral therapy can be directly applied to COVID-19 patients with anxiety, fear, and bad behavior. Treatment is mainly aimed at the signs and symptoms (target problems) of a certain disorder of patients, helping to improve their psychological, physiological, and behavioral indicators, guiding them to handle their bad emotions or behaviors and enhance their adaptability and social skills.

BIBLIOGRAPHY

1. Zhao Hongmei, Xie Yuxiao, Wang Chen. Recommendations for respiratory rehabilitation of COVID-19 patients (2nd Edition) [J]. *Chinese Journal of Tuberculosis and Respiratory Diseases*, 3(3): 308–314. [2020].
2. Xie Yuxiao. Rehabilitation treatment of patients infected with COVID-19 [J/OL]. *Journal of Rehabilitation Medicine*, 30(1): 5-6. [2020].
3. Min Rui, Liu Jie, Dai Zhe, Sun Jiazhong, Deng Haohua, Li Xin, Wu Yuwen, Huang Qi, Sun Li, Yang Miao, Xu Yan cheng. Pathogenesis and clinical research progress of COVID-19 [J/OL]. *Chinese Journal of Nosocomiology*, 30(7): 1–6. [2020].
4. Keiji Kuba, Yumiko Imai, Shuan Rao, et al. A crucial role of angiotensin converting enzyme 2 (ACE2) in SARS coronavirus -induced lung Injury [J]. *Natural Medicines*, 11(8):875–879. [2005].

5. Patrick Younan, Mathieu Iampietro, Andrew Nishida, et al. Ebola virus binding to tim-1 on T lymphocytes induces a cytokine storm [J]. *mBio*, 8(5): e00845-17. [2017].

6. Zhang Wei, Pan Chun, Song Qing. Problems that should be paid attention to during respiratory treatment of COVID-19 [J/OL]. *Medical Journal of Chinese People's Liberation Army*, 45(2): 1–6. [2020].

7. Feng Bin, Chen Zhengxian, Jin Longwei, et al. Reflections on the treatment of COVID-19 based on the nature of 'phlegm thrombus' [J/OL]. *Pharmacy Today*, 1(1): 1–7. [2020].

8. Lawrence P Cahalin, Malinda Braga, Yoshimi Matsuo, et al. Efficacy of diaphragmatic breathing in persons with chronic obstructive pulmonary disease: A review of the literature. *Journal of Cardiopulmonary Rehabilitation*, 22(1): 7–21. [2002].

9. Zhang Yuan, Wang Yuguang, Cheng Haiying. Ideas and methods of TCM rehabilitation treatment for COVID-19 discharged patients [J/OL]. *Beijing Journal of Traditional Chinese Medicine*, 39(1): 1–6. [2020].

10. Yan Li, Li Yongsheng. Recognition and management strategies for severe COVID-19 patients [J]. *Journal of New Medicine*, 51(3): 161–167. [2020].

11. Han Fang, Yang Yi. Application of non-invasive positive pressure ventilation in respiratory failure of severe acute respiratory syndrome [J]. *Chinese Journal of Tuberculosis and Respiratory Diseases*, 30(10): 795–797. [2007].

12. Zhu Lei, Hu Lijuan. Rational application of respiratory support technology for COVID-19 patients [J/OL]. *Fudan University Journal of Medical Sciences*, 47(1): 1–3. [2020].

13. Liu Xiaodan, Liu Li, Lu Yunfei, et al. Guidance of integrated traditional Chinese and Western medicine rehabilitation training for functional recovery of COVID-19 patients [J]. *Shanghai Journal of Traditional Chinese Medicine*, 54(3): 9–13. [2020].

14. Chen Xiaofeng, Guo Yi. Strategies for rehabilitation prevention and control in neurology department during the pandemic [J/OL]. *Guangdong Medical Journal*, 41(3): 1–4. [2020].

15. Huang Huai, Dai Yong. Considerations on respiratory rehabilitation of COVID-19 patients [J/OL]. *Chinese Journal of Rehabilitation Theory and Practice*, 26(3): 1–4. [2020].

16. Wang Ruiyuan, Su Quansheng. *Exercise physiology [M]*. Beijing: People's Sports Publishing House, 251–252. [2012].

17. Yu Pengming, He Chengqi, Gao Qiang, et al. Operational guidelines and recommendations for full-cycle physical therapy for COVID-19 patients [J]. *Chinese Journal of Physical Medicine and Rehabilitation*, 42: 102–104 [2020].

18. Xiaoling Huang, Yan Tiebin. *Rehabilitation medicine [M]*, Beijing: People's Medical Publishing House. [2018].

19. Dou Zulin. *Occupational therapy [M]*, Beijing: People's Medical Publishing House. [2018].

20. Tian Wei, Liu Geng, Zhang Xiaoying, et al. COVID-19 respiratory rehabilitation program with integrated traditional Chinese and Western medicine (Draft) [J/OL]. *Chinese Journal of Information on Traditional Chinese Medicine*, 27(3): 1–7. [2020].

21. Linda Nici, Claudio Donner, Emiel Wouters, et al. American Thoracic Society/European Respiratory Society statement on pulmonary rehabilitation. *American Journal of Respiratory and Critical Care Medicine*, 173:1390–1413. [2006].

22. Jadranka Spahija, Michel de Marchie, Alejandro Grassino. Effect of imposed pursed lips breathing on respiratory mechanics and dyspnea at rest and during exercise in COPD. *Chest*, 128: 640–650. [2005].
23. National Health Commission. Notice of the rehabilitation program for discharged patients with new coronary pneumonia (trial implementation) [EB/OL].2020-03-04.
24. Huang Zhijian, Chen Rongchang. The clinical application and progress of prone position ventilation in acute respiratory distress syndrome[J]. *International Journal of Respiration*, 6: 452–453+462. [2006].
25. Meng Shen. Pulmonary rehabilitation[M]. *Beijing: People's Medical Publishing House*, [2007].

Chapter 6

Traditional Chinese Medicine Rehabilitation Treatment Techniques for COVID-19

6.1 TREATMENT WITH TRADITIONAL CHINESE MEDICINE

Traditional Chinese medicine (TCM) has a long history in the prevention and treatment of plagues with its unique theory and practice. It has played an important role in the treatment of severe acute respiratory syndrome coronavirus (SARS-CoV) and Influenza A (H1N1). TCM is an effective way to treat COVID-19 by taking advantage of the body's self-regulation mechanism, enhancing immunity, and stimulating disease resistance and rehabilitation.

When the pandemic broke out, TCM experts drew on their knowledge of ancient classic prescriptions through symptom collection and clinical analysis. Then they combined them with clinical diagnosis and treatment programs, quickly put forward TCM programs, and continuously optimized them in clinical practice. According to the plan, the experts adhere to the early measures, full participation, precise measures, and TCM deep intervention in the whole process of prevention, treatment, and rehabilitation. For mild and ordinary patients, Chinese medicine is used occasionally; for severe and critically severe patients, TCM and Western medicine experts have joint consultation, and Chinese and Western medicine are used together to play the superposition effect of the two types of medicine. For the convalescent population, TCM, acupuncture, moxibustion, acupoint massage, and other methods are used to promote patient rehabilitation.

TCM has been proven effective in treating COVID-19. The newly released *Diagnosis and Treatment Plan for COVID-19 (7th Trial Edition)* contains a rich discussion of TCM treatment, including universal prescriptions, formulations for different conditions and symptoms, and proprietary Chinese medicine, which reflects the unity of syndrome and disease differentiation, theory and clinical practice, and guidance and norms. These are the vivid practices of inheriting the essence, upholding integrity, and generating innovation.

In the realm of TCM, COVID-19 is categorized as a "pandemic disease" that is due to the feeling of pestilence. The disease belongs to *yin* disease, which is the main line against *yang*. The disease is mainly in the lungs, involving the spleen, stomach, heart, brain, kidney, and other organs. In the early stage, evil *qi* invaded the lungs, which caused discord between the guard and the expression and the function of inhaling and exhaling, thus eventually leading to lung lesions. In the period of medical observation and clinical treatment, the pathogenesis is different with the changes of the disease.

6.1.1 Principles of Treatment

The symptoms of this disease are insidious in the early stage, and it progresses rapidly in the middle stage. It is generally a syndrome of asthenia in origin, and asthenia in superficiality and mixed excessiveness and deficiency. The pathogenesis is that damp evil accumulates in the lungs, leading to discord between the guards. To cure diseases, it is necessary to remove the evil, protect the lungs, and relieve the dampness. In the late stage of the disease, the lungs and spleen are both deficient, and *yin* was injured. To cure diseases, it is necessary to strengthen the vitality of breath to replenish deficiency, invigorate the spleen and lung, and nourish *yin*. In addition to direct treatment of the lung, we should also focus on general health, and pay attention to tonifying the spleen, liver, kidney, heart, etc.

The main symptoms that help to diagnose are the basis for treatment include fever, dry cough, and fatigue. A few patients had nasal congestion, runny noses, sore throats, myalgia, and diarrhea. In severe cases, symptoms such as dyspnea, wheezing, and inability to lie down were found 1 week after onset. It is worth noting that during the course of severe and critically severe cases, patients may have moderate to low fever or even no obvious fever.

6.1.2 Treatment Mechanisms

Wu Youke, a doctor in the Ming Dynasty, pointed out in his *Treatise on the Pandemic Disease* that "pandemic disease is a disease, which is caused by neither wind nor cold, nor heat nor humidity. It is a strange gas from heaven and earth", and this strange gas is also called "hostility", "pandemic", and "sickness". *Su Wen • Chi Fa Lun* stated, "All the five pandemics are easily infected, they cause similar symptoms no matter how strong they are", pointing out that "pandemics" are highly contagious. According to the available clinical data, COVID-19, mainly transmitted through respiratory droplets and close contact, is highly contagious and pandemic, and it changes rapidly. Moreover, there is no specific antiviral drug for COVID-19 at present. Tong Xiaolin et al. believe that the pandemic is a "cold and dampness pandemic", which damages *yang*, but also causes heat transfer, dryness, *yin* injury, blood stasis, and closure. The infected disease is located in the lung and stomach, and the pathogenesis is "dampness, poison, and stasis". Based on syndrome differentiation, the treatment mainly includes dispelling cold and drying the dampness, clearing away heat, detoxifying, nourishing the body, and dispelling pathogenic factors.

TCM has a long history of curing pandemic diseases, and doctors take these pandemic diseases seriously. They actively explored pandemic diseases from different levels and developed the theories of "pestilence caused by breath", "pestilence caused by pathogen", and "pestilence caused by evil poison", thus forming a complete theoretical and practical system on the etiology, pathogenesis, and treatment of pandemic diseases. Medical books on the treatment of pandemics, such as Zhang Zhongjing's *Treatise on Typhoid Fever and Miscellaneous Diseases*, Wu Youke's *Treatise on the Pandemic Disease*, and Wu Jutong's *Treatise on the Disease of Fever*, etc., were produced. The enduring classic prescriptions for the treatment of pandemics, such as maxing shigan soup, da yuan decoction, qinqiao powder, and angong niuhuang pill, were left behind. These texts serve as a good reference for the prevention and treatment of COVID-19.

The purpose of early COVID-19 intervention with Chinese medicine is mainly to delay or block the development of COVID-19. Led by academician Huang Luqi of the Chinese Academy of Engineering, the first national TCM medical team implemented the TCM treatment scheme, which enabled the cure and discharge rate of Wuhan Jinyintan Hospital to exceed 40%, far higher than that of Wuhan in the same period (about 5%). It reflects the clear clinical efficacy of TCM in the treatment of COVID-19. Active and effective TCM treatment in the early and advanced stages is the key to reduce critical illness and fatality rates. The National Health Commission (NHC) also released the TCM treatment plan for COVID-19 in *COVID-19 Diagnosis and Treatment Plan (3rd Trial Edition)*, which has been updated to the seventh edition so far, and the proportion of TCM treatment plan has significantly increased. In the plan, the contents of treatment based on syndrome differentiation and corresponding proprietary Chinese medicine treatment are recommended, especially for the usage and dosage of severe and critically severe Chinese medicine injections.

The pandemic is insidious, characterized by its rapid progress, long treatment course, and level of difficulty in curing; therefore, effective intervention should be carried out as soon as possible, i.e., prevention before disease onset, prevention of the progress of disease, and prevention of the recrudescence of disease. From the perspective of TCM, when the pathogen is not clear, as long as the etiology is clear and the syndrome type is consistent, the idea of "treating different diseases together" can still be adopted to take effect.

At the same time, clinical practice data disclosed by relevant national authorities show that integrating Chinese and Western medicine is effective in the treatment of COVID-19.

The occurrence of COVID-19 may be related to elevated inflammatory factor levels or "cytokine storm"; therefore, inhibiting the production of these inflammatory factors is essential for the treatment of COVID-19. Arachidonic acid (AA) mediates the production of various inflammatory factors and is closely related to the occurrence, development, and regression of inflammation. Inhibition of the AA metabolism pathway helps to inhibit the release of inflammatory factors in the body and alleviates cytokine storm. Through screening, Ren Yue et al. found that prescribing huoxiangzhengqi capsule, jinhuqinggan granule, lianhuqingwen capsule, qingfei detoxification decoction, xuebijing injection, retoxing injection, and tanreqing injection have potential inhibitory effects on the AA metabolism pathway and may inhibit the pneumonia caused by COVID-19 by relieving the cytokine storm.

TCM syndrome differentiation pays attention to meridian tropism. Meridian tropism refers to the orientation of drug action and efficacy in the viscera and meridians of the human body, which summarizes through long-term practice and observation of therapeutic effects. Qingfei detox decoction contains 21 Chinese medicines, of which 16 are attributed to the lung meridian, indicating that this compound medicine is specific to lung diseases. At the same time, this compound has many herbs on the spleen, stomach, heart, and kidney meridians, which can strengthen and dehumidify the spleen by transplanting spleen and stomach, in order to protect the heart, kidney, and other viscera.

Cao Xinfu et al. analyzed the drug regimens for COVID-19 prevention and control in various regions of the country and found some frequently used drug pairs, including ephedra-almond, ephedra-gypsum, ageratum-magnolia bark, rhizoma atractylodis-amomum, honeysuckle-forsythia, semen lepidii-gypsum, amomum-ephedra, etc. Ephedra-almond is considered as the most supportive drug pair, and semen lepidii-gypsum is the most reliable drug pair. This indicates that, in all regions of the country, dispelling pathogenic factors is the main approach used for the prevention and treatment of COVID-19, which roughly corresponds to the pathogenesis of the disease: "dampness, poison and blood stasis".

In addition to antivirus, the advantage of TCM intervention lies in its ability to regulate human immune function, stimulate the internal defensiveness and disease resistance ability, and achieve the combination of dispelling pathogenic factors and reinforcing the foundation of the body. This advantage allows patients with mild cases to gradually recover, prevent patients with moderate cases from progressing into severe or critically severe cases, thereby cutting off the development of the disease.

Recently, TCM has become required for all suspected cases in Hubei Province. Thus, it is clear that TCM will play an increasingly important role in the treatment of COVID-19 in the future.

6.1.3 Stages and Clinical Manifestations

6.1.3.1 Medical Observation Stage

- *Clinical manifestations*: Fatigue with gastrointestinal discomfort or fatigue with fever.
- *Recommended Chinese patent medicine*: Huoxiang zhengqi capsule (pill, water, oral liquid), jinhua qinggan granule, lianhua qingwen capsule (granule), shufeng detoxification capsule (granule).

6.1.3.2 Clinical Treatment Stage

- *Main prescription*: Lung-detoxification soup.
- *Scope of application*: Mild, ordinary, severe patients, in addition, critical patients can use it according to the actual situation of patients.
- *Basic prescription*: 9 g ephedra herb, 6 g processed licorice, 9 g almond, 15–30 g raw gesso (decocted first), 9 g cassia twig, 9 g alisma cathayensis, 9 g poria cotta, 16 g atractylodes rhizome, 6 g scutellaria baicalensis, 9 g ginger pinelliae, 9 g ginger, 9 g aster, 9 g butterbur, 6 g asarum, 12 g Chinese yam, 6 g fructus aurantii immaturus, 6 g tangerine peel, 9 g agastache rugosa.
- *Dosage*: Decocted in water. Take one dose daily, twice a day, one in the morning and one in the evening (40 minutes after meal); warm three doses for one course of treatment.

If possible, half a bowl of rice soup can be given to the patient after taking the medicine each time. More than one bowl can be given if the patient's tongue is dry and body fluid is low. (Note: If the patient does not have a fever, the dosage of raw gypsum should be reduced, and the dosage of raw gypsum can be increased for fever or strong heat.) If the symptoms improve but are not cured, then the patients can take the second course of treatment. If the patient has special conditions or other existing conditions, the second course of treatment can be modified according to the actual situation, and the drug will be stopped when the symptoms disappear.

6.1.3.2.1 Mild

1) Syndrome of cold dampness and stagnation of the lung
- *Clinical manifestations*: Fever, fatigue, body aches, cough, sputum, chest tightness, stupor, nausea, vomiting, and sticky stool.

Checking the tongue coating is a special method of diagnosing diseases in traditional Chinese Medicine. Tongues light fat tooth mark or red, with tongue moss white thick and greasy or white and greasy, and pulse is moistening or slippery.

- *Recommended prescription*: 6 g raw ephedra, 15 g raw plaster, 9 g almond, 15 g notopterygium root, l5 g lepidium apetalum willd, 9 g cyrtomium fortunei, 15 g lumbricus, 15 g paniculate swallowwort root, 15 g agastache rugosa, 9 g fortune eupatorium herb, 15 g atractylodes rhizome, 45 g poria, 30 g white atractylodes rhizome, 9 g coke malt, 9 g coke hawthorn and 9 g massa medicata fermentata, 15 g magnolia officinalis.
- *Dosage*: One dose per day, decocted in 600 mL of water; take before meals three times a day, one in the morning, one at midday, and one in the evening.

2) Lung syndrome of dampness and heat
- *Clinical manifestations*: Low fever or no fever, slight aversion to cold, fatigue, severe headache, body and muscle soreness, dry cough, small amount of phlegm, sore throat, dry mouth but unwilling to drink more, chest distress, absence of sweat or poor sweating, vomiting and distension, and loose or sticky stool. The tongue appears light red, the coated tongue is white and greasy or thin and yellow, and the pulse is smooth or moisten.
- *Recommended prescription*: 10 g areca nut, 10 g herb, 10 g anemarrhena root, 10 g scutellaria root, 10 g bupleurum root, 10 g red peony root, 15 g forsythia forsythia, 10 g artemisia annua (decocted later), 10 g atractylodis root, 10 g rhizoma atractylodis leaf, 5 g licorice.
- *Dosage*: One dose per day of 400 mL decocted in water, take twice a day, one in the morning and one in the evening.

6.1.3.2.2 Ordinary

1) Syndrome of dampness – toxic stagnation of the lung
- *Clinical manifestations*: Fever, cough produces a small amount of sputum, yellow sputum, feeling of being suffocated, abdominal distension, and constipation. The tongue is dark red and thick in size, the coated tongue is yellow and greasy or dry, and the pulse or the string is smooth.
- *Recommended prescription*: 6 g raw epepsia, 15 g bitter almond, 30 g raw plaster, 30 g raw coix seed, 10 g rhizoma atractylodis punctatus, 15 g patchouli, 12 g artemisia annua, 20 g polygonum curpa, 30 g verbena, 30 g dried reed root, 15 g semen leiocarpa, 15 g huaba, 10 g raw licorice.

- *Dosage*: One dose per day of 400 mL decocted in water, taken twice a day, one in the morning and one in the evening.

2) Syndrome of cold dampness obstructing lung

- *Clinical manifestations*: Low grade fever or normal temperature, dry cough, small amount of phlegm, fatigue, chest tightness, prion buli, vomiting, and loose stool. Tongue appears light or light red, the coated tongue is white or white greasy, and pulse is moistening.
- *Recommended prescription*: 15 g atractylodes atractylodes, 10 g dried tangerine peel, 10 g magnolia officinalis, 10 g huoxiang, 6 g Amomum tsao-ko, 6 g raw ephedra herb, 10 g notopterygium root, 10 g ginger, 10 g areca catechu.
- *Dosage*: One dose per day of 400 mL decocted in water, taken twice a day, one in the morning and one in the evening.

6.1.3.2.3 Severe

1) Lung syndrome of virus closure

- *Clinical manifestations*: Hot, red face; cough; small amount of sticky yellow phlegm; sputum with blood; wheezing and suffocation; fatigue and tiredness; dry and bitter sticky mouth; nausea and lack of appetite; The bowel movement endless feeling, few and red urine. Tongue appears red, moss is yellow greasy, and pulse is slippery.
- *Recommended prescription*: 6 g raw ephedra, 9 g almond, 15 g raw gypsum, 3 g licorice root, 10 g *Agastache rugosus* (decocted later), 10 g *Magnolia officinalis*, 15 g Rhizoma Atractylodis, 15 g amomum tsao-ko, 9 g rhizoma pinellinae praeparata, 15 g *Poria cocos*, 5 g raw rhubarb (decocted later), 10 g *Astragalus membranaceus*, 10 g semen lepidii, 10 g radix paeoniae rubra.
- *Dosage*: 1–2 doses per day, 100–200 mL for each dose decocted in water, taken 2–4 times a day via oral or nasal feeding.

2) Syndrome of flaring heat in qifen and yingfen

- *Clinical manifestations*: Fever, irritability, thirst, shortness of breath and feeling of suffocation, delirium, hysteresis, rash, vomiting of blood, epistaxis, or convulsions of limbs. The tongue is purple with little or no moss, and the pulse is either thin or frequent.
- *Recommended prescription*: 30–60 g raw gypsum (decocted first), 30 g rhizoma anemarrhenae, 30–60 g dried rehamnnia root, 30 g cornu bubali (decocted first), 30 g radix paeoniae rubra, 30 g scrophulariae, 15 g fructus forsythiae, 15 g moutan bark, 6 g coptis chinensis, 12 g bamboo leaves, 15 g semen lepidii, 6 g raw radix glycyrrhizae.

- *Dosage*: 1 dose per day, decocted in water. Decoct gypsum and cornu bubali first, followed by other medicinal materials, 100–200 mL each time. Take two to four times a day via oral or nasal feeding.
- *Recommended Chinese patent medicines*: Xiyanping injection, xuebijing injection, reduning injection, tanreqing injection, xingnaojing injection. Drugs with similar effects may be selected on an individual basis, or both may be used in combination with clinical symptoms. TCM injection can be used in combination with TCM decoction.

6.1.3.2.4 Critically Severe (Inner Blocking Causing Collapse)

Clinical manifestations: dyspnea, frequent asthma, or the need for mechanical ventilation, accompanied by dizziness, irritability, sweating, and cold limbs. Tongue appears dark purple, tongue mass is either thick and greasy or dry, and pulse is floating without root.

- *Recommended prescription*: 15 g ginseng, 10 g black prepared lateral root of aconite (decocted first), 15 g cornus officinalis, suhexiang pill, or angong niuhuang pill. If the patient has abdominal distension constipation or constipation symptoms, raw rhubarb or glaucoma 5–10 g can be used.
- *Recommended Chinese patent medicine*: xuebijing injection, reduning injection, tanreqing injection, xingnaojing injection, shenfu injection, shengmai injection, shenmai injection. Drugs with similar effects may be selected on an individual basis, or both may be used in combination with clinical symptoms. TCM injection can be used in combination with TCM decoction.

Note: The use of TCM injections in severe and critically severe patients should start from a small dose and be gradually adjusted according to the drug instructions.

6.1.3.2.5 Convalescent Period

1) Deficiency of the lung and spleen

Clinical manifestations: Shortness of breath, fatigue, poor appetite and vomiting, abdominal distension, weakness of defecation and loose stool. Tongue is light and thick in size; the coated tongue is white and greasy.

Recommended prescription: 9 g rhizoma pinellinae praeparata, 1 g pericarpium citri reticulatae, 15 g codonopsis pilosula, 30 g radix astragali preparata, 10 g roasted rhizoma atractylodis macrocephalae, 15 g poria cocos, 10 g agastache rugosus, 6 g amomum villosum (decocted later), 6 g licorice root.

Dosage: 1 dose per day, 400 mL decocted in water, two times a day, one in the morning and one in the evening.

2) Deficiency of *qi* and *yin*

Clinical manifestations: Fatigue, shortness of breath, dry mouth, thirst, palpitations, sweating, poor appetite, low or no heat, and dry cough with little phlegm. Tongue is dry with less saliva and pulse is thin or weak.

Recommended prescription: 10 g adenophora tetraphylla, 10 g radix glehniae, 15 g radix ophiopogonis, 6 g American ginseng, 6 g schisandra chinensis, 15 g raw gypsum, 10 g lophatherum gracile, 10 g folium mori, 15 g rhizoma phragmitis, 15 g salviae miltiorrhizae, and 6 g raw licorice root.

Dosage: 1 dose per day, 400 mL decocted in water, two times a day, one in the morning and one in the evening.

In COVID-19, its pathogen is the evil of dampness and poison. The main symptoms are fever, dry cough, and fatigue. A few patients have nasal congestion, runny nose, sore throat, myalgia and diarrhea. The cause of COVID-19 is exogenous infection with the virus. When the human body's security function is weakened and the strain cannot be adjusted, the virus invades the human body from the fur, mouth, nose and mucous membrane, and finally results in the disease caused by the evil attack on the lung and the healthy surface. Syndrome differentiation belongs to the deficiency of the original standard and solid. According to the syndromes, different syndromes, such as cold and dampness, dampness and heat, dampness and poison, deficiency of breath and other syndromes can be distinguished. The treatment of the deficient syndrome is to remove the pathogenic factors to benefit the lungs and relieve dryness and dampness; the treatment of the deficient syndrome is to strengthen the spleen and nourish the lungs, promote breath, and nourish the *yin*. Patients should keep warm and avoid catching a cold in daily life. Cold food should be avoided. In addition, it is recommended to supplement food with chicken, beef, mutton, fish, and so on. People can also choose appropriate indoor exercise, such as baduanjin, yi jin jing, taijiquan, and other health exercises, to improve their ability to resist diseases and pathogens.

6.2 EXTERNAL TREATMENT TECHNIQUES OF TCM

6.2.1 Acupuncture Therapy

COVID-19 belongs to category of "plague" in TCM. The disease first exploded in Wuhan. According to four analyses in Wuhan of its seasons, climate, geography, and patients, experts believe that the disease belongs to "cold and dampness plague", and its essence is *yin*. Moreover, the disease is mainly located in the lungs and spleen. Acupuncture therapy is a treasure of traditional Chinese therapy. It can be used for the treatment of COVID-19 by dredging meridians and adjusting *yin* and *yang*.

6.2.1.1 Principles of Treatment

Dredge meridian and adjusting *yin* and *yang*.

6.2.1.2 Treatment Mechanisms

6.2.1.2.1 Harmonizing Yin *and* Yang

TCM holds the belief that the human body is a whole organ, which is various organs and tissues mutually coordinated and used in physiological functions and also affects each other in pathology. According to the theory of *yin* and *yang* in Chinese medicine, all things and phenomena in nature contain two aspects of *yin* and *yang*, which are opposite to each other and mutually used. The opposition between *yin* and *yang*, which restrict and root each other, is not a static and unchanging state but in constant motion and change. In *Su Wen · To the Truth*, it is said, "I would like to observe where *yin* and *yang* are and adjust them and expect that they can exist in peace". Therefore, TCM acupuncture restores the relative balance of *yin* and *yang* by adjusting them, supplementing their deficiency, and relieving their excess. The therapeutic effect of acupuncture and moxibustion harmonizes *yin* and *yang*, which is achieved through the compatibility of meridians, acupoints, and acupuncture techniques.

In COVID-19, patients with dampness-heat lung syndrome will suffer from low fever and sore throat. This corresponds to quchi and chize; it is appropriate to clear heat clearing damp to calm *yin* and *yang* of the body. This corresponds to the combination point of the lung meridian in the hand – taiyin – and the large intestine channel of the hand – yangming, and acupuncture purgatory method to clear the large intestine meridian and the lung meridian to restore the balance of *yin* and *yang* between the large intestine and the lung. During the clinical treatment of COVID-19, hegu and waiguan were selected as the main acupoints. Because the lung and large intestine are closely related, the original point and valley of the large intestine can be used to clear the lung fire. The outer pass is the collateral point of the hand, shao *yang*, which can disperse the *yang* on the surface and relieve heat. The two acupoints, hegu and waiguan, cooperate with each other to balance the *yin* and *yang* of the lungs.

In addition, a large number of modern clinical observation and experimental studies have proven that acupuncture and moxibustion have a significant regulatory effect on the functional activities of various organs and tissues. In particular, the regulatory effect is more obvious in pathological conditions. Acupuncture also plays a comprehensive role in regulating various tissues and organs of COVID-19. Whether it is the cold dampness stagnation of the lung, the dampness and heat of the lung, the dampness-toxic stagnation of lung, or the deficiency of breath and deficiency of lung and kidney *yin* during the convalescent period, acupuncture can restore the balance of *yin* and *yang* for patients through comprehensive regulation of the lung, spleen, and kidney.

6.2.1.2.2 Nourish Good and Dispel Evil

According to the *Huangdi Neijing* (also known as *The Inner Canon of Huangdi*), "When the healthy spirit is stored inside, evil spirits cannot prosper", and "when the evil spirit gathers, healthy spirit will be weak". When the human body is vigorous, the evil spirit is not enough to cause disease; if the healthy spirit is weak, the evil spirit can invade and cause disease. The development of disease is a process in which healthy and evil spirits fight against each other. The ebb and flow of good and evil forces determines the development and outcome of disease. If the evil spirit is stronger than the healthy spirit, the disease will be worse, and if the healthy spirit is stronger than the evil breath, the disease will be alleviated. Therefore, it is essential to ensure that the disease will turn benign. Acupuncture treatment's significance lies in the support of healthy spirit and the removal of evil spirit.

Modern clinical practice and experimental studies have also proven that acupuncture can enhance the immune function of the body and resist the invasion of various pathogenic factors. The onset of COVID-19 in patients is based on low immune function, that is, the deficiency of healthy breath in TCM. Acupuncture therapy is focused on supporting the healthy factors and dispelling evil factors. It is embodied in the method of supplementing deficiency and relieving excess, which is mainly embodied in the combination of acupuncture techniques and acupoints. The clinical treatment stage involves the syndrome of cold dampness and stagnation of the lung, syndrome of damp-heat accumulation of the lung, syndrome of dampness toxicity stagnation of the lung, syndrome of virus closure of the lung, and syndrome of flaring heat in qifen and yingfen, which is the focus of dispelling the evil breath. The convalescent period involves the deficiency of lung breath and *yin*, both of which mainly support the healthy spirit. In the clinical treatment stage, the main acupoints selected are fengchi, dazhui, linque, gegu, and waiguan, which promote lung breath, relieving symptoms, and evacuating cold and dampness. When mild patients have dampness-heat lung syndrome, quchi and chize were selected, which mainly remove the dampness-heat evil spirit from taiyin, which is the lung meridian of the hand, and yangming, which is the large intestine channel of the hand. In addition, the main method used during this acupuncture manipulation is releasing. Pishu, qihai, and guanyuan were selected in the convalescent period for the syndrome of deficiency of the lung and spleen, mainly to support the healthy spirit of the lung, spleen and kidney and to supplement the method of acupuncture, which could also be benefited from moxibustion. Generally, the principle is to strengthen the healthy spirit with keeping the evil spirit out of body and eliminate the evil without hurting the healthy spirit, once the healthy spirit is recovered, the evil spirit can't invade body again.

6.2.1.2.3 Dredge the Meridian to Regulate Breath and Blood

The meridian system, throughout the body, vertically and horizontally, inside and outside, constitutes the breath and blood and their running pathway and maintains the normal physiological function of the human body. The impassable meridian can lead to stagnation or blockage of breath and blood, loss of harmony between breath and blood, and internal disharmony between *yin* and *yang*. Acupuncture can make meridians smooth and passable and restore breath and blood harmony and *yin-yang* balance. If the breath and blood and meridian are blocked, symptoms such as headache, pharynx pain, chest pain, and body pain start to show up. It is then recommended to conduct acupuncture therapy on acupoints – tiantu, lianquan, zhongfu, and danzhong – to dredge the meridian to relieve pain, smooth channels, facilitate breath and blood, so that the body will heal by itself.

6.2.1.3 Choice of Acupoints

6.2.1.3.1 Medical Observation Period

Main acupoints: fengchi, dazhui, linque, hegu, and waiguan.
Matching acupoints: choose zusanli if there is a lack of power and gastrointestinal discomfort; choose quchi if there is a lack of power and fever.

6.2.1.3.2 Clinical Treatment Period

1) Mild
   - *Main acupoints*: Fengchi, dazhui, lieque, hegu, and waiguan.
   - Matching acupoints: Choose fengmen or yin ling quan for syndrome of cold dampness and stagnation of the lung; choose quchi or chize if the lung shows signs of the syndrome of dampness and heat.
2) Ordinary
   - *Main acupoints*: Fengchi, dazhui, lieque, hegu, and waiguan.
   - *Matching acupoints*: Choose yinlingquan or quchi for syndrome of dampness – toxic stagnation of the lung; choose dazhui or yinlingquan if the lung shows signs of the syndrome of cold dampness and obstructing.
3) Severe
   - *Main acupoints*: Fei shu, zhongfu, tiantu, danzhong, kongzui, dingchuan, and fenglong.
   - *Matching acupoints*: Choose chize or quze if there is virus and lung closure; choose dazhui, 12 jing, or taixi for syndrome of flaring heat in qifen and yingfen.

6.2.1.3.3 Convalescent Period

- *Main acupoints*: Feishu, fengmen, shenshu, and dingchuan.
- *Matching acupoints*: Choose pishu, qihai, guanyuan, or taiyuan for deficiency the of lung and spleen; choose qihai, taixi for qi-yin deficiency syndrome.

6.2.1.4 Location of Points

1) Chize is located in the transverse ridge of the elbow and the indentation of the radial side of the biceps tendon.
2) Feishu is on the back, 1.5 cun* from below the third thoracic spine process.
3) Fengmen is on the back, 1.5 cun from below the second thoracic spinous process.
4) Dingchuan is on the back of the neck, 0.5 cun from the midpoint of the lower edge of the spinous process of the seventh cervical vertebra.
5) Taiyuan is located on the anterior region of the wrist, between the radial styloid process and the scaphoid bone, in the ulnar indentation of the tendon of the long extensor pollicis.
6) Zusanli is outside the lower leg, 3 cun below dubi, on the connecting line between dubi and jiexi.
7) Fenglong is on the anterolateral leg, 8 cun above lateral malleolus tip, outside tiaokou, two transverse finger anterior margin of tibia.
8) Quchi is located at the lateral end of the transverse ridge of the elbow, when bending the elbow, it is at the midpoint of the connecting line between chize and epicondylus extensorius.
9) Dazhui is at the lower part of the neck when sitting straight with head bowed, at the indentation under the spinous process of the seventh cervical vertebra.
10) Yinlingquan is located on the medial side of the lower leg and in the indentation of the medial tibia below the knee, opposite to zusanli point (or in the indentation of the posterior lower part of the medial tibia).
11) Pishu is at the eleventh thoracic spine process, next to the median line, 1.5 cun aside.
12) Qihai is located in the lower abdomen, anterior midline, 1.5 cun below the umbilicus.

---

* Cun is a traditional unit of measurement often referred to as the *Chinese inch,* for which *1 cun* is ~1.312 in.

13) Guanyuan is located in the lower abdomen, anterior midline, 3 cun below the umbilicus.
14) Taixi is the hollow between the inner side of the foot, behind the medial malleolus and the heel tendon.
15) Yongquan is located at the front third of the connecting line between the second and third toes seam head, or indentation in the front of planta pedis when bending tones vigorously.

6.2.1.5 Operation Method

In the progressive stage of the disease, acupuncture treatment should be taken twice a day. The needle was retained for 30 minutes with the method of lifting, inserting, twisting, and reducing. During the convalescent period, acupuncture treatment should be taken once a day to help stop diarrhea.

6.2.1.6 Contraindication to Acupuncture

No needling near important viscera, large blood vessels, and important joints.

Inserting needles at hegu, sanyinjiao, and quepen as well as abdominal and lumbar sacral acupoints is forbidden for pregnant women. Inserting needles at xinhui is forbidden for children. Inserting needles at shimen is forbidden for women.

6.2.2 Moxibustion Therapy

Moxibustion therapy mainly refers to the use of moxibustion fire heat and moxa to burn on acupoints or diseased parts and to warm the body. Moxibustion is an external therapy for the prevention and treatment of diseases by means of conduction through meridians. The main material of moxibustion therapy is moxa floss. Moxa floss is made of moxa leaves after removing the coarse stalk. Moxa floss is fragrant and easy to burn. Moxa floss has mild heat and can penetrate the skin directly and deeply through various channels and cure all diseases.

6.2.2.1 Principles of Treatment

Warming the meridian and dispersing cold promotes the lung, regulates breath, and enhances immunity.

6.2.2.2 Treatment Mechanism

6.2.2.2.1 Moxibustion Materials

Moxa is easy to get, as it is derived from a wide range of sources. In ancient times, moxa floss was officially recognized as the material to preserve the seeds of fire. The ancients accumulated rich application experience for us. In the *Compendium of Materia Medica*, it was said, "Mugwort leaves are slightly bitter when they are born, slightly bitter when they are ripe, and pure *yang* when they are warm and when they are ripe. Warm and hot, pure *yang* is also. You can take the sun true fire, you can turn back the Yuan Yang. ... Moxibustion is through the classics and cure 100 kinds of disease evil, the people who rise and sink are healthy, its work is also great". In *Bian Que's Book*, it was said, "Moxibustion is the first way to protect one's life, the second is the Dan medicine and the third is the aconite". Moxibustion can help warm *yang*; invigorate breath, xuanqi, and blood; promote blood movement; dispel cold and moisture; enhance the power of breath and blood circulation; and change the human internal environment.

Modern pharmacological studies have proven that artemisia argyi contains a variety of volatile oils, with disease-resistant microorganisms, and have sedative, antitussive, expectorant, antiasthma, antiallergic, and other effects. Therefore, in *Shen Jiu Jing Lun*, it is said, "taking moxa as a wick, can pass Shierjing, into Sanyin, regulate breath and blood, in order to treat all diseases easily".

6.2.2.2.2 Therapeutic Mechanism of Moxibustion

Introduction to Medicine Acupuncture and Moxibustion stated that "If the medicine and acupuncture are not enough, it must be moxibustion", which indicates that moxibustion plays an important role in clinical practice. It is often combined with acupuncture and medicine to supplement each other. *Cases of Moxibustion* also recorded, "When you go to Wu Shu, you often need three or two moxibustion on your body. Don't let the sores go temporarily, then warm malaria gas cannot go into you", which explains that moxibustion can be used to prevent the spread of plague.

Moxibustion therapy, is the fire attack of moxibustion, which can strengthen the *yang qi* and benefit the true *yin*. Artemisia argyi, which is aromatic, is a rare medicine that can pass shierjing, regulates breath and blood circulation and cures all diseases. As recorded in *New Compilation of Materia Medica*, "folium artemisiae argyi is bitter, warm, hot and pure *yang*. It can return the sun, pass Shierjing, Sanyin, combing breath and blood, expel cold and dampness ... Moxibustion fire, can penetrate all the meridional and get rid of all disease." Li Chan, in *The Introduction to Medicine*, it is said, "use moxibustion to restore Yuanyang for the weak." This shows that moxibustion has a strong role in invigorating breath and generating blood. Breath, blood, jin, fluid, and essence depend on the warmth and gasification of *yang qi*, so that the *yin* fluid of the whole body can run normally, and the water and grain can be used by people. Therefore, moxibustion can warm the *yang* and production *qi*, and warm the cold and dampness. In addition, the *yang qi* of the critically severe patients is deficient, thus gasification can be easily lost, and if coupled with various external attacks, it may lead to "*yang qi* is sudden deficient thus *xie qi* bursts out." The rise and fall of *yang qi* determines the susceptibility and prognosis of individuals with COVID-19. In this pandemic, most of the patients are based on pandemic virus, which is mixed with cold and dampness evil spirits. Therefore, it is an important method in the prevention and treatment of COVID-19 to return to the *yang* to reverse the adverse situation, restore health, and dispel the evil.

6.2.2.3 Selection of Acupoints

6.2.2.3.1 Main Acupoints
Chize, feishu, and taiyuan

6.2.2.3.2 Match Acupoints with Symptoms

1) Medical observation period
- Fatigue with gastrointestinal discomfort: Matching with zusanli.
- Fatigue with fever: Matching with quchi.

2) Clinical treatment period (not applicable for severe and critical cases)
   a. Mild cases
      i. Syndrome of cold dampness and stagnation of the lung: matching with dazhui.
      ii. Lung syndrome of dampness and heat: matching with quchi.
   b. Average cases
      i. Syndrome of dampness – toxic stagnation of the lung: matching with yinling quan or Quchi.
      ii. Syndrome of cold dampness obstructing the lung: matching with dazhui or yinling quan.
   c. During convalescent period

      i. Deficiency of the lung and spleen: matching with pishu, qihai, zusanli.
      ii. Deficiency of *qi* and *yin*: matching with qihai, yongquan.

6.2.2.4 Operation Method
Warm moxibustion box for 30 minutes at feishu, pishu, and qihai; mild moxibustion with moxa at remaining points

Mild moxibustion method: ignite one end of the moxa stick and place it about 3 cm away from the skin so that the patient experiences a warm sensation at a certain area but without any burning discomfort. Generally, conduct moxibustion for 5–7 minutes at each place until a certain degree of redness on the skin is reached. This should be done once a day for 10 days for 1 course of treatment.

6.2.2.5 Precautions

6.2.2.5.1 Posture Selection
According to the choice of acupoints for each moxibustion session, it is recommended to choose a body posture that is easy to operate, easy to maintain, and relatively safe.

6.2.2.5.2 Operation Order of Moxibustion

Moxibustion operation is generally performed in the following order: top to bottom, back to abdomen, head and main body to four limbs, the *yang* meridians to the *yin* meridians.

6.2.2.5.3 Applied Amount of Moxibustion

The applied amount of moxibustion gradually increases, from small moxa sticks to larger ones and from a mild level of burning to a stronger level, to build patients' tolerance.

6.2.2.5.4 Moxibustion Duration

Moxibustion should be controlled within 30 minutes if possible. If the moxibustion duration is too long, patients would experience dry mouth, sore throat, constipation, and other symptoms, and should drink water accordingly.

6.2.2.6 Contraindication of Moxibustion

6.2.2.6.1 Contraindicated Demographic

Moxibustion should not be performed for those who are overworked, hungry, full, drunk, frightened, terrified, angry, or are suffering from extreme exhaustion. Moxibustion should not be performed on those who suffer convulsions or are allergic to artemisia argyi or have frequent skin allergies.

6.2.2.6.2 Contraindicated Area

Moxibustion should not be performed on the lower abdomen and lumbosacral of women during pregnancy and menstruation. Moxibustion should not be performed on the failure of the fontanelle in children, facial features, heart, great vessels, joints, testicles, nipples, pudendal parts, or where the skin is broken or scarred.

6.2.2.6.3 Contraindicated Existing Condition

Moxibustion should not be performed if the patient has solid heat syndrome and displays high fever, thirst, red face, constipation, urine yellow, etc. Moxibustion should not be performed if the patient has syndrome of *yin* deficiency fever and displays hot flushes, night sweats, dry mouth, dry throat, thirst, a small amount of yellow urine, dry stools, etc. Moxibustion should also not be performed on patients who have been diagnosed with hypertensive crisis, advanced tuberculosis, organic heart disease with cardiac insufficiency, schizophrenia, scarlet fever, measles, erysipelas, infectious skin diseases, etc.

6.2.3 Acupoint (Meridian) Massage Therapy

Acupoint (meridian) massage therapy refers to the use of the hands or other parts of the body to massage specific acupoints or meridians on the surface of the patient's body, according to a variety of specific skills of movement. Acupoint (meridian) massage therapy promotes the overall metabolism through local stimulation of the body, thus adjusting the coordination and unity of the functions of various parts of the body and maintaining the relative balance of *yin* and *yang* of the body. Therefore, it can enhance the body's natural disease resistance ability, relax the muscles, and facilitate blood circulation and fitness.

6.2.3.1 Principles of Treatment

Acupoint (meridian) massage therapy helps to regulate the spleen and stomach, nourish the lung and *qi*, strengthen the immune system, and resist the virus.

6.2.3.2 Treatment Mechanism

Acupoint (meridian) massage therapy is based on the theory of TCM. Through the benign stimulation of specific meridian acupoints, it can regulate the function of the corresponding viscera and treatment can help to prevent disease by improving the immune system. Studies have shown that stimulating relevant acupoints through appropriate acupoint massage can enhance the strength of respiratory muscles, improve pulmonary ventilation and lung function, relieve anxiety and depression in patients, and significantly improve the quality of life.

6.2.3.3 Selection of Points

6.2.3.3.1 Main Points

Hegu, zusanli, fei shu, shen shu, san yin jiao

6.2.3.3.2 Match Acupoints with Symptoms

1) Medical observation period
   - Gastrointestinal discomfort: Match with tianshu.
   - Fever: Match with yuji.
2) Clinical treatment period (not applicable for severe and critically severe cases)
   a. Mild
      i. Syndrome of cold dampness and stagnation of the lung: match with dazhui.
      ii. Lung syndrome of dampness and heat: match with quchi.
   b. Moderate
      i. Syndrome of dampness – toxic stagnation of the lung: match with yinling quan, and quchi.
      ii. Syndrome of cold dampness obstructing the lung: match with dazhui and yinling quan.
   c. Convalescent period

i. Deficiency of lung and spleen: match with pishu and qihai.
ii. Deficiency of *qi*, deficiency of the lung and temper: match with qihai and yongquan.

6.2.3.4 Location of Acupoints

To find the hegu point, open one hand upside down naturally, and extend the thumb on the other hand. Place the thumb on the back of the hand near flexor pollicis brevis. Press the thumb down, and the point below the fingertip is the hegu point. Obvious soreness is expected when pressure is applied at this acupoint.

1) With the patient in the sitting position, the zusanli point is located outside the lower leg, 3 cun below dubi, on the connecting line between dubi and jiexi.
2) Feishu is located on the back, 1.5 cun from the third thoracic spine process.
3) Shenshu is located at the waist, 1.5 cun from the second lumbar spine process.
4) Sanyinjiao is located on the medial side of the lower leg, 3 cun above the tip of the medial malleolus, the posterior margin of the tibia.
5) Tianshu is at the center of the abdomen, 2 cun from the umbilicus.
6) Yuji is located at the posterior of the first metacarpal phalangeal joint, the middle point of the first metacarpal bone, the edge of the white eminence behind the metacarpal bone. Obvious soreness is expected when pressure is applied at this acupoint.
7) With the patient in the sitting position with head bowed down, the dazhui point is at the lower part of the neck, at the indentation under the spinous process of the seventh cervical vertebra.
8) Quchi is located at the tip of the transverse striation of the elbow when bending the elbow. Obvious soreness is expected when pressure is applied at this acupoint.
9) With the patient in the sitting position, the yinlingquan point is found by using the thumb to push up along the medial edge of the lower leg bone (medial tibia) to the lower knee joint. The yinlingquan point is at the indentation where tibia bends upward.
10) With the patient in the prone position, the pishu point is located in the eleventh thoracic spine process, 1.5 cun from the median line.
11) With the patient in the supine position, the qihai point is located at the anterior median line, 1.5 cun inferior umbilicus.
12) The yongquan point is at the foot acupoint of the human body. It is located at the upper third of line between heel to the junction of the second and third toes, or indentation in the front of planta pedis when bending tones vigorously.

6.2.3.5 Operation Method

1) Dazhui and feishu: Both are kneaded by the middle finger or index finger of both hands alternately for 1–2 minutes per acupoint until the patient feels soreness at certain areas.
2) Feishu and pishu: With patients' hands behind their backs in the akimbo shape, use the thumb to knead for 1–2 minutes per acupoint until patients feel soreness at certain areas.
3) Yuji: Both hands can be crossed to press yuji at both sides, rubbing back and forth for 3–5 minutes, until warmth is felt at certain areas.
4) The rest of the acupoints can be kneaded with the thumb for 1–2 minutes per acupoint until the patient feels soreness in certain areas.
5) Pat lung meridian: Pat about 30 times by palm repeatedly from the clavicle to the thumb along the medial outer edge of the upper limb.

6.2.3.6 Operation Precautions

1) Massage should not exceed 20 minutes per treatment, preferably once in the morning and once in the evening, such as getting up and before going to bed.
2) For self-massage, it is better to wear only a vest and shorts, and try to contact the body surface directly during operation.
3) Some substances can be used as lubricants during operation, such as talcum powder, sesame oil, massage milk, etc., which can enhance the curative effect and prevent skin damage.
4) In case of local skin breakage, ulcer, fracture, tuberculosis, tumor, bleeding, etc., massage is prohibited.
5) Patients who sweat after massage should avoid direct contact with wind to prevent catching a cold.
6) Do not use massage therapy on patients who are hungry, full, drunk, or overtired.

6.2.3.7 Contraindications

Acupoint (meridian) massage should not be performed on patients with severe or critically severe COVID-19 who suffer from shortness of breath, dyspnea, delirium, confusion, etc.

Acupoint (meridian) massage is also contraindicated for the following situations:

1) Patients with undiagnosed acute spinal cord injury or with spinal cord symptoms.
2) Patients with various fractures, joint tuberculosis, osteomyelitis, bone tumors, and severe senile osteoporosis.

3) Patients with severe heart, lung, liver, and kidney failure; extreme weakness; and malignant tumor.

4) All kinds of acute infectious diseases, acute peritonitis (including gastric and duodenal ulcer perforation).

5) Patients with bleeding tendency or blood diseases.

6) Patients with open soft tissue injury, water and fire scald, skin ulcer, and various sores and ulcers.

7) Women over 3 months of pregnancy should not have acupoint (meridian) massage on the abdomen, buttocks, and lumbosacral regions as well as acupoints with specific functions such as hegu and sanyin jiao.

8) When a person is mentally ill or overly stressed.

9) Patients with high fever and high fever convulsion.

6.2.4 Acupoint Application Therapy

Acupoint application therapy is an external therapy formed under the guidance of the holistic view of TCM. This method is based on the theory of meridians and collaterals of TCM and uses the acupoints on the body surface as stimulation points. Through the stimulation of applying medicine, the medicine can be absorbed through the skin to harmonize *qi* and blood, adjust the balance of *yin* and *yang*, and help to rehabilitate patients. TCM advocates that "those who are good at treating diseases should follow the rules of timing and establish the alternation of treatment as per seasons", so it emphasizes the treatment of winter diseases in summer. According to the principle of "Nourishing *yang* in spring and summer" in "The Theory of Regulating The Spirit of the Four *qi*", combined with the medicinal moxibustion and drug therapy, the drug application is applied on the acupoints of the human body to stimulate the healthy *qi* and enhance the body's ability of resist disease and cure diseases.

6.2.4.1 Treatment Mechanism

6.2.4.1.1 Medicine Acts on Pathogen

The disease evil of COVID-19 lies in the surface, the form of lung lies in the skin, and the disease evil first invades the surface. The medicine cannot only act directly on the skin striae, but also penetrate the tissue below the skin to eliminate or resist the external evil. The study shows that the permeability of acupoint skin is better than that of nonacupoint skin, and the permeation and absorption of TCM at acupoint is more obvious. Therefore, after the drug is applied to the corresponding acupoints, it can reach the disease of viscera meridian where *qi* is disordered, then the medicine's meridional effect and functional effect can be brought into play.

6.2.4.1.2 Long-Term Acupoint Stimulation

Acupoint application therapy is the embodiment of the physiological functions of acupoints themselves. The functions of acupoints are generally divided into distal treatment, proximal treatment, and special functions. In *Su Wen Five zang generation*, it is said, "people have 12 Acupuncture points ... Acupuncture points are not only the place where *yang qi* stays on the muscle surface to resist external evils, but also the breakthrough point for external evils to easily invade." This indicates that acupoints are the place that can maintain health and keep muscle surfaces resistant to exogenous evil. Moreover, it is the breakthrough point for exogenous evil to invade the human body. The acupoints are more sensitive to the warmth of the medicine, and the warming effect of the medicine can be maintained at the acupoints for a long time to further stimulate the acupoints. Li Zhen et al. believed that when medicine application stimulated acupoints, it opened up the pathway of "*yang* meridian of lung to *yin meridian of* lung" and was mediated by acupoints. The function of dredging lung collaterals, *qi* and blood through medicine can result in a long-term health effect.

6.2.4.1.3 Regulate the Body as a Whole

The meridian system communicates with the tissues and organs of the human body and maintains the relative internal relations under the physiological state; however, when the body being damaged, the meridian acupoints can stimulate the self-defense of each tissue and organ. Exogenous evil located at fur and feather firstly, connected internally, and dispersed in the stomach and intestines, indicating that exogenous pathogens, through meridian points, construct the internal and external interaction of the human body. Similarly, acupoint application therapy is not only about the effect of drugs, but also the correction of the pathological state and the imbalance of the body. Zhang Yunwei et al. adjusted and improved the physique of COVID-19 patients to a stable stage with different Chinese medicine applications, corrected the imbalance of the body, reduced the susceptibility to disease, and further changed the pathological state of the body so that the balance of viscera, *yin* and *yang*, and *qi* and blood could be achieved.

6.2.4.1.4 Effects of Immune Mechanism

Chinese medicine has made great progress in disease prevention, health care, treatment, and so on, in recent years, especially in terms of the public recognizing the concepts of "healthy qi" and "*yin* and *yang*". Healthy qi is similar to the immune function of Western medicine, and the imbalance of *yin* and *yang* is similar to the disorder of immune function in Western medicine. Chinese medicine has remarkable results in this respect. Acupoint application therapy, as an appropriate technology for the prevention and treatment of COVID-19 with TCM, can stimulate the immune function of the relevant system to the maximum extent, improve the body's vital *qi*, and fundamentally cure or control the disease. Some scholars have proposed that the determination of the body's immune function can be started from four aspects: cellular immunity, humoral immunity, mononuclear macrophage function, and natural killer cell (NK) cell activity. Other studies have shown that acupoint application therapy can further improve the level of pulmonary function of patients through cellular immunity and humoral immunity.

6.2.4.1.5 Effects of Inflammatory Mechanisms

COVID-19 is a disease composed of various factors, among which inflammation, always accompanied by disease progression, is the core factor. The lungs are the main diseased organs, but patients with increased inflammatory factors in the lungs can produce systemic inflammation and systemic effects. When external particles and bacteria enter the lungs, macrophages, neutrophils, lymphocytes, and other cells that have long existed in the lungs and trachea tissues will be activated. While playing a phagocytic role, they also release a variety of mediators.

6.2.4.2 Operation Method

6.2.4.2.1 Selection of Acupoints

- *Medical observation period*: Zhongwan, guanyuan, and zusanli.
- *Mild (syndrome of cold dampness and stagnation of the lung) and moderate (syndrome of cold dampness obstructing the lung)*: Guanyuan, hegu, zusanli, and taichong.
- *Convalescent period (deficiency of the lung and spleen)*: Dazhui, feishu, geshu, zusanli, and kongzui.
- *Convalescent period (deficiency of yin)*: Zusanli, danzhong, qihai, and yinlingquan.

6.2.4.2.2 Composition and Production of Drugs

The application medicine mainly consists of ephedra, pinellia ternata, lumbricus, sinapis alba, perillaseed, and almond. The prescription has broad-spectrum antibacterial, anticancer, and osmotic effects. It is mostly used for cold phlegm stagnation, chest full hypochondriac pain, cough, asthma, and many other diseases. Ephedra and almond are good for cough and asthma, lumbricus is good for clearing heat and asthma, pinellia ternata is good for dryness and dampness. The combination of various drugs has the effect of warming the lung, dispersing cold, eliminating phlegm, and promoting *qi*, so the application of acupoint application therapy can effectively improve the symptoms of patients' upper respiratory tracts.

Grind the medicine into a powder and mix it with honey to make a peanut-size pill.

6.2.4.2.3 Operation Steps

1) Take out the gasket.
2) Tear off the adhesive.
3) Fix it on the acupoints.
4) Take a prepared medicine mud and press to fill the entire gasket.
5) Take out the spacer moxibustion paste.
6) Tear off the silicone oil paper.
7) Align the spacer moxibustion paste with the gasket, and press it firmly.
8) After pasting, have patients rest on their backs for 40 minutes.
9) Remove it after 40 minutes.

6.2.5 Auricular Acupoint Pressing Therapy

Auricular acupoint pressing therapy, also known as auricular acupressure therapy, refers to a kind of therapy for preventing and treating diseases by pressing and stimulating the acupoints or reaction points on the auricle with granule drugs such as vaccaria segetalis and cassia seeds. According to holographic theory, the ear has a shape of an inverted fetus, with very close relationship between the ear and the viscera. The ear plays an important part in connecting body surface with viscera, through the conduction of the meridians to the corresponding viscera, in order to treat diseases of the corresponding viscera. Studies have indicated that, through percutaneous stimulation of the ear's vagus nerve, inflammatory factors can be regulated, thereby reducing the inflammatory response. Other studies have confirmed that auricular plasters can improve vital capacity, increase hemoglobin content, and relieve palpitations, chest tightness, shortness of breath, dyspnea, and other symptoms in COVID-19 patients.

6.2.5.1 Treatment Mechanism

The nerves on the auricle are extremely rich and closely related to the whole body. Because there are shallow and deep receptors in the auricle, the *qi* obtained by using different stimulation methods, such as acupuncture, auricular acupoint pressing, electric pulse, and laser and magnetic lines, may be excited by a variety of sensory devices, especially the pain receptors, which receive and transmit various sensory impulses and gather into the spinal nucleus of the trigeminal nerve. Then the nucleus transmits impulses from the reticular structure of the brain stem, thus regulating various visceral activities and various sensory functions.

The ear is closely related to the 12 major meridians. There are more than 30 records of auricular diagnosis and treatment in *Huangdi Neijing*. All 12 meridians reach the ear directly or indirectly around the eardrum. Although the six *yin* meridians do not enter the ear directly or are distributed around the ear, they all combine with the *yang* meridians through the meridians. In clinical practice, it has been found that patients receiving auricular point pressure treatment experience a slight chill, a flow within the body, or a sense of heat and warmth radiating from the ear to a certain part of the body along a certain route, which is mostly similar to running the course of the meridian.

The ear is closely related to the viscus, which is an important part of the body surface. In *Miraculous: Meridians*, it is said that "*qi* in the kidney can flow to the ear, and the kidney and the ear can get five sounds", which indicates that the ear and the kidney have a close relationship. In *Miraculous: Five Spirits,* it is said that "evil in the liver, causes pain in two ribs ... evil in the blood ... take the veins of the ear tip to clear it". This indicates the relationship between the ear and the liver. These expositions all show that the ear is closely related to the viscera. In clinical study, the effect of electroacupuncture on the gastric region of auricular point was observed. The results showed that the amplitude and frequency of electroacupuncture on the gastric region of the auricular point had a benign bidirectional effect. Therefore, acupuncture or pressing ear points have the function of regulating viscera and organ function.

6.2.5.2 Auricular Point Selection

- *Attack stage*: Lung, chest, trachea, asthma, kidney, sympathetic, shenmen
- *Convalescent stage*: Lung, kidney, spleen, stomach, endocrine

6.2.5.3 Auricular Point Positioning

1) The lung point is located around the auricular center, i.e. area 14 of the auricular concha.
2) The chest point is located at two-fifths of the anterior part of the anti-auricle, the anterior lateral auricular border of the thoracic vertebra, i.e. area 10 of the auricular concha.
3) The trachea point is located in the cavity of the auricular concha, between the heart area and the external auricle gate, i.e. area 16 of the auricular concha.
4) The pingchuan point is located at the tip of the tragus.
5) The kidney point is located at the lower bifurcation of the upper and lower crus of helix, i.e. area 10 of the auricular concha
6) The sympathetic point is located at the junction between the lower crus of helix and the inner side of the helix, i.e. the front end of area 6 of the helix.

7) The shenmen point is located at the upper part, one-third behind the triangle fossa, i.e. area 4 of the triangle fossa.
8) The spleen point is located at the posterior upper part of the cavity of the auricular concha, i.e. area 13 of the auricular concha.
9) The stomach point is located at where the crus of helix disappears, i.e. area 4 of auricular concha.
10) The endocrine point is located in the interscreen notch at the anterior lower part of the cavity of the auricular concha, i.e., area 18 of the auricular concha.

6.2.5.4 Operation Method

1) Material preparation: 75% ethanol, cotton swab, tweezers, vaccaria segetalis auricular plate.
2) With the patient in the lateral or sitting position, disinfect the relevant acupoints.
3) Seed burying: hold the auricle with the fingers of the left hand and the tweezers in the right hand to take the tape off the auricle board of the seed vaccaria segetalis, and stick it to the acupoints; gently rub it for 1–2 minutes until the partial auricle appears slightly red and warm.
4) After each operation, clean up materials and sanitize hands.
5) The left and right ears should be operated alternately, changing once every 3–5 days, 10 times for one course of treatment.

6.2.5.5 Contraindications

Ear needles are prohibited for:

1) Pregnant women who have habitual abortion
2) Patients with frostbite or inflammation of the ear
3) Patients who are overtired or extremely weak
4) Patients with severe organic lesions and severe anemia
5) Patients with eczema, ulcers, and such on the auricle

6.2.6 Cupping Therapy

Cupping therapy exhausts the air in the cup by using methods such as burning, suction, squeezing, etc., to create negative pressure, so that the cup sucks on the body surface or the affected area to cause engorgement of the skin. It is a therapy for dispelling cold, promoting blood circulation, and dredging collaterals to prevent and cure diseases. Western medicine believes that cupping can cause engorgement and edema through mechanical stimulation, thus enhance the permeability of capillaries. The negative pressure causes the microbubbles generated on the skin to overflow, accelerate blood circulation, and accelerate metabolism. In addition, cupping can reflexively stimulate the central nervous system through spinal nerve roots to improve patient fatigue, promote lymphatic circulation, and enhance immunity. Cupping is especially suitable for patients with mild cases of COIVD-19, with a syndrome of cold dampness and stagnation of the lung, and syndrome of dampness and heat of the lung. Cupping is also suitable for the moderate case COVID-19, with a syndrome of dampness – toxic stagnation of the lung, and syndrome of cold dampness and lung obstruction. It can effectively improve these symptoms by dispelling cold and removing dampness, clearing heat, and removing dampness.

6.2.6.1 Treatment Mechanism

6.2.6.1.1 Mechanism of TCM

According to TCM, the occurrence, development, and change of diseases are closely related to the physical strength of the diseased organism and the nature of pathogens. When pathogenic factors attack the human body, the healthy *qi* fights against them, which leads to a series of pathological changes.

In the treatment of COVID-19 with cupping therapy, acupoints are selected as the first and second lateral lines of the bladder of the zutaiyang passing through the back and spine. The bladder meridian of zutaiyang can control the whole body, which is the meeting place of all *yang*. Every pestilence that intrudes into it shall first transfigure the meridian of the sun. At the same time, the first lateral line of the bladder is the location of the acupoints of the viscera, and the meridians of the viscera are all injected here. Cupping here can adjust *qi* in the viscera and resist the invasion of foreign pathogens. The governor meridian is "the sea of *yang* meridians", which leads the healthy spirit of the whole body, so stimulating the governor meridian's dazhui acupoint can stimulate the human body's healthy *qi*. In addition, the stimulation of feishu acupoint can promote the lung and regulate *qi* and relieve cough and asthma.

By stimulating the meridians and acupoints, cupping therapy can nourish the healthy spirits, expel the evil spirits, balance *yin* and *yang*, and adjust the viscera and *qi*, thus successfully achieving the goal of curing COVID-19.

6.2.6.1.2 Mechanisms of Western Medicine

According to Western medicine, negative pressure suction of cupping can stimulate the formation of a large number of bubbles on the skin surface to strengthen the gas exchange in tissues. Cupping therapy is pathophysiologically a form of arterial engorgement. When arterial engorgement occurs, local arterioles dilate and substance metabolism and functional activities are enhanced. This will increase the supply of oxygen and nutrients in blood circulation, thus promoting metabolism and treating diseases.

6.2.6.1.3 Mechanism of Thermothermal Effect

Cupping can cause heat stimulation to the skin in certain areas, which will increase the skin temperature, dilate blood vessels, and increase blood flow. This promotes blood circulation, enhances metabolism, improves tissue nutrition, and ultimately improves the immune system.

6.2.6.2 Location Selection

The first and second lateral lines of the vesical of the bladder meridian, dazhui and dingchuan.

6.2.6.3 Location

1) The first and second lateral lines of the vesical of the bladder meridian is located at the back area, below the spinous process of the first thoracic vertebra to the posterior foramina of the fourth sacral, 1.5 and 3 cun from the posterior midline.
2) When sitting straight with head bowed, dazhui is at the lower part of the neck, at the indentation under the spinous process of the seventh cervical vertebra.
3) Dingchuan is located on the back of the neck, 0.5 cun from the midpoint of the lower edge of the spinous process of the seventh cervical vertebra.

6.2.6.4 Operation Methods

6.2.6.4.1 Retaining Cupping

Use the flash fire method to suck the cup to the first and second lateral lines of the bladder meridian on the back, focusing on dazhui, fengmen, and dingchuan, leaving the cup for 10–15 minutes.

6.2.6.4.2 Moving Cupping

Apply lubricant (Vaseline, moisturizer, etc.) on the first and second side lines of the bladder meridian on the back, and push and pull the cup repeatedly 5–10 times along the first and second side lines of the bladder meridian on the back until the skin appears red and engorged.

6.2.6.4.3 Bloodletting Puncture and Cupping

If the patient has the syndrome of dampness and heat of the lung, prick the dazhui acupoint until bleeding, then attach the cup to the dazhui point to remove a small amount of malignant blood.

6.2.6.5 Contraindications

Cupping is contraindicated:

1) For patients with bleeding tendency diseases such as thrombocytopenia, leukemia, allergic purpura.
2) For patients with fractures, scars, local malignant tumors, varicose veins, large vessels on the surface of the body, and poor local skin elasticity.
3) On the lower abdomen of women during menstruation.
4) On the lower abdomen, lumbosacral, and breast during pregnancy.
5) For patients with severe diseases of the heart, kidney, and liver and hyperthermia convulsions.
6) In areas affected by skin allergies, trauma, and ulcers.
7) Near areas of the five senses.
8) Near the area of the front and rear perineum.
9) For patients with excessive bleeding, excessive satiety, excessive sweating, excessive thirst, excessive hunger, drunkenness, and excessive exhaustion.

6.2.7 Scraping Therapy

Scraping therapy is a treatment based on the TCM theory of skin, using instruments (such as the horns, jade, cupping) to scrape skin areas in the related parts to dredge meridians and promote blood circulation to remove blood stasis. Due to the scrapping effect on the skin, the skin turns to the internal healthy qi to seek support. Healthy qi is promoted through the process of scrapping, and it increases the ability to protect the skin surface to resist the invasion of evil spirits from outside. Therefore, scrapping can facilitate health.

6.2.7.1 Treatment Mechanism

Each viscera has corresponding acupoints on the back area. These acupoints are the places where the viscera are injected and gathered. Scraping is an external treatment to regulate the viscera qi and remove pathogenic factors.

Most COVID-19 patients in the convalescent period are deficient in healthy qi with weakened viscera function, metabolic product retention, and abnormal immune function. Meanwhile, inflammation and connective tissue lesions can cause microcirculation disorders and the accumulation of metabolites. Scraping therapy can promote metabolism, remove toxins from the body, activate blood, and remove blood stasis, helping to unblock patients' muscles and veins. During the scraping, the downward pressure of the scraping board will make the blood containing toxins in the body leak out from the leaky capillary wall, forming a "scraping" under the skin. A small amount of scraping will not cause tissue damage but improve the local microcirculation.

Modern research shows that scraping causes a hemorrhagic change on the corresponding part of the skin. Soon after scraping, the hemorrhagic change will dilute and play the role of self-hemolysis, forming a new stimulating hormone, which can strengthen metabolism. The blood stasis caused by scraping can play a role in balancing the excitatory and inhibitory process of the brain by acting on the cerebral cortex through the centriole nerve. It has a very good regulatory effect on insomnia, autonomic nervous disorders, and other diseases. It might also effectively activate nerves and that brain to regulate the functional activities of muscles, viscera, and the cardiovascular system. Scraping can also enhance the immunity and disease resistance of the body. Scraping, through the conduction of the meridians, may enhance the metabolic function along the meridians to dredge them and prevent and treat diseases. The application of the scraping board can stimulate the deep tissue receptors and nerve fibers, stimulating the crude nerve fibers. This inhibits the pain signals transmitted by nerve fibers to achieve analgesic effect, thus treating other unpleasant symptoms caused by COVID-19.

6.2.7.2 Location Selection

Neck governor channel (dazhui to fengfu), fengchi, fengmen, feishu, and dingchuan.

6.2.7.3 Positioning

1) The neck governor meridian is located on the neck of the central line, from dazhui to fengfu.
2) When sitting straight with the head bowed, dazhui is located at the lower part of the neck, at the indentation under the spinous process of the seventh cervical vertebra.
3) Fengfu is located in the posterior cervical region, protruding from the occipital externus straight down in the indentation between the trapezius muscles on both sides.
4) Fengchi is located in the posterior region of the neck, below the occipital, between the upper end of the sternocleidomastoid and the upper end of the trapezius.
5) Fengmen is located on the back, 1.5 cun below the second thoracic spinous process.
6) Feishu is located on the back, 1.5 cun below the third thoracic spine process.
7) Dingchuan is located on the back of the neck, 0.5 cun from the midpoint of the lower edge of the spinous process of the seventh cervical vertebra.

6.2.7.4 Operation Method

1) Wipe the area to be scraped with 75% ethanol.
2) Take the scraper in your hand, and wipe the arteries and veins of the back and the bladder.
3) Focus on acupoints dazhui, fengfu, fengchi, fengmen, feishu, dingchuan, pishu, shenshu, quchi, chize, zusanli, taixi.
4) The direction of the scraper and swab is generally maintained at 45°–90° for scraping, scraping each part for 3–5 minutes, generally for no more than 20 minutes.
5) Do not force scraping on patients with red mark on the skin. The principle is to make those patients feel comfortable.

6.2.7.5 Contraindications

1) Scraping is contraindicated for patients with severe cardiovascular and cerebrovascular diseases, liver and kidney dysfunction, systemic edema, contact skin infection, and mental illness.
2) Scrapping of the abdomen and lumbosacral of pregnant women is prohibited.
3) Scraping is contraindicated near areas with boils, ulcers, carbuncles, maculae, and unexplained lumps.
4) Scraping is contraindicated near areas with acute sprain, trauma, or bone fracture.
5) Scraping is contraindicated for patients with bleeding tendencies, such as severe anemia, leukemia, aplastic anemia, and thrombocytopenia.
6) Extensive and large-area scraping is not suitable for patients with excessive hunger, excessive fatigue, or drunkenness.
7) Scraping is contraindicated near areas such as the eyes, lips, tongue, ear holes, nostrils, nipples, and umbilicus.

6.2.8 Bloodletting Therapy

Bloodletting therapy is one of the acupuncture methods, namely the meridional piercing method in *Neijing*. This refers to the treatment of diseases by puncturing blood collaterals or acupoints with three-edged needles according to different conditions to release the appropriate amount of blood. According to *Neijing*, it is said that "Asters will take them away and they will expel evil blood". Bloodletting therapy may activate collaterals, relieve heat, and remove pathogenic factors. Moreover, it can activate *qi* and blood circulation, dispel coldness, and relieve pain, invigorating pathogenic factors and preventing and treating diseases. Bloodletting therapy is especially suitable for COVID-19 patients with fever, redness of face, headache, sore throat, and poor stool.

6.2.8.1 Treatment Mechanism

The ancients had rich experience in the application of bloodletting therapy for pandemic diseases. For example, there are 72 kinds of miscellaneous diseases recorded in *Song Feng Shuo Yi*, and 42 of them were treated with bloodletting therapy. It was believed that needling and bloodletting could "bring out the evil poison with the evil blood". In *Sha Jing He Bi*, it is said that "If gas infection or foul gas phase is violated, the disease will be concurrently treated with Sha. If there is excessive phlegm and asthma, or choking in throat, or abdominal distension, irritability and fever, the disease can be treated with Sha … There are several green veins near the back of knee. If anyone falls in to a coma with phlegm and asthma, first, I stab the scarlet tendons and release their toxic blood". This suggests that the meridional piercing method can cure pandemic disease. In the *Cud for Pandemic Prevention*, it is recorded that "quick and effective method to cure the pandemic", which refers to the treatment of patting the elbow acupoints, fossa quze, and the armpit acupoint fossa weizhong. By patting the skin until red spots appear and then pricking the skin to let out black blood, diseases can "immediately heal". In the twenty-eighth year of the reign of Emperor Guangxu of the Qing Dynasty, "Hubei Province experienced a recurrence of the pandemic, and all those who performed acupuncture according to the above method also recovered". Clinical practice has proven that this method relieves heat, activates blood circulation to remove blood stasis, and dredges channels and collaterals. This method is mainly applicable to solid syndrome, heat syndrome, urgent syndrome, and so on.

When the exogenous pathogenic factors have not completely invaded, the collateral pricking and bloodletting can remove pathogenic factors from the surface. *Su wen: li he true evil theory* stated that "this new evil has not yet stand firm … Pierced out its blood, it will be cured." Congzheng put forward that "bleeding is the same as sweating, with different names but the same essence". In *Su wen: Ci Re*, it is proposed that lung fever patients should be treated by pricking taiyin and yangming. Letting out a drop of blood the size of a soy bean can cure disease. This reflects the remarkable effect of bloodletting therapy on fever. Bloodletting by acupuncture can promote the leakage of evil heat or reduce the evil heat in blood, balancing *yin* and *yang* in the body and reducing the fever. In *Su Wen: Miuci*, it was said that "People fall from evil blood staying inside". In *Lingshu: Shou Yao Gang Rou*, it is recorded that "the disease cannot be cured for a long time" would have all the syndromes of damaged meridians and collaterals, *qi* stagnation and blood stasis, all of which were treated by bloodletting. This shows that this method can activate blood circulation and remove blood stasis. Collateral puncture and bloodletting can also be used for deficiency syndrome. Simiao recorded that "Deficiency of stomach makes people sick, hungry, unable to eat, and full of support, so they need to prick the yangming and taiyang and let out the blood".

Modern research has shown that collateral pricking and bloodletting can mobilize the immune defense function of the human body and stimulate disease resistance. The positive effect on blood vessels and blood components can improve the microcirculation so that the tissue cells get more adequate blood nutrients. It can produce benign stimulation to nerve muscle and improve muscle function reflexively by stimulating peripheral receptors or nerve corpuscles on the body surface. It contributes to the secretion of various digestive enzymes, and it helps to improve the spleen and stomach weakness caused by anorexia, dyspepsia, etc.

6.2.8.2 Selection of Acupoints
Dazhui, taiyang, shaoshang, shangyang, fengmen, and feishu

6.2.8.3 Location of Acupoints

1) When sitting straight with the head bowed, dazhui is located at the indentation of the spinous process at the highest point of the neck (the seventh cervical vertebra).
2) Taiyang is located between the tip of the brow and outer canthus, at the indentation that is a finger away toward the back.
3) Shaoshang is located at the tip of the thumb, 0.1 cun from the root of the nail.
4) Shangyang is located at the tip of the index finger, 0.1 cun from above the root of the nail.
5) Erjian is located near the ear at the tip of ear when folded forward and above the auricle.

6.2.8.4 Operation Method
Wipe all points requiring bloodletting with 75% ethanol. For example, for patients with headache, acupoints dazhui and taiyang should be selected. Pricking dazhui with 3–5 three-edge needles, this process can be combined with cupping, to let out 5–10 mL blood. Prick acupoint taiyang with 2–3 needles. This process can be combined with cupping, to let out 5–10 mL blood. Prick the tip of the ear once and squeeze out 5–10 drops of blood. For patients with pharyngeal pain, acupoints shaoshang and shangyang should be selected. Squeeze the fingertips, prick once, and squeeze out five drops of blood or so; the tip of the ear can be selected as well. Bloodletting should not occur more than twice a week. One to three times is a course of treatment. If bleeding does not stop easily, use compression.

6.2.8.5 Contraindications

Bloodletting therapy is prohibited for:

1) Patients with a weak physique, anemia, puerpera, or poor blood coagulation mechanism.
2) Pregnant women.
3) Patients who have needle phobia, or blood phobia.
4) Patients with severe cardiovascular and cerebrovascular diseases, liver and kidney dysfunction, systemic edema, contact skin infection, and psychosis.
5) Patients with over exhaustion, over hunger, over full, stress, drunkenness, excessive sweating, or severe diarrhea.

6.3 TECHNIQUES OF TCM AND GUIDED THERAPY

6.3.1 Baduanjin

Baduanjin is a popular kind of gymnastics used to regulate zang, fu, *qi*, and blood; restore metabolic function; and strengthen the body. It has been compared to the exquisite brocade, composed of a total of eight movements, hence the name Baduanjin (eight brocades). Compared with other fitness methods, baduanjin is moderately intense, and its gentle and continuous movements are simple and easy to learn. It helps to regulate the spleen, stomach, and *qi* within the lung; nourishes the kidney, and absorbs *qi*, etc.

Essential actions: hold the triple focus of heaven with both hands, open the left and right arms like shooting an eagle, regulate the spleen and stomach with single arm lifting, look back after five labors and seven injuries, shake your head and wave your tail to get rid of the fire, reach your feet with both hands to strengthen the kidney and waist, gather your fists as well as anger and strength, put seven insanities behind and all sickness disappear.

6.3.2 Tai Chi Chuan

Tai chi chuan is based on the core ideas of tai chi and *yin-yang* differentiation in traditional Chinese Confucianism and Taoism philosophy. It integrates multiple functions such as temperament maintenance, physical fitness, and combat. It combines the changes of *yin* and *yang* and the five elements of the yi study, the meridian of TCM, and a kind of traditional Chinese boxing formed by the ancient daoyin technique and tuna technique, which is soft, slow, light, and flexible.

Tai chi chuan exercises have clear instructions for multiple joints of the whole body, upper limbs, lower limbs, and spine. It is a whole-body exercise.

Tai chi chuan is soft and uniform, and does not require high cardiopulmonary function. The amount of exercise can be adjusted by the height of the patient's center of gravity during exercise. It is easy to individualize and is suitable for all ages. Tai chi chuan requires practitioners to concentrate fully and has a certain regulatory effect on the patient's mind. Studies have shown that it can alleviate symptoms of anxiety and depression. The requirements for breathing in tai chi chuan are "long, even, careful, and slow", so that patients can exercise their exhalation muscles naturally while exercising their limbs. The deep and long breathing of tai chi chuan causes the lungs to expel a lot of turbid air and inhale more oxygen, which improves the ventilation efficiency of the lungs and, at the same time, enhances the elasticity of the lung tissues and the thoracic activity, thereby improving lung function.

6.3.3 Five-Animal Exercise

Five-animal exercise is China's earliest complete set of bionic guidance and one of the most representative exercises. It is a set of bionic guided health regimen created by the famous Han Dynasty doctor Hua Tuo based on the living habits and characteristics of tigers, deer, bears, apes, and birds, combined with the organizing of human meridians and viscera. In *The Hou Han Shu: Hua Tuo Biography*, it is recorded: "I have one skill, called the play of five animals: one is tiger, second is deer, third is bear, fourth is ape, and fifth is bird. It can get rid of disease, and is beneficial for foot simultaneously. It used to act as a guide." In the five-animal exercises, the individual actions focus on the mighty power of the tiger, the comfort of the deer, the calmness of the bear, the dexterity of the ape, and the lightness of the bird. Its movements are simple and easy to learn, safe and effective, and suitable for physical exercise at home. It has the effects of strengthening the body, preventing and curing diseases, pleasing the body and mind, and prolonging life.

When practicing, it is required to imitate vividly, not only in appearance but also in spirit. It should also gradually achieve relaxation of mind, body, movement and static, both rigidity and softness, inducing *qi* with the mind, permeating the body with *qi*, nourishing the mind with *qi*, ventilating with *qi*. When practicing the five-animal exercises, participants must breathe in a lot of oxygen, especially consciously exercising abdominal breathing, which can strengthen the thoracic bones and gradually develop the respiratory muscles. Strong breathing and increased lung capacity further enable the body to take in more oxygen and emit more carbon dioxide. In this way, more alveoli can be brought into work, the elasticity and permeability of the alveoli can be improved, and gas exchange can be facilitated so that the patient's lung function can be restored.

6.3.4 Yi Jin Jing

According to legend, yi jin jing was created by Dharma, the first ancestor of Chinese Zen Buddhism. It is a kind of fitness method with the purpose of changing muscles and bones. The yi jin jing meridian inherits the essence of the 12 potentials of the traditional yi jin jing meridian. It is scientific and universal. It has a primitive style and contains new ideas, highlighting the flexion, torsion, and stretching of muscles, bones, and joints, as well as the rotation, flexion, and stretching of the spine. Each movement is a coherent organic unit, and the movement pays attention to stretching the tendons, continuous stretching, and the combination of strength and flexibility. Breathing is required to be natural, continuous, and harmonious. It is guided by the flow of air, as the mind follows the flow. It is easy to learn and practice, with obvious effects on fitness levels.

Stretch the motion, stretch the tendon; gentle and symmetrical, harmonious and beautiful. Paying attention to the rotation, flexion, and extension of the spine is the characteristic of this exercise. In practice, students are required to relax in spirit and combine action and the mind, while breathing naturally throughout, strength and flexibility, the real and virtual. Gradually, individuals can add sound to each movement. Yi jin jing focuses on posture, supporting body parts with the mind, and adjusting the rhythm of breath, and it is suitable for different groups of people to take exercise. Long-term practice has a good effect on improving the function of the cardiovascular, respiratory, and digestive systems, improving balance, flexibility, and muscle strength and can reduce anxiety and depression.

6.3.5 Liu Zi Jue

Liu zi jue is the health-preserving practice of using six words that were inherited from ancient China. It strengthens the internal tissue function of the human body, fully inducing and mobilizing the potential ability of the viscera through breathing guidance to resist the invasion of diseases and prevent premature senescence that occurs with the increase of human age. It can affect the movement of *qi* and blood in different viscera, meridians, and collaterals. These effects can be achieved by the different pronunciation and power of the lips, teeth, throat, and tongue when speaking the six words: si, he, hu, xu, chui, and xi. Different forces on the lips, teeth, and larynx affect the operation of different viscera, organs, meridians, *qi*, and blood. The word xu calms the liver, the word hu replenishes *qi* within the heart, the word hu cultivates temperament, the word si nourishes *qi* within the lung, the word chui nourishes *qi* within the kidney, and the word xi has a triple effect.

The movements should be kept slow, while stretching smoothly and breathing evenly without holding one's breath. After reading each word 6 times, participants should adjust their breath once to take a break and restore nature. Practice three times in the morning and evening. Not only can it be used to rehabilitate patients with mild visceral dysfunction, but also to help healthy people regulate viscera and prevent diseases.

6.4 OTHER THERAPIES

6.4.1 Emotion Therapy of TCM

TCM believes that having seven emotions to an extreme extend can hurt people. Seven emotions refer to seven normal emotional activities, such as happiness, anger, anxiety, wistfulness, sadness, fear, and shock. They are different responses of the body's physiological and psychological activities to external environmental stimuli and belong to everyone's emotional experience. Under normal circumstances, they do not cause or induce disease. Only strong and long-lasting emotional stimulation, which surpasses the human body's physical and psychological adaptability, damages the body's visceral essence and *qi*, leading to dysfunction, or the human body's weakness of righteousness, visceral essence, and weakened ability to adapt to emotional stimulation. When a disease occurs or is induced, the seven emotions are called "seven emotions internal injuries." TCM emotion therapy is a medical psychology with traditional and cultural characteristics, reflecting the ancient philosophy of restraint of the five elements, and it is a perfect combination of classic theory and clinical experience.

In the face of COVID-19, anxiety and fear are inevitable. Wistfulness hurts the spleen; sadness hurts the lungs. And some patients even suffer from such uncomfortable symptoms as loss of appetite, restless sleep, palpitations, and chest tightness, which seriously affect their physical and mental health. Therefore, psychological intervention is essential for COVID-19 patients. In the course of thousands of years of development, Chinese medicine has accumulated a lot of scientific methods for diseases caused by seven emotions, and it can be used to treat diseases.

6.4.1.1 Ancient Chinese Medicine Emotion Therapy

The ancient Chinese medicine of emotion therapy is rich, colorful, and full of wit. Many anecdotes about diagnosis and treatment show the belief that emotions are medicine. TCM has unique emotion therapy for some difficult and strange diseases, and the magical curative effect contains rich scientific principles.

6.4.1.1.1 Anger Therapy

Legend has it that King Qi Min of the Warring States Period suffered from depression, so he asked Wen Zhi, a well-known doctor of the Song Dynasty, to treat him. After a detailed diagnosis, Wen Zhi said to the prince: "King Qi's illness can only be cured by irritating methods. If I irritate King Qi, he will definitely kill me." The prince pleaded, "As long as you can cure my father's disease, my mother and I will guarantee your safety." Wen Zhi had to agree.

Wen Zhi made an appointment with King Qi, but Wen Zhi did not come. Wen Zhi made and missed appointments with the king two more times. This made King Qi furious. A few days later, Wen Zhi suddenly appeared to meet with King Qi, but he did not abide with formality and take off his shoes. He went to King Qi's bed to start diagnosis and irritated King Qi with his profane language. King Qi was enraged, so he got up and started to curse Wen Zhi. With the mixture of anger and cursing, King Qi let out all negative emotions, and the depression was healed. Based on the principle of "anger is better than thinking" in the treatment of sentiment in TCM, Wen Zhi cured King Qi's depression by irritating his patient, leaving a typical example of sentiment therapy in the history of medical records.

6.4.1.1.2 Laughter Therapy

In the Qing Dynasty, there was a patrol man who was suffering from mental depression. He was frowning and depressed all day long. Nothing has changed even after several treatments. His condition became increasingly critical day by day. After being recommended by someone, he went to an old Chinese doctor for treatment.

The old Chinese doctor took a look and asked some questions, and said to the 1 word: patrolman, "You have irregular menstruation, just take care of it." The patrol man laughed and felt that this was a confused doctor. How could he not tell the difference between men and women? After that, whenever he thought of it, he still couldn't help but laugh secretly. As time passed, his depression got better.

A year later, the old Chinese doctor met the patrol man again, and said to him, "The disease that you had suffered in the past was *qi* stagnation. There is no good medicine, but if you are in a good mood and you often laugh, *qi* will start to flow unrestrictedly and coherently, and the disease can be healed without treatment. Your illness is cured without medicine through each and every laugh you had." The patrol man suddenly realized it and thanked the doctor immediately.

6.4.1.1.3 Pain Therapy

There was a farmer named Li Dajian in the Ming Dynasty. He had been diligent and studious since he was a child. He was admitted as an entry-level scholar.

The following year, he was admitted as a second-level scholar. In the third year, he was admitted as a third-level scholar. Good news continued to be heard year after year. His father was very happy, so he praised his son when he met everybody, and laughed at every boast. He couldn't stop laughing, and eventually became mad with laughter. Many doctors came to treat him, but they were unsuccessful. Li Dajian had no choice but to ask an imperial physician for treatment. The imperial physician thought for a long time before he said to Li, "The disease can be cured, but I may be disrespectful. Please forgive me." Li said, "I will obey the doctor's orders and dare not violate it."

The imperial physician immediately sent someone to Li Dajian's hometown to report the funeral. He said to his father, "Your son has passed away because of a sudden illness." After Li Dajian's father heard the bad news, he cried with extreme grief. Due to excessive grief, the symptoms of mad laughter stopped.

Soon, the imperial physician sent someone to tell Li's father: "After your son died, he was lucky enough to be rejuvenated by the imperial physician, and he was resurrected and saved." Li's father stopped his grief again. In this way, the mad laugh disease that lasted for 10 years was cured. Psychologically speaking, this is so-called reverse therapy.

6.4.1.1.4 Joy Therapy

According to legend, Zhang Zihe, a famous doctor in ancient times, was good at treating difficult and strange diseases and enjoyed high prestige among the masses. One day, a man named Xiang Guanling came to see a doctor and said that his wife had a strange disease. She only knew she was hungry, but she did not want to eat and drink. She vociferated every day and night, and she took a lot of medicine, but it was useless.

After hearing it, Zhang Zihe thought it was difficult to cure this type of disease with medicine. He told the patient's family to find two women, dressed as acting harlequins, and making many antics with twists and turns. This would make the patient happy. As soon as the patient was happy, the disease was relieved. Then, Zhang Zihe asked the patient's family to invite two women with strong appetites to come eat in front of the patient. The patient watched and then unknowingly began to eat. In this way, he used joy therapy to gradually calm the patient's mood, and the patient recovered without medicine.

6.4.1.1.5 Shame Therapy

Shame is a human instinct. By using this instinct, Chinese medicine has cured some difficult and strange diseases. All received a magical unexpected effect. According to legend, there was a folk woman who could not put her hands down at her side anymore because of yawning, and no medication was effective.

Taking advantage of the woman's shyness, the doctor pretended to untie the woman's belt and threatened to do acupuncture treatment for her. The woman was stunned by this sudden movement, and unconsciously hurriedly covered her lower body with her hands. Changes emerge within an emergency. The woman's hands dropped naturally and she was cured. This is the emotion therapy adopted by Chinese medicine to "besiege Wei to rescue Zhao" strategy, and it has received immediate results.

6.4.1.2 Application of Emotion Therapy in Chinese Medicine

The principle and core of TCM emotion therapy is to correct abnormal emotions, which is also the basic spirit of "emotion inter-resistance". It is the general principle of treatment to correct abnormal emotions such as anxiety and panic through a series of methods.

6.4.1.2.1 Principles of Treatment

1) Principle of acceptability: All COVID-19 patients must be treated equally and warmly. Patients must be guided with sympathetic, understanding eyes, encouragement, and heuristic questions, and their words must be patiently listened to. In fact, listening is the beginning of treatment, as patients can release emotions when they talk, and symptoms may be reduced by this. It is necessary for therapists sympathize and empathize with patients so that the patients feel that the therapists are trustworthy, making them willing to receive treatment.

2) Principle of supportability: After patients get sick, they will inevitably have a feeling of frustration and helplessness. Often they have experienced hardships or painful struggles. Some patients feel hopeless or have only a glimmer of hope, so they often ask when seeking treatment if their disease can be cured. For this reason, the therapist should continuously deliver supportive information to patients, explaining the curability of the disease, and giving examples of successful cases to relieve their anxiety caused by lack of relevant knowledge. At the same time, it will enhance patients' confidence and courage to fight the disease, with a firm, prudent, cordial, and credible attitude.

3) Principle of sincerity: Whether the disease can be cured is a matter of great concern to patients, family members, and therapists. For the treatment, it is necessary to take a sincere attitude and earnestly understand the patient's symptoms, pathogenesis, diagnosis, and response during treatment. After carefully determining the treatment plan, the therapist must continuously modify and improve it according to the specific situation. On this basis, a scientific and realistic explanation and guarantee can be made to the patient, so that the therapist's guarantee is justified. It is better to have a longer guarantee

period for the time, so as to avoid disappointment and frustration of the patient due to the failure to achieve the expected effect, and even doubt the therapist. Of course, it is also necessary to explain to the patient that any guarantee requires the patient to actively cooperate and follow the doctor's advice. Otherwise it will affect the treatment. The progress made by patients in the treatment process should also be given timely recognition and appreciation.

4) Principle of science: To conduct psychotherapy, therapists must follow the laws of psychology and be guided by scientific psychological theories. Therefore, the therapist must first have a solid professional foundation and establish an attitude of treating illnesses and saving people, and not aiming at making profits and confusing people.

5) Principle of confidentiality: Keeping the patient's name, occupation, condition, and treatment process confidential is the professional ethics that therapists should follow, and it is also an important principle for psychotherapy. Without the patient's permission, the therapist must not disclose the patient's situation to anyone, including the patient's relatives or the therapists' colleagues.

6.4.1.2.2 Major Emotion Therapies

1) Emotion interresistance: *Plain Questions · About yin and yang* and *Plain Questions·Five Movements* point out that "anger hurts the liver, grief overcomes anger", "happiness hurts heart, fear overcomes happiness", and "wistfulness hurt spleen, anger overcomes wistfulness", "sorrowfulness hurts lungs, happiness overcomes sorrowfulness", "fear hurts kidneys, wistfulness overcomes fear". This means that one emotional activity is used to control or regulate the disease caused by a certain stimulus to cure the disease.

COVID-19 patients often experience anxiety, panic, and other emotions. The visceral theory of Chinese medicine believes that fear will lead to anger, and panic will lead to confusion. These excessive emotional changes can cause the body's qi to rise and fall, and the zhong jiao mediation to become weak, resulting in the transformation of disease. In the treatment of diseases, the medical theory of panic restraint can be used to adjust the rise and fall of the qi machine and restore the body's dynamic balance of yin and $yang$.

2) Transference therapy: The purpose of transference is to distract the patient from the disease and make them less addicted to bad emotions. According to the *Clinic Guideline of Medical Records,* "The depression of emotions is due to the recessive connotation ... The depression syndrome can be transferred to the patient." Therefore, COVID-19

patients can enjoy indoor recreation and entertainment, such as reading books, listening to music, doing handicrafts, painting, playing Baduanjin, yoga, chatting, etc. They can also cultivate hobbies, relieve anxiety and tension, and maintain a positive attitude; patients should not believe rumors, amplify negative information, and increase panic; patients should not pay too much attention to information related to the pandemic before going to bed, so as not to affect sleep quality.

3) Therapy to follow one's emotions and desires: *Plain Questions: Transferring Essence and Changing Qi* pointed out that "the patients who are related to the disease should be asked about their feelings in order to follow their meanings". This is also one of the psychotherapies. When the pandemic began, the party and the government took decisive actions to treat the sick people. This action relieved the patients from financial pressure. Through collective care and social relief, the anxiety and worries of patients have been greatly eased.

4) Speech induction therapy: The therapist should treat patients equally, be patient and meticulous, and gain their trust. In addition, the therapist should take a sympathetic attitude toward the patient, ask them about their condition in detail, and use persuasion to make the patient talk truthfully and tell about the pain. It is also a "psychological counseling" method, which is conducive to the counseling of bad emotions.

6.4.1.3 Precautions

6.4.1.3.1 Understanding
Therapists should understand that patients' emotional responses are a normal stress response, and they should be prepared in advance. Therapists should not engage in arguments with the patients, even when being irritated by patients' aggressive behavior or sadness.

6.4.1.3.2 Assessment
Under the premise of understanding the patient, psychological crisis intervention should be given in addition to drug treatment, such as timely assessment of patients' risk of suicide, self-injury, or attack; positive psychological support; and direct conflict with the patient. The therapist should explain the importance and necessity of isolation treatment to the patient, and encourage the patient to build confidence in positive recovery.

6.4.1.3.3 Explanation
It should be emphasized that isolation is not only for better observation and treatment of patients but also a way to protect relatives and society. The therapist also needs to explain the main points of the current treatment and the effectiveness of the intervention.

6.4.2 Music Therapy

The role of music therapy in psychotherapy is beyond doubt. The *Yellow Emperor's Internal Classic* put forward the theory of "five-tones healing disease" more than 2,000 years ago, which believed that five internal organs can influence the five tones and the five tones can regulate the five internal organs. It gives different attributes to the five scales of traditional music, namely, jiao (wood), hui (fire), gong (earth), shang (the second tone of five scales) (mental), and yu (the sixth tone of five scales) (water). Music therapy combines the *yin* and *yang* and five elements of TCM and the theory of harmony between man and nature and music. Through five different tonal melodies of "jiao, hui, gong, shang, and yu", with different musical instruments, different sound waves and melodies played to make the body's internal organs resonate, thereby achieving the purpose of preventing diseases and regulating emotions. Patients can listen to some music they like to relax during the hospital stay. Music therapy should be taken two to three times a day, each time for about 30 minutes.

BIBLIOGRAPHY

1. General Office of the National Health Commission, Office of the State Administration of Traditional Chinese Medicine. *Notice on Issuing the COVID-19 Diagnosis and Treatment Plan (Trial Version 7)*. [2020-03-04].
2. Tong Xiaolin, Li Xiuyang, Zhao Linhua, LI Qingwei, Yang Yingying, Lin Yiqun, Ding Qiyou, Lei Ye, Wang Qiang, Song Bin, Liu Wenke, Shen Shiwei, Zhu Xiangdong, Huang Feijian, Zhou Yide. Discussion on Traditional Chinese Medicine Prevention and Treatment Strategies of Coronavirus Disease 2019 (COVID-19) from the Perspective of "Cold-dampness Pestilence". *Journal of Traditional Chinese Medicine*, 2020, 61 (6): 465–470.
3. Tong Xiaolin, Li Xiuyang, Zhao Linhua, LI Qingwei, Yang Yingying, Lin Yiqun, Ding Qiyou, Lei Ye, Wang Qiang, Song Bin, Liu Wenke, Shen Shiwei, Zhu Xiangdong, Huang Feijian, Zhou Yide. Discussion on Traditional Chinese Medicine Prevention and Treatment Strategies of Coronavirus Disease 2019 (COVID-19) from the Perspective of "Cold-dampness Pestilence". *Journal of Traditional Chinese Medicine*, 2020, 61 (6): 465–470.
4. Jin Yinghui, Cai Lin, Cheng Zhenshun, Cheng Hong, Deng Tong, Fan Yipin, Fang Cheng, Huang Di, Huang Luqi. Novel Coronavirus Pneumonia Prevention and Treatment Team in Zhongnan Hospital of Wuhan University. A rapid advice guideline for the diagnosis and treatment of 2019 novel coronavirus (2019-nCoV) infected pneumonia. *New Medicine*, 2020, 30 (01): 35–64.
5. Ren Yue, Yao Meicun, Huo Xiaoqian, Gu Yu, Zhu Weixing, Qiao Yanjiang, Zhang Yanling. Study on treatment of "cytokine storm" by anti-2019-nCoV prescriptions based on arachidonic acid metabolic pathway. *China Journal of Chinese Meteria Medica*, 2020, 45 (06): 1225–1231.
6. Cao Xinfu, Liu Zihao, Li Xiang, Zhou Mingxue, Liu Hongxu. Prevention and treatment of novel coronavirus pneumonia in various regions of China. *Beijing Journal of Traditional Chinese Medicine*, 2020, 5 (39): 418–422.

7. Bai Qizhou, Wang Bing, Jin Dacheng, Zhang Siyuan, He Xiaoyang, Yan Ning, Gou Yunjiu. Progress in the staged diagnosis and treatment of COVID-19 in traditional Chinese medicine (medical edition). *Journal of Xi'an Jiaotong University*, 2020: 1–18 [2020-03-09].

8. Chinese acupuncture and moxibustion association guiding opinions on acupuncture intervention for COVID-19 (first edition). *Chinese Acupuncture and Moxibustion*, 2020, 40 (2): 111.

9. Wu Liping, Ye Lini, Li Zhiping, et al. Current status of outpatients' awareness of COVID-19 and nursing strategies. *General Nursing*, 2020, 18 (5): 556–558.

10. Li Jiansheng, Zhang Hailong, Chen Yaolong. Expert consensus on traditional Chinese medicine rehabilitation for COVID-19 (first edition). *Chinese Medicine Journal*, 2020: 1–19 [2020-03-09].

11. Liu Qingquan, Xia Wenguang, An Changqing, et al. Thoughts on the effect of integrated traditional Chinese and western medicine in the treatment of COVID-19. *Journal of Traditional Chinese Medicine*, 2020, 61 (6): 463–464.

12. Fan Fuyuan, Fan Xinrong, Wang Xinzhi, et al. Talking about the characteristics and prevention of pneumonia caused by COVID-19 infection in Hunan from the perspective of "dampness, toxin, clip, drying". *Chinese Medicine Journal*, 2020: 1–4 [2020-02-06].

13. Zhao Hong, Li Yisong, Liu Bing, et al. Clinical observation on 9 cases of moxibustion treatment of SARS in the convalescent period. *Chinese Acupuncture*, 2003, 23 (9): 564–565.

14. Shi Renchao. Direct and comprehensive intervention of traditional Chinese medicine for SARS prevention and treatment is very useful: traditional Chinese medicine experts offer suggestions for SARS prevention and treatment. *Zhejiang Journal of Traditional Chinese Medicine*, 2003, 38 (7): 277–279.

15. Wu Jing, Cai Shengchao. The development of the theory of "heat syndrome can be moxibustion". *Clinical Journal of Chinese Medicine*, 2017, 29 (4): 455–458.

16. Wang Yin. Analysis of the feasibility and infeasibility of acupuncture treatment of SARS. *Chinese Acupuncture*, 2003, 23 (8): 498–501.

17. Zhu Bing. Thoughts on moxibustion materials and moxibustion temperature. *Acupuncture Research*, 2018, 43 (2): 63–67.

18. Chang Xiaorong, Liu Mi, Yan Jie, et al. Theoretical origin of moxibustion's warming and tonic effect. *Chinese Journal of Traditional Chinese Medicine*, 2011, 29 (10): 2166–2168.

19. Chen Tengfei. Discussion of severely ill patients with symptoms of dampness. *Emergency in Chinese Medicine*, 2018, 27 (11): 1981–1983.

20. Lan Lei, Chang Xiaorong, Shi Jia, et al. Research progress on the mechanism of moxibustion. *Chinese Journal of Traditional Chinese Medicine*, 2011, 29 (12): 2616–2620.

21. Zou Qingxuan, Lin Youbing, Zhou Yifan, et al. The characteristics of moxibustion in different schools in recent years. *Shanxi Journal of Traditional Chinese Medicine*, 2017, 33 (10): 60–62.

22. Qi Licong. Observation on the efficacy of chiropractic plus acupoint massage in the treatment of children with pneumonia and sputum symptoms. *Continuing Medical Education*, 2019, 33 (4): 160–162.

23. Zhao Yi, Wang Shizhong. *Tuina Manipulation*. Shanghai: Shanghai Science and Technology Press, 2009.

24. Xu Beichen. Chinese medicine combined with massage adjuvant treatment of 40 cases of severe viral pneumonia of wind-heat closed lung type. *Modern Chinese Medicine*, 2019, 39 (4): 33–36.

25. Liu Xia, Guo Xiucai, Lin Yuanyuan, et al. Acupoint and non-acupoint skin biophysical properties affect sinapine permeability. *Chinese Herbal Medicines*, 2013, 44 (9): 1111–1116.

26. Zhao Juanping, Zhang Qiuyue, Qi Xiao, et al. Overview of research on acupoint application of traditional Chinese medicine in the treatment of respiratory diseases. *Chinese Journal of Traditional Chinese Medicine*, 2017, 35 (7): 1780–1783.

27. Liang Fanrong. *Acupuncture and Moxibustion*. Shanghai: Shanghai Science and Technology Press, 2013: 24–25.

28. Li Chen, Zhao Qiang, Xu Yihan, et al. Theoretical interpretation of acupoint application based on the theory of collateral disease in the treatment of chronic complicated lung disease. *Chinese Journal of Traditional Chinese Medicine*, 2015, 33 (7): 1590–1592.

29. Zhang Yunwei, Zhou Yan, Liao Xiaoqin, et al. Observation on the curative effect of acupoint application on chronic obstructive pulmonary disease in stable phase. *Shanghai Journal of Acupuncture and Moxibustion*, 2016, 35 (9): 1065–1069.

30. Han Fei, Peng Zhen, Zhou Zhiyu, et al. Research progress of efficacy classification of traditional Chinese medicines on improving the immune function of the body. *Chinese Herbal Medicines*, 2016, 47 (14): 2549–2555.

31. Li Shu, Xiao Xiong, Mao Bing. The effect of acupoint application combined with acupoint injection on the immune function of patients with acute exacerbation of COPD. *Clinical Journal of Military Medicine*, 2018, 46 (2): 199–201.

32. Wang Yingying, Yang Jinsheng. Research and prospects of the clinical treatment of Gua Sha therapy. *Chinese Acupuncture*, 2009 (2): 167–171.

33. Jia Man, Feng Fen. Gua Sha therapy and its application. *Henan Traditional Chinese Medicine*, 2011, 31 (12): 1368–1370.

34. Xu Qingyan, Yang Jinsheng, Yang Li, Yang Li, Wang Yingying, Liu Xiulan. The influence of scrapping in the Weizhong acupoint area in terms of blood circulation and skin microcirculation on the meridian line. *Acupuncture Research*, 2013, 38 (1): 52–56.

35. Zhang Jiejia. Research progress of traditional health-preserving methods on rehabilitation of patients with COPD. *Journal of External Therapy of Traditional Chinese Medicine*, 2017, 26 (6): 54–56.

36. Shi Yan. The prevention research of Baduanjin Health Qigong exercise on lung function and complications of patients with tuberculosis. *Chinese Journal of Preventive Medicine*, 2019, 20 (9): 799–802.

37. Guo Guangxin, Cao Ben, Zhu Qingguang, Zhang Shuaipan, Zhou Xin, Lv Zhizhen, Wu Zhiwei, Xu Shanda, Kong Lingjun, Sun Wuquan, Cheng Yanbin, Fang Min. Application of traditional Chinese medicine methods in the prevention and treatment of COVID-19. *Shanghai Journal of Traditional Chinese Medicine*, 2020: 1–4 [2020-03-09].

38. Han Rui, Lin Hongsheng. The clinical research of Health Qigong Ba Duan Jin on the effect of intervention on lung function and quality of life in patients with non-small cell lung cancer after surgery. *Tianjin Traditional Chinese Medicine*, 2016, 33 (12): 715–718.

39. Koh TC. Baduanjin – an ancient Chinese exercise. *The American Journal of Chinese Medicine*, 1982, 10 (1–4): 14–21.
40. Pan Yi, Wang Zhenxing, Min Jie, et al. Evaluation of the curative effect of 24-style simplified Tai Qi Chuan in the rehabilitation process of chronic obstructive pulmonary disease *Chinese Journal of Rehabilitation Medicine*, 2018, 33 (6): 681–686.
41. Gao Yanfang, Ou Yanyun, Chen Miaoyuan. The effect of Wuqinxi exercise on lung function and exercise tolerance of patients with chronic obstructive pulmonary disease during the transitional period after hospital discharge. *Journal of Clinical Pathology*, 2017, 37 (5): 975–980.
42. Zhang Lin, Wei Yulong. Clinical research progress of Wuqinxi at home and abroad. *Massage and Rehabilitation Medicine*, 2019, 10 (23): 24–27.
43. Xu Haijun, Li Lizhen, Wang Jiuli. Effects of Wuqinxi combined with chemotherapy on immune function and quality of life in patients with lung cancer. *Clinical Journal of Traditional Chinese Medicine*, 2018, 30 (9): 1697–1699.
44. Xu Mengting, Li Linlin, Wang Wanhong, et al. The effect of Yijinjing combined with endurance exercise on cardiopulmonary function and quality of life in patients with coronary heart disease. *Heart Journal*, 2019, 31 (4): 447–451.
45. Dong Jingcheng, Liu Baojun, Zhang Hongying. Application of "preventive treatment" theory in chronic airway inflammatory diseases. *Chinese Journal of Integrated Traditional Chinese and Western Medicine*, 2013, 33 (7): 983–989.
46. Xiao Jian, Du Chunling. Progress in the etiology and pathogenesis of chronic obstructive pulmonary disease. *Chinese Journal of Gerontology*, 2014, 34 (11): 3191–3194.
47. Liu Tairong, Luo Biru, Yu Zheng, et al. Application of acupoint massage combined with Liuzijue breathing exercises in patients with stable chronic obstructive pulmonary disease. *Journal of Nursing Science*, 2018, 33 (5): 41–44.
48. Guo Xiuting, Zhan Xiaoping, Jin Xizhong, Jin Xizhong, Huang Quanhai, Jin Chenci, Hu Lidan, Yu Ningnig,Qi Xu. The effect of acupoint massage combined with respiratory exercises on lung function and quality of life in patients with chronic obstructive pulmonary disease in stable stage. *Chinese General Practice*, 2017, 20 (S2): 345–347.
49. Li Bingxue, Liu Jie, Lin Hongsheng, et al. *Journal of Traditional Chinese Medicine*, 2019, 60 (24): 2150–2153.
50. Guo Xiuhua. Psychological stress and the treatment of related mental diseases. *National Health Standard Management*, 2015, 6 (16): 31–32.
51. Chen Fei. Study on negative emotion and psychological defense mechanism in patients with psychosomatic diseases. *Beijing Medical Literature Electronic Journal*, 2017, 4 (69): 13506.
52. Xie GG, Zhou X. Interpretation of COVID-19 diagnosis and treatment plan (trial version 8). *Journal of Clinical Pulmonary Medicine*, 2020, 25(10): 1459–1467. doi: 10.3969/j. issn.1009-6663.2020.10. 001.
53. Koh TC, Tai Chi Chuan. *The American Journal of Chinese Medicine*, 1981 Spring, 9(1): 15–22. doi: 10.1142/s0192415x81000032. PMID: 7030051.

Chapter 7

Diagnosis and Treatment Model of the COVID-19 Rehabilitation Unit

With the constant improvement in the clinical treatment of COVID-19, as of March 17, 2020, 69,601 patients have been discharged from hospitals nationwide. The number of new cases, a rapid increase in critically severe cases decreased significantly, and patients in many provinces and cities were cleared. It indicates that the battle against the pandemic has entered a new stage. In order to better understand the hierarchical and refined management of COVID-19 patients and build an integrated diagnosis and treatment model of prevention–treatment–rehabilitation, the rehabilitation intervention of COVID-19 is required for better clinical intervention. Based on this, we have carried out the research on the diagnosis and treatment model of the COVID-19 rehabilitation unit, hoping to help patients recover from their respiratory, physical, and psychological illnesses. We hope to promote social harmony and progress and provide future response to various health crises.

7.1 CONCEPT OF THE COVID-19 REHABILITATION UNIT

The COVID-19 rehabilitation unit (CRU) refers to a working model that uses multidisciplinary teamwork to conduct rehabilitation and treatment activities for inpatients with stable COVID-19. It is a systematic rehabilitation that includes physicians, rehabilitation physicians, Chinese medicine physicians, rehabilitation specialist nurses, physical therapists, cardiopulmonary therapists, occupational therapists, psychologists, and social workers. They provide patients with combined Chinese and Western medical treatment, including posture therapy, breathing training, sports training, free-hand therapy, breathing exercises, physical factor therapy, psychological rehabilitation and health education, etc., to promote the absorption of lung inflammation and improve respiratory muscle strength, improve respiratory function, enhance exercise endurance, and physical strength. At the same time, it also helps patients to relieve anxiety and depression, improve their ability of daily living, help patients return to their social life, and improve their quality of life. In a broad sense, CRU extends the management of patients from clinical rehabilitation in the hospital to community and family rehabilitation after discharge, thus forming a comprehensive social system.

CRU is not a new treatment method, but a comprehensive, environmental, and efficient ward management model. It integrates various existing treatment methods of COVID-19 with the purpose of improving diseases and improving health. Through teamwork, it achieves a 1+1 is greater than 2 treatment effect. The focus is to take the illness and health needs of patients as the center of care to realize the transformation from a biological model to a biological–psycho-logical–social–health model, with a view to drawing a successful conclusion to the treatment of COVID-19. The World Health Organization (WHO) proposed that in the outcome of the disease, in addition to the two clinical outcome indicators of cure and death, it also includes the third clinical outcome indicator: functioning. For COVID-19 patients, we have also observed that those who meet the discharge standards, especially critically severe patients, are still unable to live on their own when they are discharged from the hospital and cannot return to social life, which has brought a heavy burden to the family and society. The emergence of CRU reflects the humanistic care for COVID-19 patients, emphasizes the value and significance of rehabilitation, and changes the clinical recovery based on negative nucleic acid tests and improved image tests. It regards the functional prognosis of patients and the satisfaction of patients and their families as important clinical goals and reflects the team-work model of the multidisciplinary team (MDT).

After COVID-19 patients enter the COVID-19 rehabilitation ward, the routine physical examination and medical history inquiry is conducted and various necessary laboratory examinations and imaging examinations are required to be completed within 24 hours. Members of the CRU team participate in the rehabilitation assessment, make a rehabilitation plan, and emphasize the early rehabilitation of lung function under oxygen monitoring. Psychologists actively guide and support psychologically, stabilize patients' emotions, reduce or eliminate negative behaviors, enhance their confidence in rehabilitation, improve their psychological adjustment capabilities, and establish new adaptive behaviors. Patients are encouraged to actively coop-erate with treatment to prevent and reduce various complications as much as possible. At the same time, it also uses various methods such as videos, WeChat, and brochures to provide community and home remote rehabilita-tion guidance and psychological and health assessment is provided to the patient after discharge for better results.

7.2 ROLE AND SIGNIFICANCE OF THE COVID-19 REHABILITATION UNIT

7.2.1 Role of the COVID-19 Rehabilitation Unit (CRU)

CRUs enable COVID-19 patients to receive comprehensive, systematic, safe, and effective rehabilitation treatment in the ward on an early basis.

CRUs can be equipped with better rehabilitation facilities and rehabilitation treatment in the isolation ward, which provides a strong guarantee for the treatment of various difficult problems. Meanwhile, accurate assessment and MDT work are more conducive to providing individual and targeted rehabilitation programs for patients.

CRUs help to reduce various complications because of the guidance of professional trainers and medical staff in the CRU. They can more sensitively pay attention to the complications of patients, such as the formation of deep vein thrombosis of the lower limbs, urinary tract infections, muscle atrophy, osteoporosis, etc., and provide early prevention and treatment. In addition, they can pay attention to patient position management and psychological counseling as soon as possible and can guide patients in comprehensive rehabilitation treatment more comprehensively and systematically. Therefore, they can reduce the healing time of lung inflammation, reduce complications, and reduce mortality.

The CRU working group can monitor patients in real-time and conduct assessment and treatment under the monitoring of blood oxygen and heart rate. This work management mode can ensure a more safe and effective rehabilitation treatment for COVID-19 patients.

7.2.2 Significance of Constructing the COVID-19 Rehabilitation Unit

7.2.2.1 Producing Effective Clinical Results

MDTs work closely to provide standardized treatment regimens for patients while adjusting treatment to individual differences and changes in the patient's condition. Early rehabilitation intervention can effectively prevent complications, shorten the course of the disease, and consolidate the curative effect.

7.2.2.2 Improving the Satisfaction of Patients and Their Families

The ultimate goal of CRU management mode is to improve the dysfunction of patients, improve the quality of life, and promote social harmony. On the one hand, the rehabilitation treatment aimed at functional disorders has significantly improved the clinical efficacy; on the other hand, it has helped the patient to overcome the stress, psychological trauma, panic, and anxiety caused by COVID-19. Additionally, it has formed a good doctor–patient relationship through multi-dimensional communication with patients and their families through medical technology and care.

7.2.2.3 Conducive to Clinical Research on the Rehabilitation of COVID-19

COVID-19, as a newly emerging infectious disease, requires further scientific and clinical research for better treatment. Currently, many treatment plans are formulated based on the experience gained during the severe acute respiratory syndrome (SARS) outbreak. Further clinical studies are needed to understand the outcome of the disease based on long-term prognosis, especially the outcome of rehabilitation treatment.

7.3 CONSTRUCTION OF THE COVID-19 REHABILITATION UNIT

7.3.1 Types of COVID-19 Rehabilitation Units

7.3.1.1 CRUs in the Ultra-Early Period

This period is mainly based on consultation. In this stage, patients with severe and critical infections live in the respiratory ward, infectious ward, or ICU and are mainly treated by other doctors, with the super-early intervention of COVID-19 rehabilitation, MDT rounds, and medical plan formulation. Such patients are contagious.

7.3.1.2 CRUs in the Early Period

Convalescent COVID-19 patients in the early period generally refers to the ordinary type of patients who are transferred from critically severe to severe, from high to moderate severity after 1–2 weeks of onset, or the ordinary type of patients who are in stable condition. Their vital signs are stable, and their condition is no longer progressing. Their lung CT absorbs more than before, and the nucleic acid test is negative or still positive, but there is dysfunction in the respiratory system, heart, and other organs as well as with motor skills and self-care ability. Therefore, rehabilitation intervention is required as soon as possible, and the hospitalization is generally a period of 15–20 days or about 2 weeks. Such patients are infectious.

7.3.1.3 CRUs in the Convalescent Period

COVID-19 patients have been clinically cured and discharged, and they have completed 14-day sentinel isolation and 14-day home isolation. However, these patients still suffer from the above dysfunctions and cannot return to the family and society. Such patients are no longer infectious.

7.3.2 Conditions for the Establishment of the COVID-19 Rehabilitation Unit

7.3.2.1 Equipment Conditions for Isolation Wards

7.3.2.1.1 Prerequisites

According to the requirements of the *Technical Guidelines for the Prevention and Control of COVID-19 Infection in Medical Institutions* (First Edition) issued by the National Health Commission (NHC), all rehabilitation doctors, therapists, and rehabilitation nursing staff who come into contact with patients should have the training and experience of social distancing and quarantine ethics. Only after passing the assessment can the CRU in the ultra-early period and early period be established.

7.3.2.1.2 Site

The building layout and working process of the CRU ward and rehabilitation treatment area should comply with the relevant requirements of the *Technical Code for Hospital Isolation* and other relevant requirements according to the national regulations. Moreover, they should be equipped with a qualified and appropriate amount of protective equipment for medical personnel.

7.3.2.1.3 Requirements

On the basis of the implementation of standard prevention, measures such as contact isolation, droplet isolation, and air isolation are adopted. The visitation system is strictly prohibited, and escorts are not allowed. Air purification is required in accordance with the *Air Purification Management Regulations*.

7.3.2.1.4 Protection of Medical Personnel

Hospital sections, rehab directors, and head nurses should strengthen the implementation of standard preventive measures and maintain ventilation management in isolation wards and rehabilitation treatment areas. Before entering the rehabilitation diagnosis and treatment area, check the body temperature of personnel. Medical staff should wear work clothes, strictly follow the requirements of the *Hand Hygiene Regulations for Medical Staff*, and wear medical protective masks (it is recommended to be replaced every 4 hours) and latex gloves. Protective measures such as contact isolation, droplet isolation, and air isolation are taken, and the protective equipment used by medical staff meets the requirements of national regulations. Medical staff must wear and take off protective equipment in strict accordance with the specifications. The medical instruments and appliances used by each patient should be cleaned and disinfected in accordance with the *Technical Standards for Disinfection of Medical Institutions.*

7.3.2.1.5 Strengthening Patient Management

Patients shall be quarantined and instructed to choose and wear masks correctly and to perform cough etiquette and hand hygiene correctly. Visitors are not allowed in the isolation ward. As per rules and safety measures, patients' activities are restricted in the isolation ward. If relevant examinations are needed, patients should wear protective clothes and masks and be guided to complete the examination and return to the isolation ward according to the specified standard route.

7.3.2.2 Setting Up Rehabilitation and Treatment Areas

In order to avoid cross-infection and reduce the flow of patients, a rehabilitation area should be set up in isolation wards.

7.3.2.2.1 Environmental Requirements

There must be enough space, a quiet environment, smooth ventilation, and air purification devices to restrict personnel access.

7.3.2.2.2 Training Equipment and Apparatus

According to the actual conditions, certain equipment should be used, such as ultra-shortwave, shortwave, microwave, and other high-frequency therapy devices, intelligent upper and lower limb training devices, aerobic rehabilitation evaluation training treadmills, aerobic rehabilitation power bicycles, and airwave pressure therapy devices, etc. At the same time, it is necessary to make full use of equipment, intelligent equipment training, physical factors, etc. Patients should focus on active rehabilitation and minimize "one-to-one" physical interaction therapy and invasive operations. Hospitals with sufficient conditions can be equipped with mobile breathing function testers, heart and lung function testers, and several finger pulse oxygen testers.

7.3.2.3 Membership of the CRU and Relevant Work

7.3.2.3.1 Principal Members of the CRU

Rehabilitation physician, cardiopulmonary rehabilitation therapist, physiotherapist, traditional rehabilitation therapist, psychotherapist, rehabilitation specialist nurse.

7.3.2.3.2 Main Responsibilities of the CRU

Rehabilitation physicians are responsible for the clinical diagnosis and treatment of patients, including receiving patients, asking for medical history, physical examination, assessing patients' respiratory function and other dysfunctions, making rehabilitation diagnosis and treatment plans, being responsible for daily rounds or consultations, and issuing medical advice and rehabilitation treatment opinions, etc. They have to complete the writing of relevant documents, weekly rehabilitation scores, and organize the therapists and nurses to discuss teamwork using video. Cardiopulmonary rehabilitation therapists are mainly responsible for the assessment of cardiopulmonary function, posture management, respiratory function training, clearance training, etc. In addition, they carry out health education for patients on COVID-19 rehabilitation. Physical therapists are mainly responsible for aerobic training, exercise prescription formulation, physical factor therapy, etc. Traditional rehabilitation therapists are mainly responsible for traditional rehabilitation treatments, such as various moxibustion methods. They guide and lead patients to perform traditional exercise treatments, such as tai chi chuan, baduanjin, etc. Psychotherapists mainly conduct psychological assessments on patients and provide psychological counseling and psychological treatment to patients with psychological disorders to relieve patients' anxiety, panic, and depression and enhance their confidence in overcoming the disease. Rehabilitation nurses are mainly responsible for guiding the patient's posture management, actively and effectively communicating with the patients, understanding the daily conditions of the patients, carrying out health education for patients with COVID-19, and education work during the isolation after discharge from the hospital and the home isolation period.

7.3.2.3.3 Work Content of the CRU

In addition to their daily medical work, the members of CRU also communicate in the form of teamwork group discussions, with the goal of solving patients' actual problems and improving clinical efficacy. They provide the multidisciplinary evaluation and make multifaceted recommendations for patients' diagnosis and treatment plans from different perspectives to develop targeted and individualized diagnosis and treatment regimens. Generally, the first CRU group meeting should be held within 3 days of the patient's admission and once a week thereafter. It is presided over by a rehabilitation physician. All members of the CRU group must participate. Generally, there are three stages of rehabilitation group meetings: initial, intermediate, and final stages.

The initial evaluation meeting is conducted before the development of a rehabilitation plan and rehabilitation treatment. It mainly discusses the patient's current status, the existing dysfunction, the degree of dysfunction, the potential for rehabilitation, the current main problems, and the factors affecting rehabilitation treatment. Each member puts forward treatment plans, programs, and goals from their own perspective. Finally, under the comprehensive evaluation and analysis of rehabilitation physicians, the rehabilitation treatment plan, short-term and long-term goals are planned and coordinated.

The intermediate evaluation meeting is usually conducted after 1 week of rehabilitation. The meeting includes in-depth discussions on the changes in the patient's status during rehabilitation, the degree of improvement of illness, the difficulties of treatment, the implementation of the rehabilitation plan, and the completion of short-term goals. Moreover, the meeting analyzes the existing problems, makes adjustments or changes to the treatment plan, and works out the next rehabilitation plan.

The final evaluation meeting is conducted when the patient has finished rehabilitation and is about to be discharged from the hospital. At the meeting, the recovery of dysfunction after rehabilitation and the improvement of the ability of daily living of patients who have undergone intervention in the CRU ward are summarized, and the effect of rehabilitation is evaluated. In addition, the meeting develops a rehabilitation guidance plan for patients' home and community rehabilitation treatment and also makes appointments for follow-up to observe the long-term effects.

7.3.2.3.4 Health Education for COVID-19

Health education on COVID-19 is one of the important functions of CRU. It can enable patients to correctly understand COVID-19, eliminate fear, promote people to consciously form healthy behavior, strengthen personal health protection, and avoid the infection of COVID-19. Through health education, the communication and exchange between patients and medical staff are increased, and the early rehabilitation of patients is promoted. It will increase people's experience in dealing with all kinds of major outbreaks in the future and reduce stress trauma. During the pandemic, health education and extended rehabilitation guidance can be provided to patients through video and WeChat by medical staff themselves.

7.3.2.3.5 Organization and Operation of the CRU Ward

CRU wards in the ultra-early and early periods contain patients who are contagious, which means personnel need to work under strict protection and isolation. During the convalescent period, the CRU will work in accordance with the routine rehabilitation medicine process. However, after the pandemic is over, future work should also strictly follow the requirements of the *Hand Hygiene Regulations for Medical Staff*. Medical staff should wear medical protective masks (it is recommended to be replaced every 4 hours) and disposable latex gloves to protect themselves and patients from cross-infection.

7.3.2.3.6 Discharge Plan

COVID-19 patients meet the discharge criteria according to *Notice of the COVID-19 Diagnosis and Treatment Plan (7th Trial Edition)* jointly issued by the NHC and the State Administration of Traditional Chinese Medicine (TCM):

1) Body temperature returns to normal for more than 3 days.
2) Respiratory symptoms have improved significantly.
3) Pulmonary imaging shows that acute exudative lesions were significantly improved.
4) Respiratory tract samples such as sputum, nasopharyngeal test paper, and other respiratory tract samples have a negative nucleic acid test (at least a 24-hour interval) before being discharged. At the same time, patients discharged from the CRU ward have significantly improved respiratory function, heart function, other organ function, and motor function and achieve basic self-care. After a period of home recuperation, they can return to work and society. It will be discussed and determined by the CRU working group.

7.3.2.3.7 Discharge Follow-Up

Members of the CRU working group will make regular visits to discharged patients, supervise patients to carry out home and community rehabilitation treatment programs, and help patients develop a healthy lifestyle and good hygiene habits to improve patients' long-term life quality.

7.4 DIAGNOSIS AND TREATMENT PLAN FOR THE COVID-19 REHABILITATION UNIT

Due to the pandemic's particularity, CRU has not been launched in other hospitals and other countries. Moreover, due to the lack of a clear understanding of the changes in COVID-19 and the characteristics of dysfunction, it is not yet possible to determine the most reasonable rehabilitation medical plan. We also tried and explored CRU's work and management model based on the stroke unit management model. At the same time, we actively drew on various expert consensus and guidance on rehabilitation during the SARS and COVID-19 pandemic to carry out related work, including the *Rehabilitation Plan for Discharged Patients from COVID-19* (Trial) issued by the General Office of the NHC, the *Expert Consensus on Rehabilitation Diagnosis and Treatment During the Pandemic of Respiratory Infectious Diseases Based on COVID-19* issued by the Chinese Society of Rehabilitation Medicine, and *Guiding Opinions on Respiratory Rehabilitation for COVID-19* issued by the Chinese Association of Rehabilitation Medicine in conjunction with the Respiratory Rehabilitation

Committee of the Chinese Association of Rehabilitation Medicine and the Cardiopulmonary Rehabilitation Group of the Chinese Physical Medicine and Rehabilitation Branch.

CRU is an integrated management system and process for diagnosis, evaluation, observation, treatment, and rehabilitation of COVID-19 patients. Patients can receive targeted and individualized rehabilitation treatment plans, including medications quickly. These programs can promote the absorption of lung inflammation in patients with COVID-19, reduce clinical symptoms related to pneumonia (cough, palpitation, chest tightness, fatigue, etc.), improve patients' respiratory function, improve heart and lung functions, and increase respiratory muscle strength. Moreover, the implementation of these programs can prevent various complications (including deep vein thrombosis of the lower extremities, pressure sores, and deterioration of skeletal muscle function, etc.) and enhance exercise endurance and physical strength. It can also relieve anxiety and depression, improve patients' activities of daily living, help patients gradually return to their families and society, and reduce the after-effects of COVID-19. It is necessary to improve the long-term quality of life of patients as a work goal and carry out targeted medical treatment.

7.4.1 Dysfunction

7.4.1.1 Respiratory Dysfunction

COVID-19 is caused by SARS-CoV-2 acting on the ACE2 receptor and enters cells through receptor-mediated endocytosis. It mainly infects ciliated bronchial epithelial cells and types II alveolar cells, causing systemic diseases with lung damage. Acute lung inflammation damages lung epithelial cells and pulmonary capillary endothelial cells, causes pulmonary interstitial and alveolar edema, affects oxygen diffusion, and causes alveolar gas exchange disorders. At the same time, the alveolar surface-active substances decrease, the alveoli collapse, and the number of alveoli participating in the gas exchange on the alveolar surface decreases. The ventilation/blood flow ratio is imbalanced, and the lung ventilation function decreases. For severe and critically severe patients, pulmonary fibrosis may also occur in the later stage, and restrictive ventilation dysfunction may occur. Therefore, COVID-19 patients have respiratory symptoms such as dyspnea, chest tightness, and wheezing. Through the results of lung function testing, it is possible to identify whether the patient is ventilator dysfunction or diffuse dysfunction, and the type of ventilatory dysfunction (obstructive, restrictive, mixed).

7.4.1.2 Physical Dysfunction

Limb weakness, wheezing, and fatigue during activity are common clinical symptoms of COVID-19, which can be the first symptoms of the onset and last for a long time. Even after returning to the community and at home, it is still the biggest problem that affects patients. Therefore, exercise training is one of the important contents of pulmonary rehabilitation. The exercise test can assess the patient's cardiopulmonary function and exercise capacity (muscle strength, exercise endurance, overall exercise level, etc.), and understand the patient's finger oxygen saturation and heart rate during exercise. It can develop safe, moderate, and individualized exercise prescriptions for patients. Studies have found that cardiomyocytes, renal proximal tubule epithelial cells, bladder epithelial cells, esophagus, ileum, etc., all have high expression of ACE2. Therefore, COVID-19 not only infects the respiratory system but also affects the circulation, urinary, and digestive systems. Critically severe patients will experience damage to multiple organs, including the heart. Heart damage may be related to hypoxemia, respiratory failure, inflammation, and viral infection that directly damage the myocardium. Abnormal blood biochemical indicators are often found in severe and critically severe patients, such as serum myocardial necrosis marker-cardiac troponin I (c*TnI*), creatine kinase isoenzyme (Cκ-MB), lactate dehydrogenase (LDH), abnormal levels of liver enzymes and kidney function. Clinical practice has found that COVID-19 patients are often accompanied by symptoms such as palpitation, hyperhidrosis, anorexia, and diarrhea. Therefore, these physical dysfunctions also require long-term attention and comprehensive intervention.

7.4.1.3 Psychological Dysfunction
COVID-19 patients often have fear, anxiety, and even depression due to their uncertainty about the disease. There are also some patients who have Post-Traumatic Stress Disorder (PTDS) brought about by a major pandemic, which all lead to psychological disorders. It is often clinically manifested as asking about one's own condition repeatedly, or being indifferent to the outside world, or full of fear and worry about the disease. In severe cases, insomnia and even suicidal tendencies occur. Therefore, active psychological intervention and guidance can help patients overcome fear and anxiety and build confidence in overcoming the disease.

7.4.1.4 Barriers to Social Participation
The basic point of recovery for COVID-19 patients is to gain enough independence, avoid dependence, and eventually return to families and society. The majority of COVID-19 patients are elderly people. Many people have multiple underlying diseases such as hypertension, diabetes, and hyperlipidemia, which aggravate the dysfunction of discharged patients. Therefore, activities of daily living (ADL) training has a certain effect and significance.

7.4.2 Work Principles

For COVID-19 patients with stable conditions and stable vital signs, after being transferred to the CRU ward, a team of rehabilitation physicians, therapists, and nurses will conduct rehabilitation treatment for them. Under certain electrocardiogram (ECG) and blood oxygen monitoring, CRU conducts a systematic and comprehensive assessment and safe and effective rehabilitation for these patients. At the same time, CRU staff should pay attention to safety protection at work to avoid infection. All rehabilitation treatments should exclude contraindications, and the basic principle is not to increase the burden of patients with clinical infection protection.

7.4.3 Work Requirements

A comprehensive, detailed, and adequate rehabilitation assessment must be developed to fully grasp the indications and contraindications.

An individualized and comprehensive rehabilitation plan with integrated Chinese and Western medicine must be formulated.

A gradual rehabilitation treatment must be carried out under the monitoring of ECG and blood oxygen.

During the entire medical process, doctors, therapists, and nurses need to follow strict infection prevention and control measures to avoid medical staff infection.

The entire rehabilitation treatment should be safe and effective, and attention should be paid to adverse reactions in the treatment process. In the course of treatment, if the person has any unsuitability, immediately terminate the treatment, report to the rehabilitation physician, complete the examination, and actively take treatment measures.

7.4.4 Workflow

Patients are transferred from the COVID-19 isolation ward to the CRU isolation ward for comprehensive rehabilitation intervention. The specific workflow is shown in Figure 7.1.

The work management model of CRU integrated Chinese and Western medicine is to adhere to the combination of Chinese and Western medicine and complement each other's advantages. In the CRU ward, it is necessary to realize the full rehabilitation of COVID-19 patients with integrated traditional Chinese and Western medicine. At the same time, formulate and improve CRU's diagnosis and treatment specifications to improve clinical efficacy on the basis of ensuring safety and effectiveness. It is necessary to integrate multidisciplinary

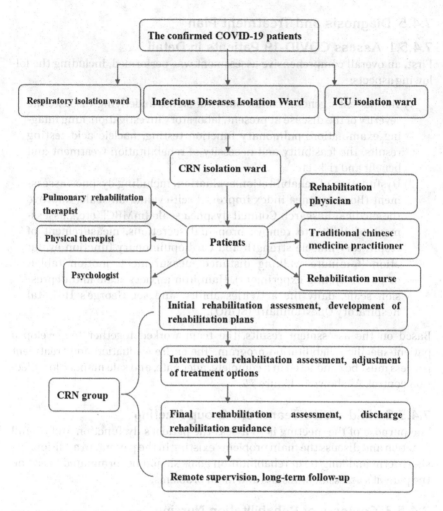

Figure 7.1   Workflow chart of a COVID-19 rehabilitation unit.

resources to establish a COVID-19 rehabilitation platform to maximize the advantages of multiple disciplines, carry out the treatment of COVID-19 in a three-in-one model of prevention–treatment–rehabilitation to achieve seamless, continuous, full-cycle management of COVID-19. Finally, remote rehabilitation guidance for patients at home and in communities is emphasized to be an effective extension. This will accelerate the achievement of national health to community work to improve the social satisfaction of patients and their families and promote social harmony and progress.

7.4.5 Diagnosis and Treatment Plan

7.4.5.1 Assess COVID-19 Patients in Detail

First, an overall comprehensive assessment was performed, including the following aspects:

1) The patient's general condition, vital signs, underlying disease, the severity of the disease at present, laboratory investigation, lung imaging examination, pulmonary function testing, nucleic acid testing results, the feasibility and necessity of rehabilitation treatment and benefit and risk, etc.

2) Dysfunction of rehabilitation evaluation, including dyspnea assessment (Borg dyspnea index improved self-evaluation scale, improve the medical Research Council dyspnea scale [mMRC], etc.), assessment of ability to remove bronchial secretions, measurement of respiratory muscle strength and cardiopulmonary function evaluation (6-minute walking distance measurement, motion tablet, or power cycling experiment), Hamilton anxiety scale and depression scale, daily life activities ability, and set George's Hospital Respiratory Questionnaire (SGRQ).

Based on the assessment results, the team worked together to develop a patient-specific rehabilitation program. The entire evaluation and treatment process must be conducted in a complete, adequate, and safe manner for infection control. As shown in Figure 7.2.

7.4.5.2 Hold a CRU Teamwork Group Meeting

The purpose of the meeting is to assess the patient's dysfunction and overall function and discuss the main problems existing in the patient. In addition, the short-term and long-term rehabilitation goals should be formulated based on the patient's assessment results and main problems.

7.4.5.3 Contents of Rehabilitation Nursing

Rehabilitation nursing mainly includes basic nursing and rehabilitation nursing of COVID-19 diseases, such as body temperature, respiration, pulse oxygen, heart rate, and blood pressure. It also needs to pay attention to patients' clinical symptoms, such as cough, sputum, throat pain, dyspnea, and other respiratory system-related symptoms. Once there is palpitation, weakness, sweating, anorexia, nausea, diarrhea, insomnia, dizziness, and other organ-related symptoms, as well as anxiety, depression, apathy, and other psychological and emotional problems, the rehabilitation nurses should report to the bedside doctor. Rehabilitation nurses should explain the requirements of the admission and isolation ward to patients. At the same time, medical staff

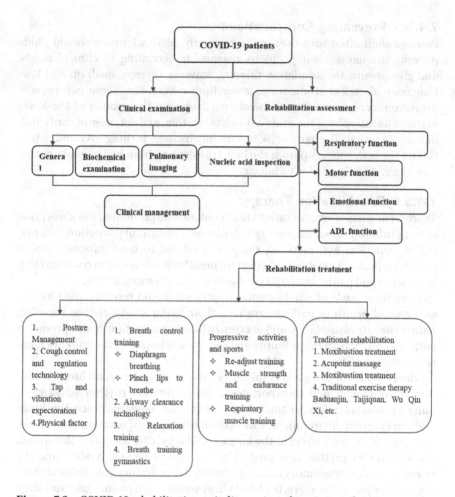

Figure 7.2 COVID-19 rehabilitation unit diagnosis and treatment plan.

should closely observe the patient's condition and monitor every 4–6 hours. They must pay special attention to changes in blood oxygen saturation and body temperature. Patients with complex conditions and many underlying diseases should be monitored at any time.

7.4.5.4 Treatment Measures

Treatment is conducted in accordance with the *Diagnosis and Treatment Protocol for COVID-19 (7th Trial Edition)* jointly issued by the NHC and the State Administration of TCM.

7.4.5.5 Preventing Complications

Patients shall often turn over and move early. Medical nurses should guide patients to change their positions reasonably according to clinical needs, and give pneumatic circulation therapy, massage therapy, medium and low-frequency electrical stimulation, lower limb robots, etc. These can prevent pressure ulcers, urinary tract infections, deep vein thrombosis of the lower extremities, atrophy of the musculoskeletal system, and decrease of cardiopulmonary function. The early activities mainly include: turning over and activities on the bed, sitting up from the bed, transferring from bed to chair, sitting on a chair, standing and walking etc.

7.4.5.6 Rehabilitation Therapy

Short-term goals of rehabilitation treatment include promoting the absorption of lung inflammation, improving the patient's respiratory function, improving oxygenation, and reducing symptoms related to lung inflammation. It also helps patients establish an effective breathing pattern, overcome anxiety, depression and panic, and build confidence in overcoming illness.

Long-term goals of rehabilitation treatment should promote the physical and mental health of patients, reshape their living ability, reduce sequelae, reduce the rate of disability, and maximize function retention. It also promotes patient's early return to the family and society and improves the patient's long-term quality of life.

The completion of a good respiratory function requires good lung ventilation, gas exchange and transportation, and respiratory rhythm adjustment. Lung ventilation refers to the process of gas exchange between the lungs and the external environment. Gas exchange and transportation refer to the exchange of gas with blood in the lungs' capillaries after air enters the alveoli. The respiratory rhythm is regulated by the central nervous system and the reflexes from the respiratory organs themselves, respiratory muscles, and other organs' receptors. Therefore, the breathing exercise pattern and the respiratory muscles' strength play an essential role in the recovery of respiratory function. It mainly includes posture management, breathing control technology, airway clearing technology, progressive activity and exercise, breathing training gymnastics, physical factor therapy, etc.

7.4.5.7 TCM Rehabilitation Therapy

TCM rehabilitation treatment includes Chinese medicine exercise training, moxibustion, acupoint application, massage, etc. These treatments can alleviate patients' symptoms, enhance resistance, and promote the recovery of cardiopulmonary function and physical strength. Moreover, they can also play an active role in alleviating patients' anxiety and depression, helping them recover their physical and mental health.

7.4.5.8 Extended Rehabilitation Therapy

Extended rehabilitation therapy is to extend patients' rehabilitation to their homes and communities after they are discharged from the hospital. When the patient is discharged from the hospital, a home and community rehabilitation treatment plan can be developed. Extended rehabilitation therapy uses the internet, such as WeChat and video, to provide remote rehabilitation guidance and supervision to continuously deepen and develop new models of rehabilitation management.

7.5 COMMON COVID-19 COMPLICATIONS AND THEIR MANAGEMENT

7.5.1 COVID-19 Associated Venous Thromboembolism

During the treatment of COVID-19, first-line clinicians found that nearly 20% of patients had abnormal coagulation functions, affecting the coagulation and fibrinolysis system through various ways. Eventually, it leads to the activation of the coagulation cascade and the inhibition of the fibrinolysis process, which promotes the formation of blood clots. It is essential to pay attention to and prevent deep vein thrombosis (deep venous thrombosis, DVT) and pulmonary thromboembolism (PTE) that occurs after formation. We made the following, with reference to *Recommendations for Prevention and Treatment of Venous Thromboembolism Related to COVID-19* (Trial).

Vein thromboembolism (VTE) refers to the abnormal coagulation of blood in the veins, making the blood vessels entirely blocked. It is a disease of venous return disorder. It includes DVT and PTE, which are often acute. DVT of the lower limbs is the most common. In severe cases, it can cause sudden death in patients with COVID-19.

7.5.1.1 VTE Risk Factors and Risk Assessment

7.5.1.1.1 Risk Factors

COVID-19 patients have symptoms of the digestive system such as diarrhea and anorexia, which lead to severe and nondominant water loss, insufficient fluid volume, and high blood viscosity due to blood concentration. Severe patients are accompanied by other infections and long-term bed rest, obesity, underlying diseases, and advanced age. Critically severe patients have slowed blood return to the limbs and blood stasis due to hypotension, shock, coma, etc. The release of a large number of inflammatory mediators, the application of hormones and immunoglobulins are also risk factors. Injury to the vascular endothelium caused by central venous catheterization and surgery are all risk factors for VTE occurrence.

7.5.1.1.2 Risk Assessment

(1) COVID-19 patients aged ≥ 40 years and confined to bed for > 3 days, such as age ≥ 75 years, severe infection or sepsis, respiratory failure, heart failure, obesity, previous history of VTE, acute exacerbation of the chronic obstructive pulmonary disease, acute cerebral infarction, acute coronary syndrome, chronic kidney disease, pregnancy or maternity.

(2) It is recommended to use the Padua rating scale for VTE risk assessment for hospitalized patients in the CRU ward, mainly including active malignant tumor (3 point), previous venous thromboembolism (3 point), immobilization for more than 3 days (3 point), a tendency to thrombosis (3 point), recent trauma or surgery (2 point), age older than 70 years (1 point), heart and respiratory failure (1 point), acute myocardial infarction and ischemia stroke, acute infection and/or rheumatic disease (1 point), obesity (1 point), receiving hormone therapy (1 point). Patients with a total score of ≥ 4 are classified as high-risk patients, and patients with a total score of < 4 are classified as low-risk VTE patients.

7.5.1.2 VTE Prevention Advice for Inpatients in the CRU Ward

As patients are treated in the isolation ward, the activity time and area of activity is reduced, and the time of sedentary or bed rest increases, which causes the lower limb venous blood flow to slow down the venous blood flow stasis is prone to lower limb DVT. Therefore, patients are encouraged to drink more water and carry out activities as soon as possible within a safe range and are instructed to perform active and passive activities in bed. Also, mechanical prevention can be implemented, such as intermittent pneumatic compression (IPC), graded compression stockings (GCS). Massage therapy on the limbs can also be given to promote blood circulation. During IPC treatment, the therapist should use IPC under monitoring and pay attention to the lower limbs' swelling and the pulsation of the dorsal ankle artery. If DVT occurs, IPC treatment should be stopped immediately. GCS is generally used as an adjuvant treatment for IPC. IPC combined with GCS is recommended to prevent DVT in lower limbs in patients with high bleeding risk.

For inpatients in the CRU ward with medical diseases and surgical conditions, such as high-risk or medium-high-risk VTE patients, drug prevention can be considered. It is recommended to choose ultra-low molecular weight heparin (LMWH) or directly remove risk factors. The use time of LMWH is 7–10 days. For patients with thrombocytopenia or heparin-induced thrombocytopenia (HIT) during heparin application, argatroban, bivalirudin, rivaroxaban, etc., are recommended.

For hospitalized patients in CRU wards, dynamic monitoring of D-dimer or other coagulation indicators should be performed as much as possible. The rise of D-dimer in early stage pneumonia may be related to acute inflammation. A sharp increase in respiratory failure indicates that an inflammatory storm may occur. With the control of the disease, the D-dimer gradually returned to normal. If the COVID-19 patient's condition is stable, and D-dimer is progressively increased or increased during the recovery process, but the original disease has not progressed, the ultrasound examination of both lower limbs should be perfected to exclude DVT of the lower limbs. If the upper extremity or superior vena cava cannulated, the upper extremity venous ultrasound examination should be perfected to exclude DVT of the upper extremity.

7.5.1.3 COVID-19 Complicated with DVT

For patients with a high clinical suspicion of DTV (symptoms such as swelling of the affected limb, increased circumference, pain or tenderness, superficial vein dilation, skin pigmentation, increased swelling of the affected limb or heaviness of the affected limb after walking), the bedside and lower limbs should be improved through intravenous ultrasound and ECG. If the protection conditions permit, it is recommended to conduct a Computed Tomography Angiography (CTA) inspection and discharge PTE.

If it is diagnosed as DTV, treat according to the following principles.

1) General treatment: The affected limb is raised, and the movement should be reduced. After the swelling of the affected limb gradually subsides after 2 weeks, the patient should wear elastic stockings to relieve symptoms.
2) Drug treatment: When the risk of bleeding is assessed as low at acute stage (within 2 weeks of onset), anticoagulant therapy is given; anticoagulant therapy for 3 months is appropriate for patients without persistent VTE progression factors. Patients can directly take anticoagulant drugs (argatroban, dabigatran, rivaroxaban, etc.), low molecular weight heparin, and warfarin. Contraindications in drug use should be noted. The preferred dose of anticoagulant may be, for example, rivaroxaban 20 mg orally, once a day; 1 low-molecular-weight heparin, subcutaneously injected once every 12 hours; the initial dose of warfarin is 1 tablet orally, and the International Normalized Ratio (INR) is tested to maintain the INR 2.0–3.0.

7.5.1.3.1 Other Treatments

During the pandemic, if the protection conditions permit, patients with a greater risk of PTE or widespread DTV or DVT patients with anticoagulation contraindications or complications after anticoagulation may consider inferior vena cava filter implantation.

Early activities and related preventive measures are the keys to reducing the mortality and morbidity of VTE.

7.5.2 Pressure Ulcers

Pressure ulcers refer to the local skin or soft tissues of COVID-19 patients being compressed for a long time due to long-term bed immobilization or other underlying diseases that restrict their activities, affecting blood circulation, resulting in damage to the skin or potential subcutaneous soft tissues. The pressure injury can be manifested as local tissue damage, but the epidermis is intact or open ulcers with pain. The tolerance of subcutaneous soft tissues to pressure and shear is affected by environment, nutrition, comorbidities, etc. It usually occurs in the bony prominences, such as the sacrum, ankle, and heel.

7.5.2.1 Stages of Pressure Ulcers

Pressure ulcers are divided into the following stages.

Stage 1 stress injury: Erythema does not disappear when pressed. The epidermis of the local tissue is intact, with non-pale redness.

Stage 2 pressure injury: Partial dermis defect. The wound bed is alive. The basal surface is pink or red and moist. Serum blisters may appear intact or ruptured, but the fat layer and deeper tissues are not exposed.

Stage 3 pressure injury: Full-thickness skin defect. The ulcer surface may show the phenomenon of subcutaneous fat tissue and granulation tissue wound edge curling.

Stage 4 pressure injury: Full-thickness skin and tissue damage. Fascia, muscle, tendon, and/or cartilage are exposed on the ulcer surface.

Unclear staging of pressure injury: full-thickness tissue is covered and tissue defect, etc.

Pressure ulcers can bring a series of harms, such as increasing the suffering of patients, prolonging the course of the disease, and even causing sepsis and endangering patients' lives.

7.5.2.2 Treatment of Pressure Ulcers

7.5.2.2.1 General Treatment

Patients can change their position regularly. Special mattresses are also used to relieve the formed ulcers and prevent the further development of pressure sores. Patients who can move on their own should move once every minute when sitting, and change positions every 1 hour. Patients who cannot move on their own should change positions every hour when sitting, and change positions every 2 hours when lying. Special mattresses include inflatable mattresses, protective foam pads and pressure regulating pads.

7.5.2.2.2 Debridement
The wounds of patients with pressure sores should be debrided and changed.

7.5.2.2.3 External Dressings
The wounds of patients are protected from contamination by using film dressings, hydrogel dressings, antibiotic dressings, biological dressings, etc. These materials can absorb exudate, fill the necrotic cavity, reduce edema, and promote the healing of pressure sores.

7.5.2.2.4 External Antibacterial Agents
When patients have infection symptoms, they can be coated with antibacterial agents such as iodide and silver.

7.5.2.2.5 Antibiotics
When ulcers are infected secondary to cause sepsis, cellulite, sepsis, etc., antibiotics can be used for treatment.

7.5.2.2.6 Analgesics
When the ulcer has severe unbearable pain, nonsteroidal antipyretic analgesics can be given to relieve the pain.

7.5.2.2.7 Growth Factors
When ulcer wounds are difficult to heal, external growth factors can be used to promote wound healing.

7.5.2.2.8 Surgical Treatment
When severe pressure ulcers cannot heal on their own, debridement or skin repair is required to promote pressure ulcer healing.

7.5.3 Urinary Tract Infections
Urinary tract infections are mainly secondary to COVID-19 patients who have been bedridden or have had indwelling catheters for a long time. The inflammation caused by the invasion of bacteria into the urothelium may be accompanied by bacteriuria and pyuria. Acute simple urinary tract infections mainly manifest as bladder irritation, such as frequent urination, urgency, and pain. In severe cases, urge incontinence, cloudy urine, and hematuria may occur. Once urinary tract infections occur, patients should promptly undergo blood routine examinations, routine urine examinations, urine bacterial cultures, and drug

sensitivity tests to guide antibiotic treatment. Long-term indwelling urinary catheters should be avoided. For example, urinary catheters should be strictly aseptic to reduce the probability of urinary tract infection.

7.5.4 Malnutrition

COVID-19 patients are in a high catabolic state due to obvious systemic inflammation. At the same time, due to the COVID-19 infection, patients often have digestive symptoms such as anorexia and diarrhea. In the isolation ward, the types and tastes of food are difficult to meet the requirements of every patient, resulting in unguaranteed nutrition. Therefore, patients are prone to malnutrition. For patients with chronic underlying diseases, the probability of malnutrition is higher. Malnutrition will weaken the function of respiratory muscles and reduce the immunity of patients, leading to further deterioration of the disease. Therefore, in the CRU ward, it is of great significance to carry out nutritional screening and assessment of patients with COVID-19 and to guide the nutritional supplement of patients.

7.5.4.1 Nutritional Screening and Assessment for COVID-19 Patients

Nutritional risk screening scores NRS2002 is recommended for nutritional risk screening. An NRS2002 score ≥ 3 indicates a nutritional risk and requires intervention.

7.5.4.2 Selection of a Nutritional Treatment Plan

The metabolic changes and energy and nutrient requirements of COVID-19 patients are in dynamic changes at different stages. Therefore, dynamic nutrition management should be conducted at different stages according to patients' different conditions. For patients who can eat on their own without the risk of vomiting or accidental inhalation, oral feeding should be given priority. The general principle is to ensure a sufficient amount of energy, high-quality protein, essential fatty acids, vitamins, and water, and avoid spicy and pungent food. For patients with poor appetite, formula foods and nutrient supplements can be provided to meet their needs. It is also necessary to ensure that such patients eat quantitatively and regularly. For patients who cannot eat or cannot meet their daily needs, tube feeding enteral nutrition can be given. If the demand is still not met, parenteral nutrition support should be given as soon as possible.

7.5.5 Disuse Muscle Weakness and Muscle Atrophy

The earliest and most significant abnormality of long-term bed rest is the muscular system. Disuse muscle weakness and muscle atrophy in COVID-19 patients refer to the phenomenon of muscle volume reduction, muscle strength reduction, and endurance reduction caused by muscle inactivity. This phenomenon is dominated by the reduction of myoglobin and myofibril protein. Due to long-term bed rest, the muscle volume is significantly reduced, which will inevitably lead to the decline of muscle function. At the same time, due to prolonged bed rest, the patient's active movement is reduced, and muscle weakness symptoms may be more pronounced. Studies have found that the decline in muscle strength is related to the decrease in muscle volume and the decline in neuromuscular innervation. The degree of muscle atrophy is related to active exercise and daily activity.

Preventive measures include getting patients to start activities as soon as possible. For example, when the patient exercises, the oxygen saturation decreases significantly, or the symptoms such as dyspnea and wheezing occur, passive exercises can be performed first, such as upper and lower limb rehabilitation robots on the bed, intermittent inflatable compression pump (IPC), low-frequency electrical stimulation, body massage, etc. The patient gradually increases the amount of active activity, starting from the exercise in bed and gradually returning to getting out of bed.

7.5.6 Joint Contracture

Joint contracture refers to the limitation of the active and passive range of joint motion due to the inactive state of patient's joints, muscles, and soft tissues. Joint contractures can be caused by pain, poor posture for a long time, fear of increased oxygen consumption by activities, and psychological factors. The pathological basis of contracture caused by any reason is the abnormality of collagen tissue. Long-term immobilization can cause inflammatory changes in the joints, resulting in intra-articular adhesions, proliferation, and bursa's fibrosis. Simultaneously, joint fixation can lead to changes in the synovium and proliferation and shortening of collagen in the joints, which can cause joint contractures. The essence of contracture is connective tissue abnormality, including abnormality of collagen and matrix, and the two influence each other. Active and passive exercises are the simplest means to deal with contractures, which have preventive and therapeutic effects.

The main measures to prevent joint contractures include getting patients to change their positions regularly, such as turning over, managing their positions, and transferring in and out of bed. Exercise should follow the principle of gradual progress and gradually expand the range and amount of exercise.

7.5.7 Disuse Osteoporosis

Osteoporosis (OP) is a bone metabolism disease caused by the loss of bone matrix and minerals. It causes a decrease in bone strength and an increase in brittleness. Even minor trauma can cause fractures. COVID-19 patients believe that long-term bed rest is the best way for recovering from the disease due to the reduced space for activities in the isolation ward or the lack of understanding of the disease. This misunderstanding causes patients to stay in bed for a long time. Patients' bones lack stimulations, such as weight-bearing, center of gravity, and muscle activity, which gradually leads to bone loss and degeneration of the fibrous structure of bone tissue. Due to the long-term lack of sunlight in the isolation ward, 7-dehydrocholesterol in the human body cannot be converted into vitamin D3, which affects calcium absorption and bone mineralization disorders. Moreover, long-term inactivity affects the patient's endocrine system and increases calcium excretion in the urine. All of the above further aggravate the patient's osteoporosis. Patients with disuse osteoporosis caused by immobilization can lose 30%–40% of their total bone mass in a relatively short period. Therefore, prevention is more important than treatment for OP.

Standing with weight and getting out of bed as soon as possible are the primary means to prevent osteoporosis. Aerobic training and endurance training can improve the degeneration of skeletal muscle function. Therefore, combining exercise therapy and food therapy can delay bone degeneration and osteoporosis.

BIBLIOGRAPHY

1. Deng Zhigao, Liu Jie, Zhao Xiaomei. *Construction and application of stroke units.* Beijing: People's Military Medical Press Club. [2011].
2. Chen LDIAN. *Practice manual of stroke unit.* Beijing: People's Medical Publishing House. [2008].
3. Chan JC. Recovery pathway of post-SARS patients[J]. *Thorax,* 2005, 60(5): 361–362.
4. Coronavirus infection prevention and control in medical institutions: Guidelines for the first version [J]. *Chinese Journal of Infection Control,* 2020, 19(02): 189–191.
5. Technical specification of hospital isolation [J]. *Chinese Journal of Nosocomiology,* 2009, 19(13): 1612–1616.
6. Li Liuyi, Li Weiguang, Gong Yuxiu, Wang Lihong, Wu Anhua, Hu Bijie, Wei Hua, Shao Lili, Jia Huixue. Collection of 2014 Henan Nursing Association Hospital Infection Management Academic Symposium [C]. 2014.
7. Manual hygiene of medical staff [J]. *Chinese Journal of Nosocomiology,* 2009, 19(12): 1463–1464.
8. WS/T 367-2012. Technical specification for disinfection of medical institutions [S].
9. General Office of the National Health Commission, Office of the National Administration of Traditional Chinese Medicine. Notice on Issuance of coVID-19 Diagnosis and Treatment Protocol (Trial Seventh Edition) [EB/OL]. [2020-03-03].
10. Yu Pengming, He Chengqi, Gao Qiang, et al. Complete cycle physical therapy exercises for patients with COVID-19[J/OL]. *Chinese Journal of Physical Medicine and Rehabilitation,* 2020, 42. [2020-03-02].

11. National Health Commission Office. COVID-19 discharged patients rehabilitation program (trial) [J]. *China Food*, 2020(07): 142–143.
12. The consensus of rehabilitation experts during the epidemic of respiratory infectious diseases based on COVID-19 [J/OL]. *Chinese Journal of Physical Medicine and Rehabilitation*, 2020(02): 97-98-99-100-101
13. Wang Chen, Fang Guoen, Xie Yuxiao, Zhao Hongmei, Yu Pengming. Coronavirus 2019 respiratory rehabilitation guidelines (1st Edition)[J/OL]. *Chinese Journal of Reconstruction Surgery*: 1–5.
14. Recommendations for the prevention and treatment of venous thromboembolism [J/OL]. *Chinese Journal of Medicine*, 2020(11): 808-809-810-811-812-813 [2021-01-06]
15. General Office of National Health Commission of the People's Republic of China, Office of National Administration of Traditional Chinese Medicine. Diagnosis and treatment of corona virus disease-19 (7th trial edition) [J]. *China Medicine*, 2020, 15(6): 801–805. doi: 10.3760/j.issn. 1673-4777. 2020. 06. 001

Chapter 8

Management of COVID-19 Rehabilitation Nursing

COVID-19 confronted rehabilitation specialists with a new challenge. With the rapid development of rehabilitation medicine, rehabilitation nursing became a new and independent discipline with its unique theories, contents, and tasks closely related to but different from basic clinical nursing. Rehabilitation nursing emphasizes the rehabilitation of patients as the main focus, mobilizing patients' subjective initiative in rehabilitation treatment, guiding them to participate actively, and attaching importance to the role of social and psychological factors. Through rehabilitation health education, rehabilitation psychological nursing, and rehabilitation extended nursing guidance, patients' rehabilitation can be accelerated.

8.1 ESTABLISHMENT AND MANAGEMENT OF THE WARD

8.1.1 Establishment of the Rehabilitation Isolation Ward

8.1.1.1 Rational and Scientific Layout

COVID-19 is mainly transmitted through the respiratory tract, droplets, and contact, and can be transmitted sustainably from person to person Therefore, according to patients' admission and treatment requirements with respiratory infectious diseases, the disease areas are strictly divided. Following the principle of "three zones and two channels", the three zones are contaminated zones, semicontaminated zones, and clean zones; the two channels are the staff channel and patient channel, and the staff and patients go in and out separately. In the meantime, set up a buffer between the two channels and the three zones with clear and well-marked boundaries between the districts. Establish two treatment areas in the ward to meet the needs of rehabilitation treatment.

8.1.1.2 Establishment of Nursing Staff

The infectious disease nature of COVID-19 and the national recommended protection plan calls for 36 beds and two treatment areas for a COVID-19 rehabilitation ward. Twenty nursing staff are deployed by the nursing department in the face of the sudden outbreak and intensive nursing work, including 12 former rehabilitation nurses and four rehabilitation specialist nurses.

8.1.2 Establishment of the Rehabilitation Isolation Ward

8.1.2.1 Management of Nursing Personnel

Divide the 20 nurses of the department into two responsible groups with three nurses and a leader in each group. The group leader should be a rehabilitation specialist nurse. Group A's working hours are from 8:00 to 14:00, and from 14:00 to 20:00 for Group B. In addition to basic care, a COVID-19 rehabilitation and nursing plan should be customized and implemented under the leadership of the team leader. The head nurse makes nursing rounds twice a week and directs the nursing work of the responsible group. The rest are the shift group, and the clerical group and shift nurses work in pairs. By taking personal ability, specialty, and age into consideration, the nurses' strength is relatively evenly matched. Each shift is 6 hours long.

8.1.2.2 Disinfection and Isolation Management in the Ward

All rehabilitation practitioners who contact patients for assessment and treatment of respiratory rehabilitation should strictly observe and implement *Technical Guide for COVID-19 Prevention and Control in Medical Institutions (First Edition)* and *COVID-19 Guidelines for Common Use of Medical Protection (Trial)* issued by the National Health Commission (NHC).

8.1.2.2.1 Air Disinfection

Air disinfection shall be carried out following the requirements of the *Air Purification Management Standard in Hospitals.*

Open the window of occupied rooms for ventilation twice a day for 30 minutes each time, or use an air sanitizer four times a day for 2 hours each time. Make general wards as isolation wards. Air conditioners can be used if the air conditioning system is set independently; otherwise, they should be shut down.

An ultraviolet lamp is irradiated once a day for more than one hour in an unoccupied room.

It is advisable to use 3% hydrogen peroxide or 5,000 mg/L peracetic acid or 500 mg/L chlorine dioxide for disinfection through an ultralow-capacity sprayer, 20–30 mL/m^2 for 2 hours. Close doors and windows during disinfection, and disinfect in strict accordance with the concentration use, dose usage, disinfection effect time, and operation method. After disinfection, rooms can be used only after full ventilation (at least 1 hour).

8.1.2.2.2 Disinfection of Articles and Ground

1) Strictly follow the *Technical Specifications for Disinfection of Medical Institutions.*
2) Ground and walls: When there are visible contaminants, remove them entirely before disinfection. When there is no visible contaminant, disinfect by wiping and spraying 1,000 mg/L chlorine-containing disinfectant or 500 mg/L chlorine dioxide disinfectant. For ground disinfection, it is first sprayed from outside to inside with a spray amount of 100–300 mL/m^2. After disinfecting the room, spray again from inside to outside. Disinfection time should be no less than 30 minutes.
3) Article surface: When there are visible containments on the surface of medical facilities and equipment, such as bed fences, bedside tables, furniture, door handles, household items, etc., completely clean them before disinfection. If there are no visible containments, spray, wipe or soak articles with 1,000 mg/L chlorine-containing disinfectant or 500 mg/L chlorine-containing disinfectant and wipe with clean water after 30 minutes.
4) Contaminants (patient's blood, secretions, vomit, and excreta)
   a. A small amount of contaminants can be carefully removed with disposable absorbent materials (such as gauze or dishcloths) by dipping 5,000–10,000 mg/L chlorine-containing disinfectant (or disinfectant wipes that can achieve a high
   b. A large number of containments should be fully covered with disinfection powder or bleach-containing water-absorbing ingredients, or completely covered with disposable water-absorbing materials and then pour enough 5000–10000mg/L chlorine-containing disinfectant on the water-absorbing materials. Then carefully remove after more than 30 minutes.
   c. Avoid contact with containments in the process of removal, and dispose of the cleaned containments as medical waste. The excreta, secretions, and patients' vomitus should be collected in a special container and soaked and disinfected for 2 hours with 20,000 mg/L chlorine-containing disinfectant in the ratio of 1:2 for patient's contaminants and disinfectant.
   d. After the removal of contaminants, the surfaces of contaminated articles should be disinfected. Containers containing contaminants can be soaked in a disinfectant solution with 5,000 mg/L of active chlorine for 30 minutes and then wiped with clean water.

8.1.2.2.3 Disinfection of Reusable Instruments and Articles

1) Use disposable medical equipment, appliances, and articles as much as possible. The cleaning, disinfection, or sterilization of reusable medical equipment, instruments and articles should be handled following the *Technical Specifications for Disinfection of Medical Institutions*.
2) Common articles such as stethoscopes, infusion pumps, and blood pressure monitors should be thoroughly wiped and disinfected with 1,000 mg/L chlorine-containing disinfectant after each use. Thermometers should be soaked in 1,000 mg/L chlorine-containing disinfectant for 30 minutes and then cleaned and dried.

8.1.2.2.4 Medical Fabric Washing and Disinfection

Reusable medical fabrics should be disposed of following the *Technical Specification for Washing and Disinfection of Medical Fabrics in Hospital* (WS/T508-2016).

1) Avoid aerosol generation during collection and incinerate medical waste.
2) If there are no visible contaminants, the medical fabric can be disinfected by circulating steam or boiling for 30 minutes if it needs to be reused; or soak in 500 mg/L chlorine-containing disinfectant for 30 minutes and then wash as usual; or use orange-red bags for air-tight packaging, and immediately transport to the washing center, and record the hand-over.

8.1.2.2.5 Treatment of Medical Waste

The disposal of medical waste shall comply with the requirements of the *Regulations on Management of Medical Waste* and *Measures on Management of Medical Waste in Medical and Health Institutions*, and shall follow the routine disposal process after the packaging of the double-layer yellow medical waste bags.

8.1.2.2.6 Precautions for Ultraviolet Air Disinfection

1) Air disinfection: Doors and windows should be closed, and rooms should be kept clean and dry when used. Start the time after the light is on for 5–7 minutes. The effective distance is no more than 2 meters. The disinfection time is 60 minutes each time; open the window for ventilation after irradiation; stop the ultraviolet disinfection lamp's exposure when there is a need to enter the room.
2) Disinfection of article surface: Spread or hang the items to expose them to direct radiation. Ultraviolet rays cannot penetrate objects.

The distance from the lamp to the contaminated surface should not exceed 1 meter. If the lamp's ultraviolet radiation intensity meets the requirements, the exposure time should be no less than 60 minutes.

3) Personnel protection: Ultraviolet radiation causes unavoidable damage to human skin mucosa and has a stimulation effect on the deep respiratory tract and eyes. When using an ultraviolet disinfection lamp, be careful not to look directly at the ultraviolet light source. After the eyes are burned by ultraviolet ray, symptoms such as red eyes, fear of light, tears, pain will appear after 5–7 hours, and the pain will last for 24–72 hours.

4) Equipment management: The surface of the ultraviolet lamp should be clean during the use. Wipe it once a week with 75% alcohol cotton balls. If there is dust or oil on the surface of the lamp tube, wipe it at any time.

8.1.2.2.7 Precautions for Using Chlorine-Containing Disinfectants

1) Skin corrosion: Chlorine-containing disinfectants should not be sprayed directly on the face for disinfection. Long-term contact with chlorine-containing disinfectants will erode the skin. Its chemical properties are very active and toxic, so personnel must wear gloves when using chlorine-containing disinfectants and wash their hands afterward.

2) Stimulation of the nerve system and respiratory tract: Do not use chlorine-containing disinfectant in an acidic environment, as it will produce toxic chlorine, and then stimulate the nerve system and respiratory tract.

3) Chronic disease induction: chlorine is a strong irritant gas, causing sore eyes and tears, throat itching, and dyspnea. Long-term inhalation may cause chronic poisoning, rhinitis, chronic bronchitis, emphysema, and liver cirrhosis.

4) Instability after water dissolving: chlorine disinfectants dissolved in water can produce substances that can inhibit microbial activity and can also kill all kinds of microorganisms, including bacterial propagator, virus, fungus, mycobacterium tuberculosis, and the most resistant bacterial spores. However, it is susceptible to light, heat, and humidity and is unstable when dissolved in water, so it can be a health hazard if not used properly.

8.1.2.3 Protection Management of Medical Staff

All rehabilitation practitioners who are in contact with patients for rehabilitation treatment and care shall strictly comply with the requirements of the

Technical Guide for COVID-19 Prevention and Control in Medical Institutions (First Edition) and *COVID-19 Guidelines for Common Use of Medical Protection (Trial)* issued by the NHC. The Office of Hospital Infection Management organizes online and offline training guidance uniformly. The head nurse assesses wearing and taking off protective equipment for all staff in the department and is responsible for the supervision and inspection of disinfection, isolation, and use of protective equipment for each person in and out of the area, especially for the therapists, cleaning workers, and other staff, giving on-site correction for existing problems.

COVID-19 is highly contagious. Strengthening the protection awareness of medical personnel should be given top priority. The health registration of all on-duty staff shall be carried out by the department's special staff at work. After work, nurses are required to take a hot bath, wash their hair and hands with running water after leaving the isolation area.

8.1.2.3.1 Protection Classification and Requirements

1) Low-risk areas: People with low probability of direct contact with patients, patients' contaminants, contaminated articles, and environmental surface.
   a. Requirements: Strictly take standard preventive measures; wear work clothes, disposable work caps, and disposable surgical masks; strictly observe hand hygiene during medical treatment and the removal of personal protective equipment.
2) High-risk areas: All medical personnel have direct or potential contact with patients, the patient's contaminants, contaminated articles, and environmental surfaces.
   a. Requirements: Strictly take standard preventive measures; wear work clothes, protective clothing, medical protective masks, goggles/face masks, disposable hats, and latex gloves, and shoe covers if necessary. When performing operations that may produce aerosols (such as endotracheal intubation and related operations, cardiopulmonary resuscitation, bronchoscopy, sputum aspiration, throat swab sampling) for patients with suspected or confirmed cases and when using high-speed equipment (such as drilling, sawing, centrifugal operation), medical personnel should take three-level protection, that is, add a comprehensive type of protective mask for secondary protection.
3) Order of putting on and taking off protective equipment (tertiary prevention):
   a. Putting on: Wash hands, wear a medical protective mask (do a tightness test), wear a disposable round cap, wear goggles/face masks, wear gloves, wear protective clothing, wear a comprehensive

protective mask or respirator, wear shoe covers, and wear a second layer of gloves.

b. Taking off: Remove the outer gloves, wash hands, remove the comprehensive protective mask or respirator, wash hands, remove the protective clothing and shoe covers, wash hands, remove the goggles/protective mask, wash hands, remove the disposable round cap, wash hands, remove the medical protective mask, wash hands, change personal clothes.

8.1.2.3.2 Hand Hygiene
The hand-washing method of medical personnel shall be strictly carried out following the "six-step washing method" stipulated in the *Hand Hygiene Standards for Medical Personnel*.

Quick-drying hand disinfectant is preferred when sanitizing hands, and other hand sanitizers can be used for allergic people. Chlorhexidine is ineffective in inactivating coronavirus, so it is not recommended. Hand disinfectants containing chlorine, alcohol, hydrogen peroxide, and other ingredients are recommended.

Wearing gloves should not replace hand hygiene. Hand hygiene should be carried out after removing gloves.

8.2 REHABILITATION NURSING OF CHINESE AND WESTERN MEDICINE

8.2.1 Objective of Rehabilitation Nursing

The first objective is to improve patients' life quality, prevent respiratory complications, improve respiratory function, and enhance mental health.

The second objective is to develop individualized nursing programs. It is essential to fully understand patients' conditions in the formulation of a rehabilitation nursing plan. Teach step by step according to the different stages of the disease and publicize rehabilitation nursing knowledge to patients. Mobilize patients' subjective initiative, actively cooperate with rehabilitation treatment and nursing, and let patients do progressive exercise to improve sports endurance.

The third objective is to use traditional Chinese medicine (TCM) nursing programs to improve fever, insomnia, gastrointestinal disorders, and other problems.

8.2.2 Rehabilitation Nursing Assessment

Based on the comprehensive collection of patients' subjective and objective data, the following contents should be emphasized in patients' nursing assessment with COVID-19.

8.2.2.1 Course of Onset and Treatment

8.2.2.1.1 Course of Illness

Understand the onset time, main symptoms, and concomitant symptoms, such as cough, sputum, dyspnea, hemoptysis, chest pain, etc., and their manifestations and characteristics; ask whether there is an inducement, symptom aggravation, and related factors or rules of mitigation.

8.2.2.1.2 Diagnostic and Therapeutic Process

Ask the patients what kind of tests they have had and the results, the names or types of drugs used, drug usage, the time of the last use, whether the drugs were used after the doctor prescribed, and the improvement of symptoms after the use.

8.2.2.1.3 Current Status

The disease impacts the patient's daily life and self-care ability, for example, dyspnea can affect the patient's daily eating, rest, and excretion, and can even decline self-care ability.

8.2.2.1.4 Relevant Medical History

Obtain patients' history of diseases related to respiratory diseases, such as allergic diseases, measles, pertussis, and cardiovascular diseases.

8.2.2.2 Psychosocial Data

8.2.2.2.1 Knowledge about the Disease

Determine patients' understanding of the occurrence, course, prognosis, and health care of the disease.

8.2.2.2.2 Psychological Status

Persistent cough, chest pain, dyspnea, and other symptoms may cause adverse emotional reactions.

8.2.2.2.3 Social Support Systems

Know necessary and basic information of patients, such as their family members, economic status, and educational background, etc. Ask the primary caregivers of patients about their understanding of the disease, the degrees of care, and their support for the patients.

8.2.3 Rehabilitation Nursing Measures

Patients with COVID-19 are at risk of respiratory dysfunction at all stages of the disease. In addition to monitoring patients' vital signs and observing the blood oxygen saturation and rehabilitation routine care closely, nursing staff can effectively help patients relieve symptoms, restore function and improve life quality by using specialized rehabilitation nursing techniques, such as respiratory function guidance, cough training, posture drainage, muscle strength, and endurance training as well as psychological rehabilitation nursing guidance.

8.2.3.1 Nursing Guidance and Training Techniques for Respiratory Function

8.2.3.1.1 Definition

Respiratory function training refers to the training methods used to ensure the respiratory tract's patency, improve respiratory muscle function, promote sputum excretion and drainage, improve blood metabolism of lung and bronchial tissues, and strengthen gas exchange efficiency.

8.2.3.1.2 Purpose

1) COVID-19 patients are prone to dyspnea during activities. Improve respiratory function through the control and regulation of respiratory movements to restore effective abdominal breathing as far as possible.
2) Increase the voluntary movements of respiratory muscles and respiratory capacity to improve oxygen inhalation and carbon dioxide emissions.
3) Improve the observance of the chest through active training and increase the abilities of patients' cardiopulmonary function and physical activity.

8.2.3.1.3 Key Points of Operation

1) Half-closed lip respiration training
   a. Position: Sit upright with hands on knees.
   b. Lips shrink into a "whistling" shape. Allow gas to enter through the nostrils as inhale inhaling. Do not exhale in a hurry after each inhalation, but hold the breath for a while and then exhale through half-closed lips. When exhaling, retract the lips to be like a whistle, and gently blow air out of lungs through a narrow mouth. Each exhalation lasts 4–6 seconds. Inhale and exhale for a ratio of 1 to 2. Practice three to four times a day for 15–30 minutes each time.
2) Abdominal breath training: Diaphragmatic breathing is emphasized to improve abnormal breathing patterns, diaphragmatic contraction capacity, and contraction efficiency and change patients' thoracic breathing into abdominal breathing. Abdominal breathing and half-closed lip respiration can be used.

    a.   Position: Patients shall be placed in the supine position or sitting position (leaning forward position); or take a forward-leaning standing position. Let the patients breathe normally and relax as much as possible. First, close the mouth and inhale deeply through the nose. At this point, the abdomen will raise and lower the diaphragm as much as possible. Hold the breath for 2–3 seconds when patients can no longer breathe in (gradually increase to 5–10 seconds after practice); then use a half-closed lip to exhale slowly, meanwhile, recover the abdomen as much as possible, and blow slowly for 4–6 seconds. Simultaneously, gradually press hands on the abdomen to promote the upward movement of the diaphragm; also, place hands over the costal arch and, during exhalation, apply pressure to reduce the thoracic cavity and facilitate gas expulsion.

    b.   Take a deep and slow breath; The exhalation time must be two to three times of the inhalation time. The frequency of in-depth breathing training is 8–10 times per minute, lasting 3–5 minutes, and should be done several times a day. After proficiency, increase the number of times and length of time of the training.

3) Respiratory muscle training

    a.   Inspiratory resistance training: (a) Patients hold the handgrip resistance trainer to inhale. The trainer has tubes of various diameters. (b) Pipes with different diameters have different airflow resistance during suction. The narrower the pipe diameter is, the more excellent the airflow resistance will be. (c) On the premise that patients can accept, first select the pipe with a thick diameter for inspiratory training and start the training for 3–5 minutes per time. After training three to five times per day, the training duration can be gradually increased to 20–30 minutes per time.

    b.   Expiratory muscle training: (a) Abdominal muscle training requires patients to be placed in the supine position, with a 1–2 kg sandbag placed on the upper abdomen. Keep the shoulders and chest still while inhaling and try to hold out the abdomen while exhaling. Do lower limb flexion, hip flexion, and knee flexion while in the supine position and keep knees as close to the chest wall as possible to strengthen abdominal muscles. (b) For candle blowing training, place a lit candle 10 cm in front of the patient's mouth, and blow out forcefully after inhalation to extinguish the flame. Rest for a few minutes after 3–5 minutes' training each time, and then repeat. (c) Patients do expiratory training by holding a resistance trainer to improve the expiratory muscle capacity.

8.2.3.1.4 Cautions

1) Education and cooperation of patients
   a. Examine and provide the patients with health education and explain the significance and purpose of respiratory function training before training. Try to avoid causing patients emotional tension during training by explaining well and obtaining their cooperation.
   b. The training plan should vary from person to person, step by step in the training process, and encourage patients to persevere.
   c. Evaluate patients and make specific training plans. The training is scheduled between meals.
   d. Material preparation: Simple breathing trainer and candle.
2) Position exercise
   a. Position selection: Choose a relaxed and comfortable position. Proper position can relax the auxiliary respiratory muscle group, reduce the oxygen consumption of respiratory muscles, relieve dyspnea symptoms, stabilize the mood, fix and relax the shoulder band muscle group, reduce the upper chest activity, and facilitate the diaphragm movement, etc.
   b. Low head position and forward position: (a) Allows patients to lie on their back on a bed or flat bed that has been adjusted to tilt, with the foot of the bed raised (postural drainage in the same position). (b) Forward leaning refers to keeping the torso tilted 20°–45° when the patient is sitting. To maintain balance, the patient can support their knee with their elbow or on the table. When standing or walking, the patient can also take the forward-leaning position, or they can also use a walking stick or walk assisting car for support.
3) Precautions during respiratory function training
   a. The frequency of abdominal breathing should not be too much each time, that is, after practicing two to three times, take a rest and then practice again. Let patients gradually get used to abdominal breathing in activities. Each training is generally 5–10 minutes to avoid fatigue.
   b. Relax and exhale passively to avoid abdominal contraction. Place both hands on the patient's abdominal muscles to determine whether the abdominal muscles have contracted.
   c. Pay attention to the patient's response. There should be no discomfort symptoms during training. The patient should feel normal when they get up the next morning. If they feel tired, weak, dizzy, and other discomforts, stop the training temporarily.

d. When the condition changes, the training program should be adjusted in time to avoid respiratory acidosis and respiratory failure induced in the training process.

e. Give oxygen appropriately during training. Doing activities while inhaling oxygen can enhance the patient's activity confidence.

8.2.3.2 Nursing Guidance and Training Techniques for Effective Coughing

8.2.3.2.1 Definition

Patients should be guided through effective cough precautionary measures, which is conducive to the discharge of secretions at the far end of the airway, so as to improve lung ventilation, keep the respiratory tract open, reduce repeated infections, and improve the patient's lung function.

8.2.3.2.2 Purpose

1) Keep the respiratory tract unobstructed and avoid sputum accumulation.
2) Discharge of airway secretions effectively and promote disease recovery.
3) Prevent infection and reduce postoperative complications.

8.2.3.2.3 Key Points of Operation

1) Instruct patients to take a comfortable and relaxed position. Guide them to inhale slowly and deeply, close the glottis briefly, and increase the pressure in the pleural cavity. Then tell them to quickly open the glottis and force the abdomen to expel gas, which will also cause coughing. Inhale once and cough three times continuously.
2) Stop coughing and exhale the rest of the gas in the half-closed lip as far as possible.
3) Inhale slowly and deeply again and repeat the above actions. Rest and breathe normally after doing this two to three times in a row. Start again after a few minutes, combined with the back clapping technique if necessary. (To perform the back clapping technique, close the fingers into a cup, and tap evenly and rhythmically with the strength of the wrist, from bottom to top and from outside to inside. The intensity should be appropriate, so as not to make patients feel pain).
4) Patients should be instructed to cover the sputum with tissue to avoid splashing. After sputum excretion, let them take a comfortable position and conduct pulmonary auscultation.

8.2.3.2.4 Precautions

1) Education and cooperation of patients
   a. Explain the significance and purpose of respiratory function training before training. Try to avoid causing patients emotional tension during training by explaining well and obtaining their cooperation.
   b. Tell the patients to be prepared.
2) Effective coughing and right position
   a. According to the needs of the disease, take comfortable positions. Take five to six deep breaths first and hold the breath at the end of deep inhalation, then cough several times to bring sputum to the pharynx, and cough hard to expel it.
   b. Let the patients take a sitting position with a pillow on both legs and positioned against the abdomen to promote diaphragm elevation. Lean forward and bend head and neck when coughing, and cough with mouth open to expel sputum.
   c. Ask patients to take a lateral position with knees bent that is conducive to the diaphragmatic muscle, abdominal muscle contraction, and increased abdominal pressure. Frequently change the position, which benefits sputum coughing.
3) Precautions for effective cough training
   a. Avoid paroxysmal coughing and keep quiet breathing for a while after coughing for three times. People with a history of cerebrovascular rupture, embolism, or hemangioma should avoid coughing vigorously.
   b. Based on the patient's body shape, nutritional status, cough tolerance degree, select an effective cough training mode, time, and frequency. In general, it should be arranged 1 to 2 hours before or 2 hours after the patient's meal. Patients with continuous nasogastric feeding should be discontinued 30 minutes before operation.
   c. Check the patient's chest and abdomen for wounds and take appropriate measures to avoid or relieve the pain caused by cough. Ask the patient to gently press the wound area or use a pillow to press the wound so as to counteract or resist the local pull and pain in the wound caused by coughing.
   d. Follow the principle of labor-saving and safety. Closely observe the changes in patients' consciousness and vital signs during operation.
   e. The operator should keep a distance of 1–2 meters from the patient and instruct them to use tissue paper.

f. Evaluation indexes of effective cough and sputum excretion: Decreased sputum volume per day < 25 mL; respiratory sounds are improved at the lesion site, without moist rales; patients' good response to the treatment; improved blood oxygen saturation and chest radiograph.

8.2.3.3 Nursing Guidance and Training Techniques of Postural Drainage

8.2.3.3.1 Definition

Postural drainage refers to gravity drainage of secretions combined with thoracic manipulation, such as back clapping and tremor, most of which can achieve obvious clinical effects.

8.2.3.3.2 Purpose

Changing patients' positions by using the principle of gravity is conducive to secretion discharge. It can also improve pulmonary ventilation, increase ventilation blood flow ratio, prevent or reduce pulmonary infection, maintain the patency of the respiratory tract, reduce repeated infection, and improve the patient's lung function.

8.2.3.3.3 Key Points of Operation

1) Postural drainage is conducted by different postures according to the lesion site. If the lesion is in the upper lobe of both lungs, take the sitting position or other appropriate posture; if the lesion is in the anterior segment of the upper lobe of the left lung and the middle lobe of the right lung, the head can be taken with a height of 30° lower than the foot; if the lesion is in the left lower lobe and right lower lobe, the head can be taken with a height of 45° lower than the foot to facilitate drainage.

2) If the secretions do not come out after 5–10 minutes of drainage, perform the next position. The total time should not be more than 30–45 minutes, generally once in the morning and afternoon.

8.2.3.3.4 Precautions

1) Education and cooperation of patients
   a. Explain the purpose and method of postural drainage before sputum discharge. Eliminate the patient's tension so that they can cooperate well.
   b. Inform the patients and family members in a precise manner. Tell the patients to drink warm water during sputum discharge, to dilute the sputum and discharge efficiently.

2) Precautions for postural drainage
   a. Postural drainage and sputum excretion: It is suitable for patients with broncho-pulmonary disease who have large amounts of sputum. The principle of this activity is that it elevates the affected lung's position, makes the opening of drainage bronchus downward, and takes the corresponding position according to the lesion site and the patient's own experience. Drain the area with the most sputum first, then move on to another area. During drainage, encourage patients to breathe deeply and cough effectively, supplemented by percussive tremors. Perform drainage for 15 minutes each time, one to three times a day. Nurses or family members should assist in the drainage process to prevent falling out of bed. Pay attention to the patient's reaction during the drainage, and stop immediately if the patient experiences hemoptysis, dizziness, and cyanosis dyspnea, sweating, fine pulse speed, fatigue, and other conditions.
   b. During drainage, try to make the patients comfortable and relaxed, and guide them to breathe easily without excessive ventilation or shortness of breath. The drainage position should not be performed rigidly, for example, adopt the positions that are acceptable to the patients and that easily discharge sputum. Observe the patient's face and expression, and adjust the posture or stop the drainage at any time if the patient is not in good condition. The specialist should prepare sputum aspirator and stay with patients during treatment to avoid suffocating and falling from bed. Allow patients to sit up slowly and rest for a while after drainage to prevent postural hypotension.
   c. Avoid paroxysmal cough during the training process and pay attention to calm breathing for a while after coughing three times. People with a history of cerebrovascular rupture, embolism, or hemangioma should avoid coughing vigorously.
   d. Drainage should be arranged in the morning after waking up because the bronchial ciliary movement is weakened at night, and airway secretions are prone to retention during sleep.

8.2.3.4 Nursing Guidance and Training Techniques for Enhancing Muscle Strength and Endurance

8.2.3.4.1 Definition
Enhancing muscle strength and endurance training techniques refers to the rehabilitation techniques that use various rehabilitation training methods to gradually enhance muscle strength and endurance, improve the body's motor function, and promote muscle function recovery.

8.2.3.4.2. Purpose

The physical dysfunction of COVID-19 patients is usually characterized by general fatigue, easy fatigue, and muscle soreness, some of which may be accompanied by muscle atrophy and decreased muscle strength. Strengthen the original decreased muscle through muscle strength training. Enhance muscle endurance so that the muscle can maintain long-term contraction. Functional training enhances muscle strength through muscle training, which prepares the patient for functional training for balance and coordination gait in the future.

8.2.3.4.3 Key Points of Operation

Use sandbags, dumbbells, elastic bands, or bottled water for progressive strength and resistance training for limbs, with 15–20 movements per group, one to two groups per day, 3–5 days per week. Do it when exhaling because building muscle endurance is more important than muscle strength in COVID-19 patients. The load should be carried out at high frequency and low tension.

8.2.3.4.4 Precautions

1) Select the appropriate training method. The effect of improving muscle strength is directly related to the selected training method. Before training, assess the range of motion of the joint and the extent of muscle strength at the training site and select a training method according to the existing muscle strength level.

2) Make reasonable adjustments to exercise intensity. The intensity includes weight and repetition rate. Adjust the intensity and time of training at any time according to the patient's condition, and record the patient's training condition, including their adaptability to the exercise load during the training, whether the amount of exercise is suitable for the training, the patient's condition during the training, and the progress of muscle strength test at any time before and after the training. The maximum resistance weight for patients should be appropriate, less than the maximum contractile force of their muscles. The weight or resistance applied should be constant to avoid sudden violence or increased resistance.

3) Avoid overtraining. Muscle training should be done painlessly. Training is advisable when patients do not feel tired or sore the day after training. The increase of pain or fatigue the next morning indicates that the exercise is excessive. According to patients' general condition (quality, physical strength) and local condition (joint activity, muscle strength), select an appropriate training method. Patients can train one to two times a day for 20–30 minutes each time. They can be trained in groups with 1–2 minute breaks. The nursing staff should

explain the exercise well and ask for the patient's reaction at the time of training and the next morning to adjust the training plan.

4) Pay attention to cardiovascular reactions. There will be different degrees of a stress reaction in the cardiovascular system during exercise. When the isometric resistance is considerable, it has an obvious reaction of raising blood pressure, and isometric exercise is accompanied by extra load on the cardiovascular system. Therefore, patients with hypertensive heart disease or other cardiovascular diseases should be contraindicated from excessive exertion or breath-holding during the exercise of equal length of strength, including weight resistance.

8.2.3.5 Psychological Rehabilitation Nursing

COVID-19 patients are often accompanied by a series of different psychological dysfunction degrees, such as fear, anxiety, anger, depression, even post-traumatic stress disorder and other pressures and burdens. Improving patients' psychological problems and promoting psychological rehabilitation are important links in the diagnosis and treatment of COVID-19. Nurses at work should analyze patients' psychological needs with existing or potential psychological problems, grasp their psychological state, and find out their psychological problems. Use the theory, method, and technology of psychology to provide care, support, and help to patients; reduce or eliminate negative emotions; enhance the ability to adapt to the disease state; and encourage their belief that they will overcome the disease to promote patients' recovery.

8.2.3.5.1 Psychological Rehabilitation Nursing Goals

Psychological rehabilitation nursing goals can be divided into a phased goal and ultimate goal. The phased goal is establishing a good nurse–patient relationship to achieve effective communication so that patients can gradually have beneficial changes in cognition, emotion, and behavior. The ultimate goal of psychological nursing is to promote the development of patients, including their self-realization, self-acceptance, and self-respect; improve their self-confidence and personal perfection; enhance their ability to establish harmonious interpersonal relationships and meet their needs; and acquire personal goals of adaptation. The specific objectives are as follows:

1) Improve patients' adaptability.
2) Establish a harmonious doctor–patient relationship, nurse–patient relationship, and relationship among patients.
3) Accept the role of the patient, recognize the disease, and treat it correctly.
4) Reduce or eliminate patients' adverse emotional reactions, such as tension, anxiety, pessimism, depression, etc.; mobilize their subjective

initiative; establish their confidence to overcome the disease; and fight against the disease with a positive attitude.

5) Meet the practical needs of patients.

8.2.3.5.2 Common Methods of Psychological Rehabilitation Therapy

1) Supportive psychotherapy.
2) Music relaxation therapy.
3) Rational emotion therapy.

8.2.3.5.3 Psychological Rehabilitation Nursing Measures

1) Do well in supportive psychological care.
2) Make full use of psychological and social support to help patients develop a positive emotional state to participate in group activities and outdoor sports so that they can realize their social value. Help patients resolve the psychological crisis by applying active psychological defense mechanisms.
3) Create a good rehabilitation environment to promote the rehabilitation of patients. A good environment, including physical environment, psychological environment, social environment, and medical environment, can positively impact patients' psychological activities.
4) Strengthen communication with the patient's family members, encourage them to accompany the patient more, and guide them to give more care and comfort to them. It is commonly recognized that family care is the best way to arouse the patient's survival awareness.

8.2.4 TCM Nursing

8.2.4.1 Instructions for Taking TCM Decoctions

Instruct patients to take COVID-19 TCM prescriptions twice a day. Pay attention to the reaction and effect after taking medicine.

8.2.4.2 Appropriate TCM Nursing Techniques

8.2.4.2.1 Acupoint Application

The purpose of acupoint application is to improve patients' symptoms, such as loss of appetite, fever, and fatigue.

1) Operational steps and precautions
   a. Keep everything ready. Let patients take an appropriate posture, fully expose the application site, select the right acupoints, and keep them warm.

b. The operators should wash hands, disinfect, and dry the patient's skin, stick cold moxibustion on the acupoints, and pay attention to prevent the plaster from falling off after sticking the medicine. If necessary, add paper tape for fixation. If patients are allergic to paper tape, use transparent tape instead (plaster on thoracic and abdominal acupoints are not easy to fall off, but should be fixed appropriately on leg acupoints).

c. During and after application, observe and ask the patient if there is any local skin discomfort. If there is severe itching and intense burning sensation, remove it immediately.

d. It is recommended to treat once every 3–5 days and apply for 8 hours each time according to the instructions. If there is discomfort, shorten the application time. The specific time should be determined according to the patient's constitution.

e. Small blisters that appear on some patients after treatment can be absorbed by themselves. Puncture the bottom of the blister with a sterile needle and apply gauze externally to prevent infection; if there is a large area of severe skin erythema or itching, stop the treatment, and apply local skin disinfection or antiallergic treatment.

2) Acupoint selection

a. A box of two plasters can be applied to two acupoints. After clinical trial application by colleagues, it is suggested that the acupoints of limbs, chest, and abdomen should be mainly used, which is safer and simpler because this moxibustion paste will cause heat, and it is difficult to deal with the back and waist after being burned. Additionally, because there are no extensive heating facilities in the ward, having patients put on and take off clothing causes them to easily catch a cold, which is not conducive to recovery.

3) According to *Diagnosis and Treatment Protocol for COVID-19 (7th Trial Edition)*, the clinical syndrome types are promulgated:

a. Medical observation period: Zhongwan, gunagyuan, and zusanli.

b. Mild (syndrome of the cold-damp stagnating the lung), moderate (syndrome of cold-damp obstructing the lung): gunagyuan, hegu, zusanli, and taichong.

c. Convalescent period (syndrome of *qi* deficiency of the lung and spleen): Dazhui, feishu, geshu, zusanli, and kongzui.

d. Convalescent period (syndrome of *qi* and *yin* deficiency): Zusanli, danzhong, qihai, and yinlingquan.

4) Acupoints location

a. Zusanli is located on the outside of the lower leg, 3 cun on the connecting line below dubi and jiexi.

b. Yinlingquan is inside the lower leg and in the posterior depression of the medial condyle of the tibia.
c. Danzhong is between the nipples, on the midline of the sternum, and it levels with the fourth intercostal space.
d. Zhongwan is located at the upper abdomen and on the anterior median line, 4 cun above the umbilicus.
e. Qihai is located 1.5 cun below the umbilicus in the anterior midline.
f. Guangyuan is located 3 cun below the umbilicus in the anterior midline.

8.2.4.2.2 Auricular Plaster Therapy

In auricular plaster therapy, vaccaria beads or press-needle sticks are applied to the corresponding auricular point followed by a little pressure to the acupoint to produce a feeling of sour, numb, swelling, or fever. This method improves insomnia, gastrointestinal disorders, endocrine disorders, and other symptoms caused by excessive pressure.

1) Acupoint selection: Endocrine, shenmen, sympathetic, occipital acupoint, spleen and large intestine, etc.
2) Operation method: Choose vaccaria segetalis beads or press-needle stick to make the patient's auricle feel sore, numb, or hot. After sticking, press the acupoints several times a day, 3–5 minutes each time, alternating ears, three to five times a day for 2–3 days.

8.2.4.2.3 Precautions

Patients with skin ulceration, skin allergy, and scar constitution are forbidden.
Strictly follow the operation method to the extent that patients can tolerate the treatment.
Strictly disinfect to prevent infection. Ear disinfection should be done according to the operation specifications before an operation.
It should be operated by personnel with solid knowledge of TCM.

8.2.4.3 Emotion Nursing

Emotion nursing has existed since ancient times. Remove psychological pressure of patients, try to persuade patients not to rely too much on drugs, strengthen mental care, pay attention to their emotional changes, eliminate their doubts, enlighten, inform, comfort, and keep their mood positive and comfortable to help them to recover their psychological and physiological functions and promote the rehabilitation of the disease. Meanwhile, the TCM method of tempering should be combined.

8.2.4.3.1 Therapy of Calming the Mind

In addition to creating objective conditions (such as a quiet living environment) for patients to be calm and refreshed, remind patients to maintain a spotless mind, think less, and be spiritual and calm. Qigong therapy plays a leading role in regulating the spirit. Its emphasis on tranquility can achieve the tranquil state of "true *qi* follows tranquil nothingness and the internal defense keeps disease away" described in *Huangdi Neijing*.

8.2.4.3.2 Therapy of Emotions and Depression Relieving

This method has a certain effect on some diseases of internal injury. Only patients who reveal their inner depression can allow *qi* to be relaxed.

8.2.4.3.3 Therapy of Emotion Being Diverted

This therapy is also called empathy therapy or transference therapy, with specific methods and measures, in which the patient's mood and will are transferred or changed, freeing them from bad emotions. Hobbies such as music, dance, piano, chess, calligraphy, and painting can help ease the mind and benefit patients' physical and mental health. There is also a sports transference method, such as making friends in tourist attractions, flowers planting, and fishing.

8.2.4.3.4 Therapy of Doubt Analysis

This therapy removes patients' misunderstanding and avoids disease aggravation because of reticence and personality depression impeded *qi*. Also, avoid patients' extreme suspicion.

8.2.4.3.5 Therapy of Emotion Interresistance

This form of therapy focuses on how one kind of emotion suppresses another to harmonize emotions. It is also called the emotional restriction method. For example, the disease caused by excessive anger can be treated with bitter words, sudden mental shock and joy can create mood swings, and excessive thinking can provoke anger.

8.3 DISCHARGE GUIDANCE AND HEALTH EDUCATION

8.3.1 Attention to Diet

The chosen diet should be nutrient rich, high calorie, high protein, high vitamin, and easily digestible. Patients should be encouraged to eat more fresh fruits and vegetables and increase their intake of nutrients through the supplement and adjustment of diet, to improve the nutritional status and respiratory muscle function.

8.3.2 Adherence to Breathing Training and Activities

Arrange appropriate activities according to specific situations. Combine abdominal breathing exercises with general systemic exercises, such as qigong, tai chi chuan, medical walking, etc., and stick to rehabilitation exercises during remission.

8.3.3 Disease Prevention

Measures can be taken to prevent colds and respiratory infections.

1) Cold-resistant exercise: Before the winter, wash the nose with cold water two to three times a day for 2–3 minutes each time. Cold water can also be used to wash the face, and prevent cold by self-massaging the nose, Yingxiang acupoint, kneading fengchi acupoint, etc.
2) Improve respiratory and immune function by regularly practicing good living habits, such as balanced nutrition, combining work with rest, exercising regularly, ceasing smoking, and restricting alcohol, etc.

BIBLIOGRAPHY

1. Cheng Caie, Li Xiuyun. *Practical Rehabilitation Nursing* [M]. 2nd edition, Beijing: People's Medical Publishing House, 2012.
2. Zhang Longhao, Li Baihong, Jia Peng, Pu Jian, Bai Bei, Li Yin, Zhu Peijia, Li Lei, Zeng Guojun, Zhao Xin, Dong Shanshan, Liu Menghan, Zhang Nan. Novel coronavirus (SARS-COV-2) global research status analysis [J]. *Journal of Biomedical Engineering*, 2020, 37(2): 1–6.
3. Miao Xue, Gu Bo, Jiang Yan, XUE Miao, GU Bo, JIANG Yan, YUAN Li, HUANG Hao, LI Lingli, WU Xiaoling, XIANG Xi, ZHANG Yao-zhi, LUO Lan. Establishment and management of isolation wards for suspected COVID-19 patients [J]. *Journal of Nursing Advancement*, 2020, 35(8): 727–728. [2020-03-12].
4. Zhang Y, Zhang Y, Wang Y. Coronavirus infection in the Chinese medical hospital [J]. *Chinese Journal of Infection Control*, 2020, 19(02): 189–191.
5. The use of medical protective equipment for prevention and control of coronavirus infection [J]. *Chinese Journal of Nursing Management*, 20, 20(02): 164.
6. WS/T 368-2012, Hospital Air Purification Management Practice [S].
7. Li Liu-yi, Zhang Liu-bo, Yao Chushui, Chen Shunlan, Ban Haiqun, Hu Guoqing, Zhang Yu, Ding Yanming, Lu Qun, Qian Liming, Liu Kun, Xing Shuxia, Ren Wuai, Huang Jingxiong, Jia Huixue, Yao Hui, Huang Huiping. Technical specification for disinfection of medical institutions [A]. Henan Provincial Nursing Association. Proceedings of 2014 Henan Provincial Nursing Association Hospital Infection Management Professional Academic Symposium [C]. *Henan Provincial Nursing Association*, 2014: 40.

8. Technical specification of hospital medical fabric washing and disinfection WS/T 508-2016 [J]. *Chinese Journal of Infection Control*, 2017, 16(07): 687–692.

9. Medical waste management regulations [A]. Henan Province Nursing Association. Compilation of the senior seminar and academic conference on the construction and management of modern disinfection supply center (room) of Henan Nursing Association [C]. *Henan Nursing Association: Henan Nursing Association*, 2007: 2.

10. Measures for the management of medical waste in medical and health institutions [J]. Bulletin of the State Council of the People's Republic of China, 2004 (18): 30–35.

11. Practice of hand hygiene for medical personnel [J]. *Chinese Journal of Nosocomiology*, 2020, 30(05): 797–800.

12. You Liming, Wu Ying. *Internal Nursing Science [M]*. 5th edition, Beijing: People's Medical Publishing House, 2012.

13. Cheng Caie, Li Xiuyun. *Operation Rules of Rehabilitation Nursing Technology [M]*. Beijing: People's Medical Publishing House, 2018.

14. National Health Commission, National Administration of Traditional Chinese Medicine. Notice on Issuance of Advice on Chinese Medicine Rehabilitation Guidance during COVID-19 Convalescent Period (Trial) [EB/OL]. [2020-02-22].

15. Yue Yang. Clinical application characteristics, influencing factors and Prospects of TCM Nursing Technology [J]. *Journal of Traditional Chinese Medicine Management*, 2019, 27(7): 72–73.

16. General Office of the National Health Commission, Office of the National Administration of Traditional Chinese Medicine. Notice on Issuance of coVID-19 Diagnosis and Treatment Protocol (Trial Seventh Edition) [EB/OL]. [2020-03-03].

17. Zhang Li. On the emotional nursing method of traditional Chinese medicine [J]. *Guangming Chinese Medicine*, 2011, 26(9): 1904.

Chapter 9

Clinical Rehabilitation of COVID-19

9.1 GUIDING PRINCIPLES AND CONNOTATIONS OF REHABILITATION INTERVENTION

Due to systemic inflammatory response and immune system dysfunction caused by a viral infection, COVID-19 patients may suffer different degrees of damage in various systems of the human body. Most patients' symptoms can be gradually alleviated after active treatment, but patients often suffer from respiratory, physical, psychological, and social dysfunction to varying degrees. Therefore, active rehabilitation intervention is needed to promote patients' comprehensive rehabilitation and improve their quality of life. *Comprehensive Guidance on Rehabilitation and Diagnosis during COVID-19 (Second Edition)* formulated by the Chinese Association of Rehabilitation Medicine makes it clear that, on the premise of safety protection, appropriate and feasible rehabilitation intervention should be provided to patients with different stages of COVID-19 according to their psychological state, cardiopulmonary function, physical ability, and other conditions.

9.1.1 Guiding Principles of Rehabilitation

9.1.1.1 Adherence to the Whole-Course Psychological Intervention

Provide patients in different stages of the disease and their families with psychological counseling through WeChat, videos, science popularization, and other means. Through appropriate musical intervention and relaxation meditation, relieve their fear of disease and learn to relax themselves to bravely face the difficulties in reality and overcome the disease.

9.1.1.2 Safe and Effective Improvement of Cardiopulmonary Function

Instruct patients to master the correct breathing methods and adopt various respiratory function training methods to improve their respiratory function to the maximum extent.

9.1.1.3 Gradual and Steady Improvement of Physical Fitness

Patients often have a decline in physical function due to dyspnea and reduced activity. All kinds of rehabilitation activities should be carried out according to local conditions and individual condition to improve patients' physical ability. Adjust the treatment in time based on the change of the patient's condition. Give appropriate physiotherapy under strict prevention and control measures.

9.1.2 Connotations of Rehabilitation Intervention

9.1.2.1 Improvement/Enhancement of Cardiopulmonary Function

Instruct patients to master correct breathing methods to improve respiratory function to the maximum extent, such as appropriate body position, effectual breathing patterns, various types of breathing exercises, and a decline in respiratory function. Carry out traditional Chinese medicine (TCM) rehabilitation actively and selectively practice tai chi chuan, baduanjin, and five-animal exercise to improve patients' respiratory function and please their bodies and minds according to patients' condition and location. The intensity is based on the patient's absence of worsening symptoms or discomfort. Selectively use targeted physical factor therapy; use the microthermal ultrashort wave to reduce lung inflammation; adopt the chest air pressure device with the special liner to assist the thoracic movement and improve respiratory function.

9.1.2.2 Enhancement of Activity/Physical Strength

Guide patients to carry out active physical activities according to their conditions to improve their bodies immunity and promote their body function to return to the normal level gradually. Methods include various types of medical gymnastics, walking training underweight loss, flat walking, and so on. Carry out rehabilitation in combination with TCM's characteristics and select traditional exercises such as tai chi chuan, baduanjin, five-animal exercise, etc., that are suitable for patients' physical fitness. Combine breathing training and dynamic and static exercise to improve patients' physical fitness and enhance their immunity. Additionally, add various physical therapy that are suitable for patients' physical strength, for example, use an electric stand-up bed to help a frail person practice standing, use intermediate frequency electrical stimulation to prevent limb muscle atrophy, use low-frequency electrical stimulation to strengthen the limbs muscles, improve joint movement with the help of a functional treadmill and limb linkage devices, and so on.

9.1.2.3 Positive Health Education, Rehabilitation Guidance, and Psychological Treatment

Educate patients about the clinical characteristics and rehabilitation of COVID-19 to enhance their confidence in overcoming the disease and improve their treatment compliance. Help patients to have regular rest and a balanced diet. Conduct psychological intervention and guidance to patients regarding their negative emotions such as fear, anxiety, anger, depression, or psychological problems such as noncompliance and abandonment of treatment.

9.2 CLINICAL MANAGEMENT OF REHABILITATION DIAGNOSIS AND TREATMENT

9.2.1 Relevant Policies and Basis in Rehabilitation Diagnosis and Treatment

COVID-19 has been included in the Category B infectious diseases stipulated in the *Law of the People's Republic of China on the Prevention and Treatment of Infectious Diseases*, and preventive and control measures are taken for Category A infectious diseases. Rehabilitation and treatment work must be in strict accordance with the requirements of the NHC on such documents as *COVID-19 Prevention and Control Plan, Technical Guide for COVID-19 Prevention and Control in Medical Institutions (First Edition), COVID-19 Guidelines for Common Use of Medical Protection (Trial), Air Purification Management Standard in Hospitals, Technical Specifications for Disinfection of Medical Institutions, Technical Specification for Washing and Disinfection of Medical Fabrics in Hospitals, Clinical Waste Management Ordinance, Regulations on the Management of Medical Waste in Medical and Health Institutions* and other documents.

9.2.2 Process Management of Rehabilitation Diagnosis and Treatment

Rehabilitation diagnosis and treatment are the same as that of other diseases. The treatment process requires the participation of medical personnel from different specialties. Even the rehabilitation field alone involves various treatment methods with strong professional characteristics in the field of rehabilitation medicine, which requires close cooperation and collaboration among medical professionals in the form of treatment groups; because COVID-19 is a highly infectious disease, it is necessary to strengthen the process management of rehabilitation diagnosis and treatment.

9.2.2.1 Working Principles

1) The diagnosis and treatment of COVID-19 rehabilitation must be in strict accordance with the requirements of the relevant documents promulgated by the NHC.

2) Attach importance to assessing patients' dysfunction so that the rehabilitation treatment process is safe, targeted, and benefits patients.

3) Targeted rehabilitation diagnosis and treatment should be carried out following local and individual conditions, with equal emphasis on traditional Chinese and Western medicine. Video, WeChat, and other methods can be used for distance rehabilitation guidance, psychological rehabilitation consultation, and rehabilitation popularization education.

9.2.2.2 Safety Precautions

1) Protection must be taken during diagnosis and treatment. Level 1 protection is necessary for assessment and guidance in which the patient is 1 meter away. Level 2 protection is required if assessment and treatment requires coming within 1 meter of contact with the patients. Level 3 protection is required for sputum aspiration.

2) Strictly enforce hand hygiene to prevent nosocomial infections. Monitor the temperature of medical staff and other related symptoms and make record it.

3) Patients need to take their temperature and wear a medical mask during rehabilitation. Avoid clustering when patients are scheduled for treatment.

4) Give priority to active rehabilitation. If necessary, intelligent equipment can be considered to improve the training effect while minimizing virus contact.

5) Pay attention to timely disinfection and disposal of the articles with which patients come in contact.

9.2.2.3 Overall Objective

The overall objective of COVID-19 rehabilitation is to promote the absorption of pulmonary inflammation and reduce the clinical symptoms of pneumonia in COVID-19 patients, improve the patient's respiratory function, enhance athletic endurance and physical strength, prevent complications (deep venous thrombosis of lower extremities, pressure sores and skeletal muscle function degradation, etc.), relieve anxiety and depression, improve the ability of daily life and to reintegrate into the family and society, reduce sequelae, and improve long-term quality of life.

9.2.2.4 Job Description

Patients with COVID-19 may have different clinical symptoms and functional disorders, and rehabilitation diagnosis and treatment may also be different. In general, the rehabilitation and diagnosis work for COVID-19 patients include the following aspects.

1) According to the disease condition, cardiopulmonary function, and physical fitness assessment, respiratory function may be improved by position therapy, breathing pattern training, free-hand therapy, and breathing exercises. Regulate *qi* and repair viscera function through acupoint massage, moxibustion, moxibustion paste, and other TCM treatments. Improve patients' physical ability through traditional exercises such as tai chi chuan, baduanjin and five-animal exercise, and the combination of dynamic and static movement.
2) Improve joint activity and endurance with the help of a functional treadmill and limb linkage equipment. If the patient cannot exercise actively, use an electric standing bed to help them stand up and low/intermediate frequency electrical stimulation to prevent limb muscle atrophy.
3) Carry out active physical activities, such as medical gymnastics, walking training underweight loss, flat walking, etc., to promote gradual physical function recovery.
4) Provide targeted psychological counseling to relieve patients' fear, help them learn to relax by themselves, and bravely overcome the disease.

9.2.2.5 Diagnosis and Treatment Procedures

The rehabilitation process for COVID-19 patients includes in-hospital rehabilitation procedures, outpatient rehabilitation procedures, and home rehabilitation procedures (Figure 9.1–Figure 9.3).

9.2.2.6 Precautions

1) Comprehensively evaluate the patient's respiratory function, physical function, daily life ability, and social participation disorders and their severity to provide a basis for rehabilitation development programs.
2) Master the indications and contraindications of rehabilitation treatment and strengthen treatment safety and pertinence.
3) Focus on functional monitoring in rehabilitation treatment to ensure the safety and effectiveness of treatment.
4) Immediately terminate the treatment if patients have maladjustment. Report to the rehabilitation physician and adjust the examination in a timely manner.

9.2.2.7 Prerequisites for Intervention

In the rehabilitation treatment, pay attention to rehabilitation timing. It is necessary to comprehensively assess patients' benefits and risks and master the

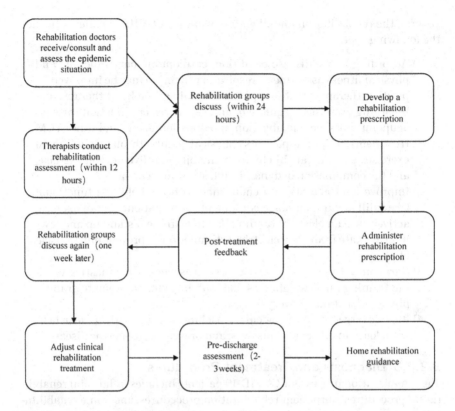

Figure 9.1   In-hospital rehabilitation procedures.

prerequisites for their rehabilitation treatment, especially for severe/critically severe patients and moderate patients.

1) Severe and critically severe patients:
   a. Temperature $\leq$ 38.5 °C
   b. Respiratory frequency $\leq$ 40 times/min
   c. Systolic blood pressure $\geq$ 90 mmHg and $\leq$ 180 mmHg; mean arterial pressure (MAP) $\geq$ 65 mmHg and $\leq$ 110 mmHg
   d. Heart rate: $\geq$ 40 times/min and $\leq$ 120 times/min
   e. Pulse oxygen saturation (SpO_2) $\geq$ 90%; forced inspiratory oxygen (FiO_2) $\leq$ 0.6
   f. Positive end-expiratory pressure (PEEP) $\leq$ 10 cm H_2O
   g. Richmond agitation-sedation score (RASS) –2 to +2
   h. Intracranial pressure < 20 cm H_2O

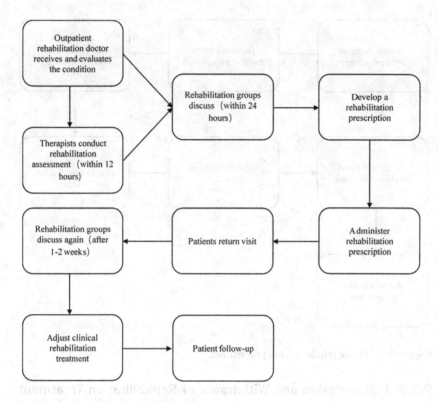

Figure 9.2   Outpatient rehabilitation procedures.

    i. No unsafe airway hazards
    j. No confrontation between ventilator and human

The following are excluded: Emerging arrhythmias and myocardial ischemia accompanied blood lactic acid ≥ 4 mmol/L, shock, emerging unstable deep vein thrombosis and pulmonary embolism, aortic stenosis, unstable limb, spinal fractures, severe hepatorenal basal disease, new and progressive hepatic and renal dysfunction, and active bleeding.

  2) Moderate patients:
    a. Time from onset to dyspnea > 3 days
    b. Initial diagnosis time > 7 days
    c. Temperature: < 38° C
    d. Static blood pressure > 90/60 mmHg (1 mmHg = 0.133 kPa) and < 140/90 mmHg
    e. Blood oxygen saturation > 95%
    f. Chest imaging progress < 50% within 24–48 hours

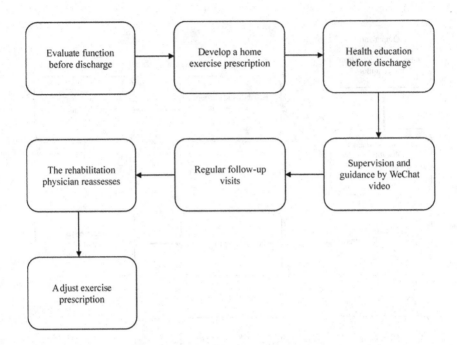

Figure 9.3   Home rehabilitation procedures.

9.2.2.8 Suspension and Withdrawal of Rehabilitation Treatment

During the rehabilitation treatment, monitor COVID-19 patients' vital signs and other relevant clinical indicators and detect the disease's aggravation in a timely manner. Once the changes in disease conditions are detected, the rehabilitation treatment can be suspended or even withdrawn.

1) Stop the treatment of severe and critically severe patients immediately when the following situations occur:

   a. Respiratory frequency > 40 times/min
   b. Systolic blood pressure: < 90 mmHg or >180 mmHg; mean arterial pressure (MAP) < 65 mmHg and > 110 mmHg; or more than 20% change from the baseline
   c. Heart rate: < 40 times/min and > 120 times/min
   d. Decreased consciousness or irritability
   e. Palpitation, dyspnea, aggravation of shortness of breath, or intolerable fatigue
   f. Blood oxygen saturation: < 90% or > 4% decreasing from baseline
   g. Confrontation between and man and machine, and the artificial airway disengages or shifts

    h. Newly developed arrhythmia and myocardial ischemia

    i. Any treatment disconnects monitoring lines

2) Stop the respiratory rehabilitation of moderate patients immediately when one of the following situations occur:

    a. Borg dyspnea score > 3 (10 points in total);

    b. Patient experiences chest tightness, suffocation, dizziness, headache, blurred vision, palpitation, sweat, the inability to maintain balance, and other conditions.

9.3 DIFFERENT CLINICAL TYPES AND STAGES OF REHABILITATION TREATMENT

9.3.1 Rehabilitation for Hospitalized Patients with COVID-19

As the conditions of COVID-19 hospitalized patients vary, the possible dysfunction may also vary. In clinical practice, make comprehensive rehabilitation assessments according to patients' characteristics and classify them accurately. In a timely manner, detect patients' functional impairment and its severity, and conduct corresponding comprehensive rehabilitation treatment.

9.3.1.1 Rehabilitation Treatment for Mild Patients

Mild patients meet the diagnostic criteria for suspected/confirmed cases of *Notice on Issuance of COVID-19 Diagnosis and Treatment Protocol (7th Trial Edition)*. Patients with mild symptoms and no imaging manifestations are taken in single rooms for isolation and medical observation.

9.3.1.1.1 Objectives of Rehabilitation Treatment

The main objectives are to improve patients' clinical symptoms, establish a correct cough mode, improve their immunity, prevent cold, prevent pneumonia and pulmonary function decline, and establish their confidence to overcome the disease.

9.3.1.1.2 Rehabilitation Treatment Methods

1) Position management: The primary purpose is to reduce respiratory work, increase effective lung volume by adjusting the patient's position, and reduce the adverse effects of supine posture on lung ventilation and perfusion. Patients can raise the head of their beds to 60° or they should lean forward while sitting or standing.

2) Cough training: Inhale deeply and quickly, and the forcefully contract the abdominal muscles and exhale the breath vigorously with the sound of "ha", to cough effectively and expel sputum. It should be

noted that the expectoration should be covered with a closed plastic bag, and the airway secretions should be placed in a special container to avoid infecting others.

3) Exercise therapy: The primary purpose is to improve muscle strength, relieve fatigue, improve daily activities, eliminate depression, reduce anxiety, and help sleep. In the choice of exercise therapy, strength training and endurance training of upper and lower limbs can be carried out. It is advisable to have no fatigue on the second day. Exercise should be for 15–45 minutes at a time and should occur two times a day. Specific forms can be cross-walking training, breathing rehabilitation exercises, and tai chi chuan, etc., to maintain motor function as much as possible to meet the needs of independent daily life activities. Exercise can be divided into small sections to facilitate self-observation and strictly avoid fatigue. If the patient cannot stand, they can choose a sitting/semirecumbent/recumbent position. Under the guidance of educational videos and brochures, perform light exercises on the limbs and torso.

4) Physiotherapy: At present, there is no precise evidence-based medicine to prove the therapeutic effect of physiotherapy on this disease; however it can be attempted.

   a.   Ultrashort wave therapy: Lung antithesis with no heat or micro heat for 10–15 minutes each time, once a day, and 10 times for a course of treatment. Patients whose body temperature exceeds 38 °C should not use this therapy.

   b.   Ultraviolet therapy: Irradiate chest or back skin by weak erythema, once a day, and four times as a course of treatment.

5) Occupational therapy: The purpose is to block the vicious circle of shortness of breath caused by mental and muscle tension, reduce the consumption of body energy, and improve the state of hypoxia as well as improve the patient's anxiety, tension, fear, and other emotions. Self-relaxation activities should be the foremost choice, specifically, slow and deep breathing, natural swinging of the upper limbs while sitting or standing, music therapy, etc.

6) Patient education: Conduct publicity and education on the cause, clinical manifestations, prognosis, the importance of rehabilitation treatment, methods, purposes, precautions, etc., of COVID-19, in order to help patients, understand the knowledge of the disease, enhance their confidence in overcoming the disease, and maximize compliance. Help patients to work regularly, get enough sleep, have a balanced diet, and quit smoking.

7) Psychological intervention: Because patients do not understand the disease, they often experience fear, anxiety, anger, depression, and

insomnia, or they do not cooperate, give up treatment, and other psychological problems. Intervene in these psychological problems by seeking a mental health professional or a psychological hotline.

9.3.1.2 Rehabilitation Treatment for Moderate Patients

Moderate patients are those who meet the diagnostic criteria for suspected/confirmed cases of *Notice on Issuance of COVID-19 Diagnosis and Treatment Protocol (7th Trial Edition)*. Patients are those with fever, respiratory symptoms, and imaging manifestations of pneumonia.

9.3.1.2.1 Objectives of Rehabilitation Treatment

The main objective are to treat clinical symptoms and clean the airway; establish a good breathing pattern, reduce respiratory energy consumption, and reduce breathing work; maintain or improve the patient's respiratory function; prevent the occurrence of acute respiratory distress syndrome; avoid deep vein thrombosis and other complications, and improve their exercise endurance and daily activity ability; adjust their psychology and build up the confidence to overcome the disease.

The intensity of exercise activities during the rehabilitation of patients should not be too large, and the timing of intervention and withdrawal should be carried out under the guidance of rehabilitation physicians.

9.3.1.2.2 Rehabilitation Treatment Method

1) Position management: This helps diaphragm activity and reduces the adverse effects of supine position on lung ventilation and perfusion. Proper positioning helps to optimize arterial oxygenation and Ventilation to blood perfusion (V/Q) ratio. The method is the same as mild ones. It is feasible to use sputum retention techniques to perform postural drainage for the affected lung (perform corresponding postural drainage according to the different parts of the lung that are affected).

2) Airway cleaning technology: Using the expansion method during deep inspiration can be adopted. At this point, avoid using vibration expectoration machine to not cause blood oxygen saturation and the risk of arrhythmia.

3) Respiratory control training: Patients with dyspnea in bed can sit in a 60° position on the bed, and a pillow can be placed under the knee joint to ensure the knee joint is bent and slightly higher than the hip joint. Patients who can get out of bed can do the activity in the sitting position. Relax the auxiliary inspiratory muscles of the shoulder and neck. Inhale slowly through the nose, exhale slowly through the

mouth, and observe the chest expansion. The intensity is between rest and light physical activity, two times a day. It should take place 1 hour after meals for 15–45 minutes per time. It can also be intermittent.

4) Position change training: During the position change training, first left, then right, from the supine position to lateral position, prone position, and then return to the supine position. Next, the patient should move from the supine position to the long sitting position on the bed, from the long sitting position on the bed to the bedside sitting position, and finally from the bedside sitting position to the bedside standing position. The patient should stay in each position for about 5 seconds and then walk around the bed. Complete the above five changing positions as a group two to three times a day, step by step, gradually changing the position movement. Patients should start with one group per time and move up to three groups per time. Patients with shortness of breath and Borg score > 3 should stop to rest and then proceed again after the feeling of fatigue disappears.

5) Progressive activities and exercise training: Patients who cannot stand can choose sitting/semirecumbent/recumbent position and perform activities such as clenching, arm raising, ankle pump, heel sliding, leg raising, quadriceps and gluteus isometric contraction under the guidance of educational videos and brochures. When the patient's condition is stable, exercises such as sitting up, standing up, waist stretching, leg lifting, striding, and cross-walking can also be arranged and broken into small self-observation sections. Strive to accumulate more than 1 hour of daily activity and strictly avoid fatigue.

6) Physiotherapy: It can be continued to improve the disease condition.
   a.   Ultrashort wave therapy: Lung antithesis with no heat or microheat, 10–15 minutes each time, once a day, and 10 times for a course of treatment.
   b.   Ultraviolet therapy: Irradiate chest or back skin by weak erythema, once a day, and four times as a course of treatment

7) Occupational therapy: The designed selective self-relaxation activity can block the shortness of breath caused by mental and muscle tension, help to break patients' vicious circle, and improve their hypoxia state. Methods can be slow and include deep breathing, natural swinging of the upper limbs while sitting or standing, music therapy, etc.

8) Patient education: Continue to strengthen publicity and education so that patients can have a further understanding of the disease knowledge, enhance their confidence in overcoming the disease, and maximize compliance.

9) Psychological intervention: In this type of patient, the clinical symptoms and dysfunction are more severe than those in patients with mile

cases. Patients with more obvious psychological problems such as fear, anxiety, anger, depression, insomnia etc., or failure to cooperate or abandon treatment should be given attention in a timely manner and psychological intervention. If necessary, continue to seek psychological professionals or psychological hotline intervention.

9.3.1.3 Rehabilitation Treatment for Severe/ Critically Severe Patients

Severe/critically severe patients meet the diagnostic criteria for suspected/confirmed cases of *Notice on Issuance of COVID-19 Diagnosis and Treatment Protocol (7th Trial Edition)*.

Severe types are adult patients who have any one of the following:

1) Respiratory distress, RR $\geq$ 30 times/min
2) At rest oxygen saturation $\leq$ 93%
3) Partial pressure of blood oxygen (PaO_2)/fraction of inspiring oxygen (FiO_2) $\leq$ 300 mmHg (1 mmHg = 0.133 kPa)
4) Lesions with significant progression within 24–48 hours in pulmonary imaging examination are treated as severe

Critically severe types are patients with any one of the following:

1) Respiratory failure and mechanical ventilation is required
2) Shock
3) Patients with other organ failure should be monitored in ICU

9.3.1.2.1 Objectives of Rehabilitation Treatment

The objectives are to promote the discharge of respiratory secretions; improve alveolar ventilation, improve respiratory function, prevent complications, such as muscle atrophy, joint contracture, decreased cardiopulmonary function, and deep vein thrombosis.

Exercise should not be too intense during rehabilitation treatment, and the rehabilitation physician should prescribe the time of intervention and withdrawal. If the patient has anemia or abnormal blood clotting function, check hemoglobin and blood clotting function indicators before respiratory rehabilitation treatment to avoid tissue hypoxia and bleeding caused by activities. For bedridden patients, guide them to exercise ankle pump or use elastic stockings to prevent the occurrence of deep vein thrombosis of the lower limbs.

9.3.1.2.2 Rehabilitation Treatment Methods

1) Position management: Patients undergoing respiratory rehabilitation therapy should be guided to change position after discussion by the clinical treatment team. By raising the bed head to the half-lying

position, gradually transition to the sitting position. Position therapy lasts for 30 minutes, three times a day. Patients with acute respiratory distress syndrome (ARDS) can use prone position > 12 hours a day to improve ventilation blood flow ratio, reduce pulmonary edema, increase functional residual volume, and reduce the possibility of intubation. Consider extracorporeal membrane oxygenation (ECMO) for poor prone ventilation. Turn over regularly, once every 1–2 hours. Lung recruitment is recommended for patients with severe ARDS.

2) Airway cleaning: The "ha" coughing technique and deep inhalation stage expansion are adopted, and personnel should take care not to cause severe irritating and increased breathing work in patients. It is also possible to use positive pressure expiratory therapy/oscillatory positive pressure expiratory therapy, high-frequency chest wall vibration, and other methods, making it easier for patients to discharge airway secretions and improve lung function and prevent pulmonary complications. Pay attention to avoid causing or exacerbating bronchospasm. Patients with impaired consciousness or sedation are usually treated with three different frequencies of 10 Hz, 12 Hz, and 14 Hz for 10 minutes each. After treatment, the nurse should suck sputum.

3) Respiratory control training: Ensure adequate oxygen supply. Apply rehabilitation treatment techniques that avoid disconnecting patients from the ventilator. Patients with clear consciousness can also be under chest expansion breathing training. If necessary, terminally ill patients should receive palliative medication to relieve dyspnea.

4) Early activity: Ensure patients are given sufficient oxygen during activities. Prevent the pipeline connecting the patients from detaching and monitor vital signs throughout the process. If SpO_2 <88%, terminate the rehabilitation treatment. Bedridden patients can perform progressive active limb movements or passive instrumental movement on the bed, turn over and regularly move on the bed, and receive active/passive whole-joint exercise training. With the help of breathing control technology, patients who can get out of bed can sit up from bed, move from bed to chair, sit on a chair, stand up and march on the spot. Perform these exercises one to two times per day without increasing fatigue. All activities should not cause oxygen saturation or blood pressure to drop. For those with transfer disorders, this can be done with a walker, a sturdy chair or a bed file, or a therapist's assistance. Patients with sedative use or cognitive impairment or physical limitations, choose passive power for lower limbs by the bedside, passive joint movement and stretching, and neuromuscular electrical stimulation. The total training time should not exceed 30 minutes at a time, so as not to cause aggravation of fatigue.

5) Exercise therapy: Patients can proceed with active body movement step by step when they are conscious. According to patients' specific conditions, progressive strength training, and endurance training of upper and lower limbs can be carried out in the choice of exercise therapy without causing fatigue.

6) Lung recruitment therapy: This therapy refers to ventilator hyperinflation (VHI) technique, recruitment maneuver (RM), and intense breathing training. It can effectively increase lung volume, improve lung compliance, optimize ventilation and blood flow ratio, and reduce pulmonary edema by recruiting collapsed alveoli to correct hypoxemia and ensure the positive end-expiratory pressure (PEEP) effect. It is particularly essential for patients with ARDS.

7) Muscle strength training: This method adopts the bedside passive power cycling training for upper and lower limbs.

8) Patient education: Continue to educate and comfort patients so they understand the outcome of disease development, maximize their compliance, and reduce their mental burden.

9.3.2 Rehabilitation Treatment of COVID-19 Patients after Being Discharged from the Hospital

For COVID-19 patients, after relieving the symptoms and achieving the clinical recovery, they may face different dysfunctions and have different needs for rehabilitation after discharge. It is necessary to give corresponding rehabilitation treatment according to their different clinical rehabilitation needs to promote further dysfunction improvement and quality of life.

Most discharged patients with mild and moderate infections have slight or no persistent residual lung function problems. Their hospital stays are shorter and the possibility of physical dysfunction is less, but the adverse psychological effects of the disease on the patient may exist longer. The objective of post-discharge rehabilitation is to restore physical fitness and adjust psychology, principally in the form of home-based rehabilitation under the guidance of professionals. The specific content of rehabilitation treatment is based on step-by-step aerobic exercise. Choose the exercise form that patients preferred in the past or choose the appropriate exercise form according to their wishes and realistic conditions. Make an aerobic exercise prescription, pay attention to the scientific nature and implementability of the movement, and gradually help patients recover to the activity level they were at before the onset of the disease and to return to society as soon as possible.

For discharged patients with severe/critically severe disease, it is necessary to make a targeted assessment of the patient's lung function impairment and develop a long-term progressive, comprehensive, and personalized respiratory rehabilitation plan in terms of exercise, psychology, nutrition, and other aspects according to the assessment results, with particular emphasis on the evaluation of comprehensiveness, scientificity, and pertinence. Rehabilitation assessment must identify the type and severity of postdischarge disorders in respiratory, physical, daily life, and social participation of COVID-19 patients, and provide a treatment framework for appropriate rehabilitation programs. The assessment project shall be based on the patient's existing functional impairment, including but not limited to the following aspects.

Perform a detailed examination and assessment of patients' vital signs, respiratory system signs, breathing patterns, respiratory muscle strength, aerobic activity ability, limb muscle strength, joint mobility, limb circumference, nutritional status, psychological status, and other aspects.

Assess patients' respiratory symptoms, musculoskeletal symptoms, pain score, balance function, activity function, quality of life, nutritional status, and psychological status through the questionnaire.

Improve supplementary examination based on chest imaging, lung function, and blood biochemical indexes, and arrange auxiliary examination items such as diaphragmatic ultrasound, cardiopulmonary exercise function test, bone density, muscle nuclear magnetic, and other auxiliary examination items according to actual conditions and dysfunction types.

It is important to note that even if the patients are clinically cured, the reinfection possibility is not excluded; therefore, it is imperative that patients strengthen protection, ask them to observe rehabilitation physicians' medical advice, and pay attention to the prevention of colds and other infectious diseases.

9.3.2.1 Rehabilitation Treatment for Mild/ Moderate Discharged Patients

9.3.2.1.1 Objectives of Rehabilitation Treatment
The rehabilitation treatment objectives are to reduce breath shortness, increase athletic endurance, improve and restore respiratory function, prevent recurrence, and restore the patient's ability of daily activities, occupational adaptability, psychological adaptability, and social participation.

9.3.2.1.2 Rehabilitation Treatment Methods

1) Patient education: Patients continue to conduct self-health monitoring for 14 days after discharge. They should wear masks and live in well-ventilated single rooms when conditions permit. They should reduce close contact with family members, eat separately, practice good hand hygiene, and avoid going out. They should prevent cold and continue to do an excellent job in self-protection and recurrence prevention.

2) Aerobic exercise training: Cross-walking, walking, fast walking, jogging or swimming, and breathing exercises should be done three to five times a week for 20–30 minutes each time. Patients should stop exercise if their Borg score is no more than 3 points or if the patients feel short of breath. It is possible to gradually increase activity intensity to moderate intensity while monitoring blood oxygen.

3) Power bicycle: Patients can perform this activity three to five for 20–30 minutes each time. The exercise intensity is the same as above.

4) Strength training: Patients can perform muscle strength training for target muscle groups three to five times a week.

5) Rehabilitation of TCM: Under the condition of eliminating contraindications, for example, limb dysfunction and abnormal consciousness, training such as baduanjin, tai chi chuan, respiratory guidance exercise, and six words breathing exercise can be conducted.

6) Activities of daily living (ADL) intervention: For discharged patients with mild disease, their ability to perform daily activities, such as transfer, grooming, toileting, and bathing, must be evaluated to see if there is any impairment caused by pain, dyspnea, and weakness during these daily activities. Within 2 weeks after discharge, possible daily life disorders can be treated with targeted rehabilitation. At the same time, it is necessary to evaluate the patient's social participation and other higher-level daily activities. Giving targeted treatment to the tool-based daily activities includes shopping, going out, cooking, doing housework, washing clothes, taking medicine, using communication equipment, handling finances, etc. During the treatment process, comprehensively consider patients' mental and physical abilities in completing these activities. By simulating the actual scene, conduct the training to find out the obstacles of task participation, and carry out targeted intervention under occupational therapists' guidance.

9.3.2.2 Rehabilitation Treatment for Discharged Patients with Severe/Critically Severe Disease

9.3.2.2.1 Objectives of Rehabilitation Treatment

The rehabilitation treatment objectives are to further improve symptoms, restore muscle strength and endurance, improve lung and motor function, reduce the risk of readmission, and restore daily activities, social participation, and psychological adaptation.

9.3.2.2.2 Criteria Exclusion and Motion Termination

At the beginning and during the rehabilitation of discharged patients with severe/critically severe disease, pay special attention to observing their vital signs and treatment response, and master the exclusion criteria and exercise termination criteria for rehabilitation.

1) Exclusion criteria:
   a. Heart rate > 100 beats/min
   b. Blood pressure < 90/60 mmHg or > 140/90 mmHg
   c. Blood oxygen saturation ≤ 95%
   d. Other diseases that are not suitable for exercise
2) Exercise termination criteria:
   a. Temperature fluctuates, > 37.2 °C
   b. Respiratory symptoms and fatigue are aggravated and are not relieved after a rest
   c. Stop exercise and consult a doctor if the following symptoms occur: Chest tightness, chest pain, dyspnea, severe cough, dizziness, headache, blurred vision, palpitations, sweating, unstable standing, and other symptoms

9.3.2.2.3 Rehabilitation Treatment Methods

1) Patient education:
   a. Help patients understand lung consolidation after virus infection and preach on the physical and psychological changes that may occur after severe patients are discharged from the hospital. Instruct patients about the importance of regular follow-up visits, precautions, nutrition support, oxygen therapy, the significance of respiratory muscle training, energy-saving ways in daily life, etc., which can be carried out through manuals or videos to improve patients' mastery of disease knowledge.
   b. Help patients understand respiratory rehabilitation treatment and its importance to increase their compliance. Introduce to patients the role of respiratory rehabilitation in patients after being discharged from the hospital, specific contents of respiratory rehabilitation, effects of respiratory rehabilitation, precautions in respiratory rehabilitation, etc.
   c. Inform patients that follow-up visits will ask about their participation in respiratory rehabilitation, progress, and benefits, as well as their participation in family and social activities.
2) Respiratory training:
   a. Active circulatory breathing techniques include breath control, thoracic expansion, and forced exhalation.
   b. Respiratory pattern training techniques include position management, breathing rhythm adjusting (inhalation: exhalation = 1:2), thoracic activity training, respiratory muscle groups activating, and abdominal breathing training, etc.

  c. If there is inspiratory muscle dysfunction, patients are recommended to perform inspiratory muscle training by using a breathing trainer with a 30%–50% MIP* load seven times a week, 30 inhalations each time, and each inhaling interval should be no less than 6 seconds. ④ For sputum excretion training, when cleaning the airway, use the "ha" coughing technique to reduce patients' sputum excretion and energy consumption. Devices such as positive expiratory pressure (PEP)/OPEP can also be used to assist patients. Train for 5 minutes three times a day. The patient should exhale for more than 3 seconds each time.

3) Aerobic training:
  a. This adopts the FITT (frequency, intensity, time, type) principle. For details, refer to the relevant chapter on rehabilitation treatment technology.

4) Strength training:
  a. For those with decreased muscle strength, progressive resistance training is recommended for target muscle groups. The training load of each target muscle group is 8–12 repetition maximum (RM) (i.e., each group repeats 8–12 movements of the load), completing one to three groups each time, with each group's training interval at 2 minutes, and the frequency is 2–3 times/week. Train for 6 weeks with a weekly increase of 5%–10%.

5) Balance training:
  a. Patients with balance dysfunction should be involved in balance training, such as free-hand balance training and balance training equipment under rehabilitation therapists' guidance.

6) Occupational therapy mainly improves necessary activities of daily living within 2–4 weeks upon being discharged from hospitals. The main concerns are contractures caused by bed immobilization, pain caused by soft tissue damage, and limited joint movement. Comprehensive treatment including drugs, physical factors, braces and stretching are mainly given. For patients with joint disorders of essential daily activities caused by weak limbs,strength training and occupational therapy training are mainly carried out to improve their muscle strength and endurance. As for the disorder in ADL caused by dyspnea, it is necessary to assess patients' respiratory function, aerobic activity ability, body strength, and other factors and then intervene with training on using energy-saving techniques or compensatory energy-saving assistance devices.

---

* The maximum inspiratory oral pressure is the maximum inspiratory oral pressure that can be generated with the maximum inspiratory effort when the airway is blocked at the residual air level or the functional residual air level.

It mainly improves patients' instrumental activities of daily life at more than 4 weeks upon being discharged from hospitals. It is necessary to evaluate patients' instrumental daily activities at more than 1 month upon being discharged from hospitals, to know patients' social participation and other higher-level daily activity abilities. It is also necessary to comprehensively consider patients' psychological and physical function capabilities when they complete these activities, find out the obstacles to task participation, and take targeted treatment. It can be carried out by simulating the actual scene.

BIBLIOGRAPHY

1. General Office of the National Health Commission, Office of the National Administration of Traditional Chinese Medicine. *COVID-19 Diagnosis and Treatment Protocol (Trial Version 7) [EB/OL]*. [2020-03-03].
2. General Office of the National Health Commission, Hospital Administration and Hospital Authority. *Notice of The General Office of the National Health Commission on Follow-Up and Follow-Up of CoVID-19 Discharged Patients [EB/OL]*. [2020-02-17]
3. Chinese Rehabilitation Medical Association. *Comprehensive Guidance on Rehabilitation and Diagnosis during COVID-19 Pandemic (Second Edition) [EB/OL]*. [2020-02-18].
4. *Novel Coronavirus Infection Prevention and Control Technical Guide (first edition) in Medical Institutions [EB/OL]*. [2020-01-22].
5. General Office of the National Health Commission, Hospital Administration. *Guidelines on the Scope of Common Medical Protection in Novel Coronavirus Infection Prevention (Trial) [EB/OL]*. [2020-01-26].
6. General Office of the National Health Commission. *Notice of the General Office of the National Health Commission on the Issuance of the Novel Coronavirus Prevention and Control Plan (Third Edition) [EB/OL]*. [2020-01-28].
7. Novel Coronavirus 2019 (Second Edition) [J/OL]. *Chinese Journal of Tuberculosis and Respiration*, 2020(04): 308–314.
8. Yu Pengming, He Chengqi, Gao Qiang, He Hongchen, Wei Quan. Guidelines and recommendations for full cycle physical therapy for COVID-19 patients [J]. *Chinese Journal of Physical Medicine & Rehabilitation*, 2020, 42(2): 102–104.
9. The General Office of the National Health Commission issued a notice on the issuance of the Rehabilitation Plan for coVID-19 discharged patients (Trial), medical Letter [2020]189 (4 March 2020) of the State Health Office.
10. Respiratory Critical Care Medicine Group, Respiratory Critical Care Medicine Branch, Chinese Medical Association, Critical Care Medicine Working Committee, Respiratory Physicians Branch, Chinese Medical Doctor Association. Airway management recommendations for adult patients with severe COVID-19 (trial) [J]. *Chinese Journal of Medicine*, 2020(10): 729-737.
11. National Health Commission. *Notice on the Issuance of Novel Coronavirus Outbreak Emergency Psychological Crisis Intervention Guidelines [OL]*. [2020-01-26].

12. Chinese Rehabilitation Medical Association. Expert consensus of rehabilitation diagnosis and treatment during coVID-19 outbreak of respiratory infectious Diseases [J]. Chinese Journal of Physical Medicine and Rehabilitation, 2020, 42(2): 97–101.

13. Li Dekun, Zou Yucong, Jin Kai, Dai Jian. Chinese Medicine combined with modern rehabilitation for coVID-19 patients [J/OL]. Clinical Journal of Chinese Medicine,: 2020, 32(05):832-836.

14. Xu Cheng, Cheng Yanqi, Tang Ling, Li Shaobin, Wu Yinyin, Fang Song. Pulmonary rehabilitation strategies for patients with severe/critically severe COVID-19 mechanical ventilation [J/OL]. *Shanghai Journal of Traditional Chinese Medicine*, 2020, 54(05): 1–4.

15. The Standing Committee of the National People's Congress of China. Law of the People's Republic of China on the Prevention and Treatment of Infectious Diseases.[EB/OL].[1989-02-12].

Chapter 10

Psychological Rehabilitation of COVID-19

10.1 ASSESSMENT OF PSYCHOLOGICAL DISORDERS

As a deadly and rapidly spreading global infectious disease, COVID-19, like severe acute respiratory syndrome (SARS), has caused great psychological stress to humans. A series of psychological dysfunctions often accompany COVID-19 patients to different degrees, such as fear, anxiety, anger, depression, loneliness, shame, even acute stress disorder, post-traumatic stress disorder, suicide, and other psychological crises and secondary trauma, which seriously affects their physical and mental health and the recovery of pneumonia. On January 27, 2020, the National Health Commission (NHC) released the *COVID-19 Emergency Psychological Crisis Intervention Guiding Principles*, which includes psychological crisis intervention into the pandemic prevention and control system, and the first step of psychological intervention is to carry out the scientific psychological assessment. Psychological assessment is a general term for comprehensive, systematic, and in-depth analysis of individual or group psychological phenomena (psychological, behavioral and spiritual values) through the integrative use of conversation, observation, and tests under the standard guidance of biological, psychological, social, and medical models. Psychological assessment helps medical staff assess patients' psychological processes during the occurrence and development of the disease and to find out existing or potential psychological or mental health problems, which is an essential prerequisite and basis for psychological intervention. This chapter mainly introduces the commonly used assessment methods of psychological disorders to quickly identify psychological problems in clinical practice and evaluate the treatment effect.

10.1.1 Role and Purpose of Psychological Disorder Assessments

10.1.1.1 Role of Psychological Disorder Assessments

1) Screening target intervention population is an important prerequisite and basis for psychological intervention and evaluation of the effect and prognosis of psychological rehabilitation. Determine patients' mental state, level of ability, and the risk of injury to themselves or others to prepare for further intervention.
2) Psychological assessment can judge the effect of psychological intervention.
3) Psychological assessment should cooperate with diagnosis and treatment of other diseases and assist the clinical diagnosis alone or with assistance.
4) Provide patients' information for clinical intervention and treatment.
5) Psychological assessment is an important means of medical science research and psychological research.
6) The role of a psychological assessment in other aspects of medical psychology.
7) Psychological assessment helps determine possible solutions, coping methods, support systems, and other resources.
8) Forecast post-disaster mental health problems and demand for services.
9) The psychological assessment itself is also an intervention process.

10.1.1.2 Purpose of Psychological Disorder Assessments

1) Understand in detail the psychological problems of those assessed during the pandemic, the causes and development of the problem, possible influencing factors, their early life experiences, family background and current adaptation, interpersonal relationships, etc.
2) Have an in-depth understanding and assessment of some special issues and key issues.
3) Analyze and process the collected data.

10.1.2 Appropriate Population for Assessment of Psychological Disorders and Their Psychological Characteristics

1) The pandemic affects a wide range of populations and requires timely mental health assessment and intervention. The *Guidelines for Public Psychological Self-help and Counseling of COVID-19* divides the

population affected by pneumonia into four levels. Its intervention focus starts at the Level I population and gradually expands. This is where the assessment's focus begins.

  a. Level I population: Confirmed COVID-19 patients (hospitalized patients with severe disease or above), frontline medical personnel, disease control personnel, management personnel, etc., are key targets for the assessment and intervention of psychological disorders.

  b. Level II population: Mild patients isolated at home (close contacts, suspected cases) and patients with fever visiting hospitals.

  c. Level III population: People related to people in the Level I and Level II populations, such as family members, colleagues, friends, and rear rescuers participating in pandemic prevention and control, such as on-site command, organization, management personnel, volunteers, etc.

  d. Level IV population: The population in the pandemic area affected by the pandemic prevention and control measures, the vulnerable population, and the general public.

2) In the face of COVID-19, people may experience various emotional, physiological, cognitive, and behavioral changes, and even mental problems, such as acute stress response, acute stress disorder, and post-traumatic stress response. These psychological and psychiatric issues are also crucial in the assessment of COVID-19 patients.

  a. Emotional reactions: Anxiety, fear, depression, anger, doubt, sadness, guilt, volatility, exhaustion, numbness, and "heroic", etc.

  b. Physiological reactions (somatic symptoms): Various physiological discomfort (decreased digestive function, fatigue, pain), insomnia (difficulty in falling asleep, nightmares, etc.), autonomic nervous dysfunction (dizziness, dry mouth, sweating, chest tightness, palpitations, shortness of breath, etc.).

  c. Cognitive changes: Paranoia, catastrophic thinking, impulsive thinking, sensitiveness, and doubt, etc.

  d. Behavior changes: Escape and avoidance behavior, degeneration and dependence, hostility and aggression, helplessness and self-pity, panic, compulsive behavior, sleep change, material aid, and interpersonal change.

10.1.3 Psychological Assessment Methods

Psychological assessment is the systematic analysis of information collected using the following methods.

10.1.3.1 Interview

Interview, also called interaction and face-to-face conversation, is the most commonly used method of psychological assessment. The interview method assesses the client's psychological function through the two-way, face-to-face interaction between the consultant and the visitor to develop appropriate treatment plans. Interviews can be conducted as a freestyle interview or a structured interview. Interview techniques include verbal communication and nonverbal communication, such as expressions and gestures.

10.1.3.2 Observation

Observation is a common means to obtain information in psychological counseling. It is a psychological assessment method through direct or indirect observation (through photographic video equipment) of the behavior of the person being assessed. Observation can be divided into natural observation and controlled observation. The former refers to the observation in natural situations (such as family, school, or work environment) in which the evaluated person's behavior is authentic and not interfered with by observers. The latter refers to the observation made in a preset situation.

10.1.3.3 Work Analysis

Work analysis, also known as product analysis, is a method to analyze and study various works of the survey subject (make clear the overall population and samples), such as notes, assignments, diaries, articles, etc., to understand the situation, find problems, and grasp characteristics, and rules. This method helps to understand people's knowledge, skills, techniques, attitude to things, intelligence, level of ability, etc. It can also reflect patients' psychological development level, psychological characteristics, behavioral pattern, and psychological state.

10.1.3.4 Psychological Tests

The psychological test refers to the objective and standardized measurement of people's psychological state and behavior performance by using psychological theories and techniques, to determine the psychological phenomenon in nature and degree of difference. These include tests for specific cognitive, emotional, and behavioral responses related to certain disorders and broader tests that measure personality traits. The test to detect psychological disorders must meet strict standards, including that they be credible, effective, and standardized, that is, meet the requirements of reliability, validity, and standardization. Such tests mainly include the following types.

10.1.3.4.1 Personality Tests

A personality test, also called an individual test, measures the peculiarity and tendency of an individual's behavior. The most commonly used methods are

questionnaires and projection techniques. Standard personality questionnaires include the Eysenck Personality Questionnaire (EPQ), the Minnesota
Multiple Personality Test (MMPI), and the Cattle 16 Factor Personality Test
(16PF). The central projection techniques include the Rorschach Inkblot Test,
the Adversity Dialogue Test, the Sentence Completion Test, and the House-
Tree-Person test.

10.1.3.4.2 Rating Scales

Rating scales help the evaluator to determine a score by observing a person's
behavior or traits. The standardized procedure used to express the evaluation
results is called a rating scale.

1) Mental state rating scale: The mental state is the psychological condition of the person being evaluated at that time. COVID-19 patients
   often suffer from fear, anxiety, depression, etc. Available assessment
   scales include self-rating scales, such as the Symptom Checklist 90
   (SCL-90), Self-Rating Depression Scale, Self-Rating Anxiety Scale, and
   nurse-administered rating scales, including the Hamilton Depression
   Scale (HAMD) and Hamilton Anxiety Scale (HAMA).
2) Rating scale related to stress and coping: Some COVID-19 patients will
   suffer from stress dysfunction. The trait coping style questionnaire, life
   events scale, and Perceived Social Support Scale (PSSS) can be used.
3) Other rating scales that may be used include the adaptive behavior
   rating scale, neuropsychological test, etc.

10.1.3.4.3 Other Scales

Other scales that may be used include ability tests, also known as an intelli-
gence test, such as Raven's Standard Progressive Matrices (SPM), revised by
Chang Houcan; Wechsler Intelligence Scale, revised by Lin Chuanding and
Chang Houcan; and the neuropsychological assessment.

10.1.3.5 Medical Tests

10.1.3.5.1 Physical Examination

Heart rate, pulse, and respiration, etc.

10.1.3.5.2 Laboratory Investigations

Ensure whether there is a hormone metabolism disorder because the abnormal physical condition is sometimes related to the psychological disorder. For
example, hyperthyroidism (an overactive thyroid gland) may produce symptoms similar to generalized anxiety disorder; while hypothyroidism (an under-
active thyroid gland) can produce symptoms similar to depression.

10.1.3.5.3 Physiological and Psychological Assessments

Physiological and psychological assessments can provide much information about the individual's physical response to a given situation. For example, an electrocardiogram (ECG) measures various stress-related levels that affect cardiovascular system conditions; an electromyographic scanner measures the level of electrical activity in muscles, evaluates and treats tension-related disorders. Other instruments, such as electroencephalogram (EEG) and event-related potentials (ERPs), detect changes in the brain's electrical activity. EEG activity, for example, reflects an individual's alertness, rest, sleep, or dreaming, as well as specific brain wave patterns when the individual is engaged in specific mental tasks. ERPs can reflect the brain's electrophysiological changes under different stress stages to evaluate the human cognitive process.

10.1.3.5.4 Brain Imaging Technology

Brain imaging allows neuroscientists to see "inside the living brain" through the latest technology. These brain imaging methods can help neuroscientists understand the relationship between specific brain regions and their functions, localize the brain areas affected by neurological disease, and invent new ways to treat brain diseases. Now, mature brain imaging technology mainly include computed tomography (CT), positron emission tomography (PET), magnetic resonance imaging (MRI) and functional magnetic resonance imaging (fMRI).

10.1.4 Psychological Assessment of COVID-19 Patients

10.1.4.1 Assessment of Emotions and Feelings

Anxiety, fear, depression, etc., are common in COVID-19 patients. Therefore, it is crucial to establish dynamic assessment and early warnings for a psychological crisis.The interview method can be adopted to evaluate emotions and feelings. Other methods include observing and measuring the external manifestations and physiological changes of patients' emotions and feelings. Evaluate patients using a rating scale. Because COVID-19 is infectious, Jiang Xixi et al. reported on psychological crisis intervention (PCI) to help medical workers, patients, and other affected people overcome any psychological difficulties through remote (telephone and internet) and/or on-site medical services. Fang Yiru et al. also suggested using remote networks and telephone consultations or services to reduce the risk of cross-infection during the pandemic.

Two commonly used emotion assessment scales include the Self-Rating Depression Scale (SDS) and the Self-Rating Anxiety Scale (SAS). These two scales are very similar from the form of scale construction to the specific evaluation methods, which is a relatively simple clinical tool to analyze patients' subjective symptoms. With a wide range of applications, they are suitable for adults with symptoms of depression and anxiety.

10.1.4.2 Assessment of Stress

10.1.4.2.1 Interview

1) Stressors: Ask the following questions to understand whether the patient has experienced significant life events and daily disturbances in the past year and the order of the impact on the individual.
   a. What are the things that make you feel stressed or nervous right now?
   b. How has your life changed recently?
   c. What stress have you experienced due to illness, hospitalization, life change, or family event?
   d. Is your environment making you nervous or upset? What is the reason?
   e. How is your relationship with your family? Is there any discordance? Does your family relationship make you feel pain or annoyance?
   f. Do you feel overwhelmed by the pressure of your job?
   g. What is your financial situation? Do you feel unable to make ends meet?
2) Psychological mediators of stress
   a. Cognitive evaluation of stressors
      i. What does this mean to you?
      ii. What do you think of it?
      iii. Do you think you have the ability to handle this, and how would you feel if you could not control it?
   b. Coping styles
      i. What do you usually do to relieve tension or stress?
      ii. Tell me which of the following measures best describes your coping style: talking to someone, trying to solve a problem, complaining about someone, asking for help, engaging in physical activity, praying, trying to forget, using drugs or alcohol, sleeping, doing nothing, become resigned, or whatever.
   c. Social support
      i. Who in your family, friends, and colleagues can help you when you are in trouble?
      ii. When you are in trouble, do you take the initiative to seek help from family, friends, relatives, or colleagues?
      iii. Are you satisfied with the help of your family, friends, or colleagues?
   d. Personality characteristics
      i. What kind of attitude and behavior do you usually adopt when facing difficulties?

      ii. Do you do things and make decisions on your own or rely on others?

     iii. When you are unhappy, do you like to talk about it or keep it to yourself?

3) Stress response

    a. Can you usually solve your problems and troubles?

    b. Are the measures you have taken useful?

    c. Do you feel tired physically and mentally?

10.1.4.2.2 Evaluation of Rating Scale

1) Assessment of stress source intensity:

    a. Life change unit (LCU): Social Readjustment Rating Scale developed by Holmes and Rahe (1967), also known as a stress rating scale, is divided into an adult and a juvenile version. This scale uses LCUs to reflect the stress intensity that may be caused by life events, evaluates the impacts of different types of life events on individuals in the past year, and predicts the possibility of individual health problems. The evaluation criterion used for this scale is the life event unit. Total > 300 scores, 80% chance of developing a disease (serious health risk); a total of 200–299 scores with a 50% chance of developing a disease (moderate health risk); a total of 150–199 points with a 30% chance of developing a disease; total < 150 scores indicates no significant problems and negligible risk of illness.

    b. Life Event Scale (LES): This scale was developed by Desen and Yalin (1986), and it is suitable for people over 16 years old. This scale affects the cause analysis of patients with neurosis, psychosomatic disorders, various somatic disorders, and severe mental illness. It can effectively understand subjects' mental load and quality of life, identify high-risk groups, and guide psychological treatment and crisis intervention. The higher the total score of LES evaluation criteria, the greater the individual mental stress is.

    c. Stress rating scale for hospitalized patients: This scale is used to evaluate the stress experienced by inpatients. The evaluation criterion is that the higher the cumulative score is, the greater the stress is.

2) Assessment of psychological stress mediators:

    a. Coping style rating scale.

    b. Social support scale.

    c. Personality test.

10.1.4.2.3 Assessment of Stress Response

Because stress often causes anxiety and depression, the scale for measuring anxiety and depression can be used as a useful tool for measuring stress response.

10.1.4.3 Observation and Medical Testing

10.1.4.3.1 General State and Behavior

Observe whether there are physiological responses caused by stress, such as anorexia, stomach pain, polyphagia, fatigue, insomnia, excessive sleep, headache, or chest pain. Also observe whether there are cognitive changes caused by stress, such as memory decline, confusion, and decreased problem-solving ability; whether there are emotional responses, such as anxiety, depression, helplessness, and anger; and whether there are behavioral reactions caused by stress, such as behavior degradation or hostility, substance abuse, suicide, or violent tendencies.

10.1.4.3.2. Changes in Various Systems throughout the Body

Observe whether there are changes in heart rate, heart rhythm, blood pressure, respiratory rate and morphology, digestive tract function (with or without complaints, such as anorexia and abdominal pain), muscle tension and physical activity, and the temperature, humidity, and integrity of the skin.

10.1.5 Prospects

COVID-19 is an infectious disease, a public health crisis, and a severe threat to public health. It is urgent and essential to assess psychological disorders in the Level IV population during the pandemic. However, there are specific difficulties in the assessment and research on them, such as the risk of cross-infection in the interview, methodological problems during the research under the natural state, and ethical problems. Therefore, online remote consultation and assessment can be applied to lay a solid foundation for psychological intervention. In addition to the COVID-19 pandemic, the SARS outbreak in China in 2003, the Wenchuan earthquake in 2008, and the H7N9 avian influenza in 2013 are all public emergencies in which similar psychological dysfunction occurred; therefore, some references can be drawn from these events.

10.2 TREATMENT OF PSYCHOLOGICAL DISORDERS

Rehabilitation treatment for psychological disorders is a process of providing psychological help for patients with chronic diseases or disabilities by rehabilitation therapists who have been professionally trained based on a good therapeutic relationship. People actively infected with COVID-19 are capable of spreading it to a wide range of the population, causing different levels of fear, anger, anxiety, depression, and other emotional problems in multiple groups. Promoting psychological rehabilitation for the vast population affected by COVID-19 is also an essential part of COVID-19 prevention and control efforts.

10.2.1 Objectives of Psychological Rehabilitation

Stabilize the emotions of rehabilitation subjects, reduce or eliminate harmful behaviors, enhance confidence in rehabilitation, improve interpersonal relationships psychological adjustment capabilities, and establish new adaptive behaviors to help rehabilitation subjects to better return to their families, reintegrate into society, and improve their quality of life.

10.2.2 Objects of Psychological Rehabilitation

People affected by COVID-19 are classified into four levels (as described in Section 10.1), and rehabilitation techniques for mental disorders should be actively and effectively applied to these four levels' mental health protection.

10.2.3 Principles of Psychological Rehabilitation Treatment

1) Medical staff shall strictly follow the documents of the NHC on COVID-19 prevention and control in terms of protection.
2) Maintain a good doctor–patient relationship, which is the basis of psychological treatment.
3) Stabilize patients' emotions and enhance their confidence as the primary purpose.
4) Rehabilitation therapists should unconditionally accept patients' abnormal emotions and behaviors and fully respect and understand their psychological feelings.
5) Rehabilitation should be patient-centered. Rehabilitation doctors, therapists, and nurses as well as patients' families should actively participate in the rehabilitation process.
6) Focusing on the principle of confidentiality is the requirement of professional quality and the basis of ensuring effective psychological rehabilitation treatment for patients.
7) Pay attention to language communication skills and adopt flexible methods to communicate on sensitive issues.

10.2.4 Psychological Rehabilitation Treatment Methods

10.2.4.1 Psychological Support Therapy

Psychological support is based on psychodynamic theory, using advice and encouragement to treat patients with severe mental impairment. The basic principle is to improve symptoms directly and maintain and rebuild self-esteem, or improve self-confidence, self-function, and adaptive skills. The therapist's goal is to maintain or enhance the patient's sense of self-esteem, minimize or prevent the recurrence of symptoms, and maximize the patient's ability to adapt.

This can be done in the following ways:

1) Listening: Understand and master the psychological problems and psychological obstacles of the patient. Let the patient use verbal/non-verbal methods to vent negative emotions, release their painful inner experience, and pay attention to skills, such as using more open-ended questions and fewer closed-ended questions. Respond to the conversation promptly with simple affirmative words and body language.

2) Explanations: Use straightforward and easy-to-understand language to explain truthfully to patients. Clearly explain the cause, nature, extent, treatment plan, and outcome of the problems to eliminate the psychological pressure caused by their lack of disease knowledge. For those who are stable, cheerful, and strong-willed the therapist can be honest about the patient's illness to maximize their enthusiasm to cooperate with the treatment and let them know the impact of a bad personality and mental state on rehabilitation. Methods of nonverbal communication include body posture, body movement, eye contact, facial expression, skin contact, verbal expression, etc.

3) Encouragement: Encourage patients according to their specific situation. It is not advisable to encourage them to do things that cannot be done.

4) Guarantees: Therapists can try to objectively and clearly state the possible prognosis of the disease in order to arouse the hope of the patient but can only make a limited guarantee based on their condition of the disease and must not easily make promises or unrealistic guarantees. According to the patient's examination and treatment results, make acceptable assurances to strengthen their confidence in overcoming the disease. If some patients are concerned about whether their disease can be cured, tell them with certainty that, as time goes by, the function will be further restored and the disease can be recovered, but it will take a long time. At the same time, cite some typical, miraculous recoveries and rehabilitation cases to enhance their confidence.

5) Guidance: To reduce psychological pressure, give directions and instructions to patients on what to do and how to do it.

6) Environment improvement: Improve the living environment that is not conducive to the solution of patients' psychological problems, especially interpersonal relationships.

10.2.4.2 Focus Solution Mode

The focus solution mode, also known as solution-focused brief therapy, refers to a short-term psychotherapy technique centered on finding solutions to problems. It is a psychotherapy model developed in the context of positive psychology that fully respects individuals and believes in their own resources and potentiality. It is widely used in the areas of family services, public and social services, community treatment centers, child welfare, and schools and hospitals and has received positive recognition. Therapists need to be time-sensitive and make consultations time-effective and treat each session as the last one. The treatment method is goal-oriented rather than problem-oriented. It emphasizes finding ways to solve problems rather than discovering the causes of problems and promotes changes with a positive, future-oriented, and goal-oriented positive attitude.

Find the problem of focus mainly through a variety of questions. For example, preset questioning techniques use some language to create cues that can influence or change the patient's thinking and lead them to think positively. Use calibrated interrogation techniques (scoring techniques) to help patients describe some abstract concepts or experiences in a more concrete and visual way. In the process of psychotherapy, when the patient has positive changes or the therapist finds positive factors, give patients heartfelt praise. The first signs of change; Miracle inquiry; Exception inquiry helps patients to find exceptions, and causes patients to think about solutions through exceptions, thus increasing patients' confidence. Relationship inquiry, response to inquiry, etc.

10.2.4.3 Music Therapy
Music therapy refers to the psychological, and social therapy utilizing music and art, and it is also a kind of rehabilitation, health care, and educational activity. It can be divided into passive and active modes, which can improve patients' physical and mental state, and play a role in emotional release and relaxation of the sympathetic nervous state to achieve the effect of nonverbal communication.

The choice of specific music should be tailored to individual conditions. Choose different music for people with different occupations. People with different emotional states are also suitable for different music. For example, people working in noisy factories should choose the classical symphony; impatient people are better to listen to slow-paced and thought-provoking music, which can adjust their mentality; negative people should listen to more majestic and exciting songs to enhance their confidence; lying-in women should listen to more poetic and confident music.

The light in the music therapy room should be bright and soft, with fresh air, and lush and vibrant plants. It is recommended to wash and clean before listening to music, keep a clear mind, massage the face with both hands, and perform a simple head massage. Music therapy can be combined with simple rest exercises or deep-breathing exercises before listening to music.

10.2.4.4 Cognition Therapy
Cognitive process is the mediation between behavior and emotion. Maladaptive behaviors and emotions are associated with maladaptive cognition. Emotions are based on people's cognition, and emotional problems

often result from incorrect cognition. Emotional problems may be alleviated by changing bad cognition.

Specific treatment methods are as follows:

1) Problem-solving: This is the central part of cognitive adjustment.
2) Hierarchical task arrangement: This is particularly important for depressed patients.
3) Activity monitoring: Patients are required to record what they do every hour and grade and score their emotions and happiness during the activity.
4) Make activity plans.
5) Psychological education: This is a key element of cognitive adjustment.
6) Enhance confidence.
7) Comparison of self-function is a very important skill for people with depression.
8) Conductive findings: The purpose of this method is to correct patients' bad cognition. Dysfunctional thought recording allows patients to record their thoughts and respond to them systematically.
9) Behavioral experiments: This helps patients test automatic thoughts that appear in a predicative form.
10) Respond to patients' true thoughts: Sometimes, patients' thoughts are true.
11) Weighing the pros and cons: When patients are confused and do not know how to choose something, the therapist can help them distinguish, record, and weigh the pros and cons.
12) Develop coping cards.
13) Imagination exercise: Therapists can use visualization techniques to help ease patients' distress, especially for those who experience automatic imagination in the way of images.
14) Relaxation exercise: This is instrumental for anxious patients to have relaxation exercises, such as muscle relaxation, breathing control, etc.
15) Gradual exposure: This is often used in patients with anxiety. Patients build a fear registration form in advance and expose themselves to the scary situation step by step, and then use the learned cognitive and behavioral techniques to reduce anxiety and gain a sense of control.

Note: It is best to use cognitive psychotherapy after the rehabilitated patients have a relatively stable mood. This method is not suitable for children with low cognitive function. The effect may be better if cognitive therapy is best combined with behavioral therapy.

10.2.4.5 Behavior Modification Therapy

Behavior modification therapy teaches and trains patients to adjust and change their original abnormal behaviors and replace them with new healthy behaviors, thus curing the disease. Through the assessment, work with the patients to determine the misconduct that needs to be corrected and establish corrective goals. For different people and problems of a different nature, use various ways to solve and choose the appropriate application method to achieve the selected goal.

Theoretically, behavior modification therapy can be carried out using the following methods:

1) Reinforcement: After a behavior occurs, if a reinforcement stimulus follows it, the behavior will happen again. For example, positive reinforcement gives a pleasant stimulus, whereas negative reinforcement gives an aversive stimulus.

2) After the patients have a bad behavior, immediately give them some kind of punishment or take away the positive reinforcement that they are enjoying. The behavior being punished should be specific, not general. Choose an effective punishment that should vary from person to person and have an appropriate intensity. Create a good educational situation and give timely punishment. When using punishment, be sure to find good behaviors that oppose bad behaviors, replace bad behaviors with good ones, and give a lot of positive reinforcement to the replaced good behaviors to accelerate the natural disappearance of bad behaviors.

3) Regression method: Reduce the incidence of bad behaviors by weakening or removing the reinforcing factors of certain bad behaviors. Reduce and eliminate bad behavior by ignoring and neglecting in general.

   The therapist should first demonstrate to the patient a correct behavior, equivalent to correct action. During the demonstration, the following should be done:

   a. Get the attention of patients, so patients have the ability to imitate.
   b. Give an appropriate description of the actions demonstrated. Note: Perform every movement accurately, and give patients repeated instructions throughout the demonstration.
   c. Arrange a large number of practice opportunities for patients, which is a vital link to ensure they master the skills.
   d. Provide feedback, including the reinforcement of the correct behavior imitation behavior and weakening the wrong behavior. Attention should be paid to correct any errors in the patient's imitation.

4) Other common methods include systemic desensitization therapy, exposure therapy, aversion therapy, behavior modeling training (affirmative training, assertive training), relaxation training, etc.

10.2.4.6 Relaxation Therapy

Relaxation therapy, also known as tension-lessening therapy and relaxing training, refers to learning to consciously control or adjust one's psychological and physiological activities according to a certain practice program to reduce the arousal level of the body and adjust all aspects of functions that are disordered due to stress.

It includes the following methods:

1) Muscle relaxation training: The most commonly used is progressive muscle relaxation training. The rehabilitative subjects can feel the difference when their muscles are tense first and then relaxed. Instruct patients to clench their fists, then tense their arms, shoulders, chest, abdomen, buttocks, and legs, etc., then relax at each step. Finally, the whole body is relaxed by gradually relaxing each muscle group.

2) Breath control training and abdominal breathing: Inhale through the nose, and exhale through the nose (mouth), and use the abdomen to breathe. Drop the shoulders naturally, slowly close eyes, place one hand on the abdomen and the other on the chest. The expiration time is twice the inhalation time. Experience the feeling of inhaling deeply and exhaling slowly.

3) Imagine relaxation: Imagine the most comfortable, coziest, and most relaxing situation, usually at the sea.

4) Other therapies include meditation, self-hypnosis, relaxation assisted by biofeedback, etc.

Several relaxation therapies can be combined, such as abdominal breathing and muscle relaxation. Also, relaxation therapy is often used in combination with systematic desensitization or other psychotherapy, or it can be used alone. Relaxation therapy is also widely used in the treatment of various anxiety neuroses, phobias, and so on.

10.2.4.7 Group Psychotherapy

Group psychotherapy is a kind of psychotherapy in which therapists organize patients with similar psychological problems. Generally, patients are divided into several groups, and each group comprises several or more than a dozen patients, then the group leader is chosen.

The main methods of group psychotherapy are lectures, activities, and discussions. The therapist explains the related symptoms, etiology, treatment, and prognosis to the patients in a simple and profound way based on the common psychological factors and viewpoints of the patients. Make the patients understand the law of occurrence and development of problems, eliminate their worries, and build confidence, or organize group members to carry out activities, and then discuss in groups.

It should be noted that the limitations of collective psychotherapy, such as personal deep-seated problems are not easy to expose, and the group leader's cognition is limited, etc. Thus, collective psychotherapy is not suitable for all rehabilitation subjects.

10.2.4.8 Family Psychotherapy

In this form of therapy, the family as a whole is treated with psychotherapy. Through the purposeful contact and conversation with all family members, the therapist can promote changes in the family and affect the patient through family members to alleviate or eliminate the symptoms of the patient.

The family-oriented group psychotherapy model to treat patients' symptoms aims to help families eliminate abnormal, pathological conditions to perform healthy family functions.

General procedures for family therapy:

1) Collect family data and understand family background: Evaluate family dynamics, family interaction pattern, social and cultural background, family intergenerational structure, etc.
2) Establish therapeutic objectives: Eliminate the usual pattern of avoiding conflict in the family, introduce good coping styles, change the intergenerational communication among family members, and provide new ideas and choices for the family.
3) Treatment time: The therapist should communicate with family members frequently, 1–2 hours each time with an interval of about 1 week or make arrangements according to specific circumstances.

10.2.4.9 Biofeedback Therapy

Process biological information such as electromyography, electroencephalography, heart rate, and blood pressure, and then show patients how they can recognize changes, such as vision and hearing. In other words, use electromyographic feedback instrument, skin electrical feedback instrument, and EEG feedback instrument, etc., to assist patients in relaxation training.

The biofeedback method generally includes two aspects: first, the rehabilitation subjects learn relaxation training, to reduce excessive tension and make the body reach a certain degree of relaxation; second, after relaxation training, they can understand and master the information about the physiological function changes in their body by the use the biofeedback device, and further strengthen the study of relaxation training. Until they form the operational conditioned reflex and relieve the normal physiological activities or pathology, their normal physiological functions are restored.

10.2.4.10 Physical Factor Therapy

Repetitive transcranial magnetic stimulation (rTMS) is a highly safe, non-invasive neuromodulation technique. A large number of studies have shown that rTMS has a good alleviating effect on mental symptoms such as depression, anxiety, sleep disorders, and compulsions. In 2008, the US Food and Drug Administration (FDA) officially approved rTMS for the treatment of depression, especially in patients who do not respond well to medication. For example, high frequency ($\geq$ 5 Hz) rTMS stimulation of the left dorsolateral prefrontal lobe or low frequency (1 Hz) stimulation of the right dorsolateral prefrontal lobe can relieve depressive symptoms. In addition, many studies have shown that transcranial direct current stimulation can also significantly promote psychological rehabilitation.

10.2.4.11 Exercise Training

Different types of exercise, such as aerobic exercise, anaerobic exercise, individual/team exercise, are beneficial to the improvement of mental disorders. Exercise training programs with different intensity, frequency, duration, and intervention time can be formulated according to the individual's own culture, physical fitness, mood state, etc.

10.2.4.12 Occupational Therapy

Occupational therapy is a patient-centered therapy that promotes patients' health and improves their happiness through occupational activities, allowing them to participate in daily life activities to support and help them return to their families and society. Gradually help patients to improve self-confidence and reduce the sense of self-defeat and powerlessness. Simultaneously, occupational activities can improve cognitive impairment, help patients improve cognitive ability, increase knowledge and skills, improve self-life ability, and enhance self-awareness and problem-solving ability. Therefore, occupational therapy can be used to improve the self-care ability of injured and disabled patients and treat mental illnesses. Design the occupational therapy activities that can produce a pleasant effect and divert attention to achieve the purpose of adjusting mood and relieving pressure. Individualized occupational therapy programs can be formulated according to personal hobbies, work, and family environment to promote physical and mental health.

10.2.4.13 TCM Therapy

Studies have shown that TCM acupuncture and moxibustion therapy, electroacupuncture, and TCM prescriptions can help regulate depression and insomnia symptoms and have the effect of strengthening psychological counseling. In recent years, acupuncture combined with Chinese and Western medicine, Chinese medicine combined with psychotherapy, acupuncture combined with psychological counseling, and other joint treatments for psychological disorders have made some progress.

10.2.4.14 Traditional Exercise Therapy

Qigong, five-animal exercise, baduanjin, tai chi chuan, and yi jin jing are traditional exercise therapies with Chinese characteristics, and they all contain different levels of intensity of exercise programs, which are widely applicable to people. They not only enhance physical fitness but also contribute to physical and mental health.

10.2.4.15 Pharmacotherapy

Drugs for improving mental disorders are classified according to the main indications: antipsychotics, antidepressants, antimanic or mood stabilizers, antianxiety medications, and psychoactive stimulants. Develop a psychiatric drug treatment program by consulting a professional psychiatrist and conducting a professional psychological assessment.

10.2.4.16 Health Education

Provide mental health education for the rehabilitation subjects, and guide them to learn psychological self-help and grooming methods, for example, decompress and relax their bodies through breathing relaxation (such as slow abdominal breathing) and changing body postures (such as finger exercises, neck exercises, baduanjin, yoga, a hot bath, etc.). Encourage patients to do their favorite things, enrich their lives, and divert attention; strengthen communication with relatives and friends by using the telephone, text messages, WeChat, or video; and maintain a normal diet, sleep quality, etc.

10.2.5 Determination of Psychological Rehabilitation Treatment Prescription

10.2.5.1 Confirmed COVID-19 Patients

10.2.5.1.1 Initial Isolation Treatment

Patients' main manifestations include numbness, denial, anger, fear, anxiety, depression, disappointment, complaint, insomnia, or aggression. The principle of psychological intervention is to support and comfort as the mainstay. Treat patients with tolerance, stabilize their emotions, and assess the risk of suicide, self-harm, and aggression early. Use comprehensive rehabilitation treatment programs such as psychological support therapy, short-term treatment for anxiety resolution, and occupational therapy. If necessary, consult a psychiatrist to determine whether patients need psychiatric medication.

10.2.5.1.2 Isolation Treatment Period

In addition to the mentality that may appear in the initial stage of treatment, patients may also be lonely, do not cooperate, give up treatment due to fear of the disease, or even show excessive optimism and have high expectations for treatment. The principle of psychological intervention is to actively communicate information and consult a psychiatrist if necessary. Adopt comprehensive rehabilitation treatment programs, such as psychological support therapy, short-term anxiety treatment, music therapy, occupational therapy, cognitive intervention, etc. If necessary, consult a psychiatrist to determine whether psychiatric medication is needed.

10.2.5.2 Patients with Respiratory Distress, Extreme Restlessness, and Difficulty in Expression

The main manifestations of these patients are near-death, panic, despair, and so on. The principle of psychological intervention is to comfort, calm, focus on emotional communication, and enhance their treatment confidence. Psychological support therapy, cognitive intervention, behavior correction, and other comprehensive rehabilitation programs can be used. If necessary, consult a psychiatrist to determine whether psychiatric medication is needed.

10.2.5.3 Mild Patients for Home Isolation and Patients with Fever for Treatment

The main manifestations of these patients are panic, restlessness, loneliness, helplessness, repression, depression, pessimism, anger, nervousness, pressure to be alienated and avoided by others, grievance, shame, or not paying attention to the disease. The principle of psychological intervention is to provide health education and get the patient to cooperate and adapt to changes. Comprehensive rehabilitation programs such as exercise therapy, music therapy, and health education can be used. If necessary, consult a professional psychiatrist online.

10.2.5.4 Suspected Patients

The main manifestation of these patients are fluke psychology, avoidance of treatment, fear of discrimination, anxiety, excessive seeking treatment, frequent hospital transfer, etc. The principle of psychological intervention is to educate in a timely manner, correct protection, obey the overall situation, and reduce pressure. Exercise therapy, music therapy, relaxation training, health education, and other comprehensive rehabilitation treatment programs can be used. Consult a professional psychiatrist online if necessary.

10.2.5.5 Medical Staff and Related Personnel

The main manifestation of these patients is excessive fatigue and tension, even exhaustion, anxiety, insomnia, depression, sadness, grievance, helplessness, repression, frustration, or self-blame in the face of patients' death. Additionally, they are often worried about being infected, worried about family members, and fear that family members worry about themselves. They are excessively hyperactive, refuse to take reasonable rest, and cannot guarantee their health, etc. The principles of psychological intervention are to regulate rotation, self-regulate, and seek help when there are problems. Psychological support therapy, relaxation training, exercise therapy, music therapy, health education and other comprehensive rehabilitation treatment programs can be used. Consult a professional psychiatrist online if necessary.

10.2.5.6 People Who Are in Close Contact with Patients (Family Members, Colleagues, Friends, etc.)

The main manifestations of these patients are avoidance, restlessness, anxiety while waiting, blind courage, refusal to protect themselves, and refusal of home observation, etc. The principles of psychological intervention are to educate, comfort, and encourage the use of network communication. Comprehensive rehabilitation treatment programs include psychological support therapy, relaxation training, exercise therapy, music therapy, health education, etc. Consult a professional psychiatrist online if necessary.

10.2.5.7 People Who Are Reluctant to Seek Medical Treatment in Public

The main manifestations of these patients are fear of misdiagnosis and isolation, lack of awareness, avoidance, neglect, anxiety, etc. The principles of psychological intervention are to explain and persuade, not criticize, and support health-seeking behavior. Psychological support therapy, relaxation training, exercise therapy, music therapy, health education, and other comprehensive rehabilitation treatment programs can be used. Consult a professional psychiatrist online if necessary.

10.2.5.8 Susceptible Groups and the General Public

The main manifestations of these patients are panic, afraid to go out, blind disinfection, disappointment, fear, irritability, aggressive behavior, over-optimism, giving up, etc. The principles of psychological intervention are to provide health education, guidance of positive response, elimination of fear, scientific prevention. Psychological support therapy, relaxation training, sports therapy, music therapy, health education, and other comprehensive rehabilitation treatment programs can be used. Consult a professional psychiatrist online if necessary.

10.2.6 Forms of Psychological Rehabilitation Counseling

There are various forms of psychological rehabilitation counseling applicable to all kinds of people to ensure that people at all levels can get effective psychological support.

1) According to the number of counseling subjects, it can be divided into individual counseling and group counseling.
2) According to psychological consultation, it can be divided into outpatient consultation, on-site consultation, telephone consultation, letter consultation, thematic consultation, internet consultation, online outpatient service, etc.

BIBLIOGRAPHY

1. Ko CH, Yen CF, Yen JY, Yang MJ. Psychosocial impact among the public of the severe acute respiratory syndrome pandemic in Taiwan [J]. *Psychiatry and Clinical Neurosciences*, 2006, 60(4): 397–403.
2. Xiang YT, Yang Y, Li W, Zhang L, Zhang Q, Cheung T, Ng CH. Timely mental health care for the 2019 novel coronavirus outbreak is urgently needed [J]. *Lancet Psychiatry*, 2020, 7(3): 228–229.
3. Huimin Han, Guangcheng Cui, Ameng Zhao, Na Wang, Zhilei He, Jidong Ma. Relationship between early awakening of depression and event-related potentials [J]. *Psychology Science*, 2011 (6): 242–245.
4. Hui Ma, Zhihong Wang, Jin Yan, Taosheng Liu. Progress in the application of event-related potential in psychological stress-related diseases [J]. *Chinese Journal of Behavioral Medicine and Brain Science*, 2006, 15(5): 477–478.
5. Meyer BM, Rabl U, Huemer J, Bartova L, Kalcher K, Provenzano J, Brandner C, Sezen P, Kasper S, Schatzberg AF, Moser E, Chen G, Pezawas L. Prefrontal networks dynamically related to recovery from major depressive disorder: A longitudinal pharmacological fMRI study. Translational psychiatry[J]. *Transl Psychiatry*, 2019, 9(1): 64.
6. Xu K, Cai H, Shen Y, Ni Q, Chen Y, Hu S, Li J, Wang H, Yu L, Huang H, Qiu Y, Wei G, Fang Q, Zhou J, Sheng J, Liang T, Li L. Management of corona virus disease-19 (COVID-19): The Zhejiang experience [J]. *The Medical Version of Zhejiang University Journal*, 2020, 49(1): 0. 32096367
7. Jiang X, Deng L, Zhu Y, Ji H, Tao L, Liu L, Yang D, Ji W. Psychological crisis intervention during the outbreak period of new coronavirus pneumonia from experience in Shanghai [J]. *Psychiatry Research*, 2020, 286: 112903.
8. Experts' Suggestions on the diagnosis and treatment procedures and routes of mental disorders during the prevention and control of major infectious diseases (COVID-19) [OL]. *Psychiatry Branch of Chinese Medical Association*. 2020. doi: 10.3760/cma.J.c.n113661-20200219-00039.
9. Lau JT, Yang X, Tsui HY, Pang E, Wing YK. Positive mental health-related impacts of the SARS on the general public in Hong Kong and their associations with other negative impacts [J]. *Journal of Infection*, 2006, 53(2): 114–124.

10. Chen XY, Chen J, Shi X, Jiang M, Li Y, Zhou Y, Ran M, Lai Y, Wang T, Fan F, Liu X, Chan CLW. Trajectories of maternal symptoms of posttraumatic stress disorder predict long-term mental health of children following the Wenchuan earthquake in China: A 10-year follow-up study [J]. *Journal of Affective Disorders*. 2020, 266: 201–206.

11. Shibata A, Okamatsu M, Sumiyoshi R, Matsuno K,Wang ZJ,Kida H,Osaka H,Sakoda Y. Repeated detection of H7N9 avian influenza viruses in raw poultry meat illegally brought to Japan by international flight passengers[J]. *Virology*. 2018, 524: 10–17.

12. Shuangyi Qi, Handsome Xi, Xin Ma. A review of Chinese mental health research [J]. *China Journal of Health Psychology*, 2019, 27(6): 947–953.

13. Tan J R. Progress of occupational therapy in the treatment of depression [J]. *China Sanatorium Medicine*, 2019, 28(1): 50–53. (Chinese).

14. Aihua Wang, Juan Wang, Bowen Gan. Research progress of TCM treatment of depression [J]. *Chinese People's Liberation Army Medical Journal*, 2019, 31(6): 112–116.

15. Downar J, Daskalakis ZJ. New targets for rTMS in depression: A review of convergent evidence [J]. *Brain Stimulation*, 2013, 6(3): 231–240.

16. National Health Commission. *Novel Coronavirus Infected Pneumonia Self-help and Counseling Guide for Public Psychology [OL]*. [2020-02-03].

17. National Health Commission. *Notice on the Issuance of Novel Coronavirus Outbreak Emergency Psychological Crisis Intervention Guidelines [OL]*. [2020-01-26].

18. Holmes TH, Rahe RH. The Social Readjustment Rating Scale. *Journal of Psychosomatic Research* 1967 Aug; 11(2): 213–218. doi: 10.1016/0022-3999(67)90010-4. PMID: 6059863.

19. Yalin Zhang, Desen Yang. Pathogenicity of life events-Data analysis of 72 cases of hysteria [J]. *Chinese Journal of Neuropsychiatric Diseases*, 1988 (02): 65–68.

Chapter 11

Assessment and Treatment for Malnutrition of COVID-19 Patients

11.1 OVERVIEW

Malnutrition is a state of insufficient macronutrients and micronutrients and insufficient protein and energy reserves due to disease or aging.

Malnutrition can be divided into the following three categories according to types:protein-deficient malnutrition, protein-calorie deficiency malnutrition, and mixed malnutrition. Protein-deficient malnutrition is seen in patients who are in good nutritional status before illness but suffer from a sudden serious illness. Patients' catabolism is significantly increased, and the nutrient intake is relatively insufficient, resulting in the reduction of plasma albumin and transferrin, accompanied by the decline of the body's immune function. But the body weight and triceps skinfold thickness are average. Protein-calorie deficiency malnutrition is caused by the long-term lack of protein-calorie intake, and the body's muscle tissue and fat are gradually consumed. This is characterized by a significant decrease in body weight, while plasma protein can still maintain normal. Mixed malnutrition is caused by the long-term malnutrition, and it has the characteristics of the above two types of malnutrition. There is a significant decrease in the protein of skeletal muscle and internal organs and a decrease in endogenous fat and protein reserves, accompanied by impaired functions of multiple organs, which is a severe state of malnutrition.

According to the currently reported pathophysiological manifestations of patients with COVID-19, many critically severe patients have and show signs of obvious systemic inflammatory reactions, even inflammatory storms, and lung, spleen, liver, heart, kidney, and other multiple organ dysfunctions. Disease conditions and inflammatory reactions cause the body's catabolism to increase, which leads to the body's metabolic disorders and increased consumption of the body's tissues, causing clinical malnutrition in patients with COVID-19. Malnutrition in patients with COVID-19 can lead to many adverse consequences, such as increased mortality, prolonged hospitalization, increased medical expenses, and decreased quality of life, especially for some elderly people with poor basic conditions and low immunity and patients with multiple chronic diseases. After infection, the condition becomes more critical, and the risk of death is higher.

The imbalance between supply and demand causes malnutrition in COVID-19 patients. According to the pathophysiological characteristics of the patients, malnutrition may occur for the following reasons:

1) Patients develop symptoms such as infection and fever, and some progress to acute respiratory distress syndrome (ARDS). The body is in a state of high catabolism, leading to increased gluconeogenesis and insulin resistance, followed by increased catabolism of protein, negative nitrogen balance of the body, and further increased demand for energy and protein an imbalance between energy supply and demand.

2) In critically severe patients, the body's oxygen supply is less than oxygen consumption, which leads to impaired intestinal function and malabsorption of nutrients.

3) The intestinal tract is also one of the target organs invaded by COVID-19. Clinically, many patients have gastrointestinal symptoms, such as diarrhea. Meanwhile, antiviral drugs, such as arbidol, lopinavir, and ritonavir tablets, can also cause gastrointestinal symptoms, such as anorexia and diarrhea.

4) Many severe and critically severe patients receive noninvasive mechanical ventilation. Such patients often have severe gastric bloating, increasing intra-abdominal pressure, causing intestinal nutritional intolerance and risk of aspiration. Additionally, it can also lead to changes in respiratory mechanics and affect the efficacy of noninvasive ventilation.

Malnutrition in patients with COVID-19 will affect ventilation, respiratory muscle structure and function, and the body's immune response. Among them, the malnutrition in severe and critically severe patients will cause more severe damage to their respiratory muscle function, gradually weaken their respiratory muscle strength, affect patients' ventilation function, make infection control difficult, and increase the risk of organ failure. Currently, there are no specific drugs for COVID-19 patients. In addition to respiratory and circulatory support, symptomatic support treatment for patients has become an important part of the overall treatment, of which a very important part is nutritional support treatment. Nutritional support can effectively ensure the needs of cell metabolism in the body, maintain the structure and function of tissues and organs, and improve patients' immunity.

This chapter mainly discusses the nutritional assessment and nutritional support treatment of COVID-19 patients, aiming to enhance the awareness of a balanced diet and nutrition for COVID-19 patients and assist clinicians in providing high-quality nutritional assessment and treatment for COVID-19 patients, thereby improving the therapeutic effect of COVID-19 patients, especially to improve the cure rate of critically severe patients and reduce mortality.

11.2 ASSESSMENT OF MALNUTRITION

At present, malnutrition has become a non-negligible complication in COVID-19 patients, especially in severe patients. For COVID-19 patients, the causes of malnutrition include insufficient intake and increased demand. Malnutrition caused by insufficient intake of nutrients can be corrected through nutritional support; however, in the period of enhanced disease catabolism, the negative energy balance and negative nitrogen balance cannot be corrected by nutritional support alone, even if a large amount of nutrients are taken in, they cannot be corrected. Only when the primary disease is effectively controlled, the infection is controlled, the inflammatory response subsides, and the human tissue enters the anabolic stage can the body's nutritional status be effectively improved and obtain good clinical outcomes. Scientific and reasonable nutritional support can effectively improve the nutritional status of COVID-19 patients, reduce complications, enhance immunity, and improve patients' prognosis. Through nutritional assessment, patients suffering from malnutrition or at potential risk of malnutrition can be identified in time to provide timely nutritional support. Therefore, early and systematic nutritional assessment is particularly important to guide individualized nutritional support treatment.

The purpose of nutritional assessment is to:

1) Determine whether the patient is at risk of malnutrition or potential malnutrition.
2) Assess the severity of malnutrition.
3) Provide the basis for nutritional support treatment.

The first nutritional assessment is nutritional screening, which is the most basic step. Patients at risk of malnutrition after screening need further nutritional assessment to make an accurate diagnosis of malnutrition.

11.2.1 Nutrition Risk Screening

Nutrition risk screening begins with the patient's medical history, such as weight loss and food intake. For the screening of the risk of malnutrition in patients with COVID-19, Nutrition Risk Screening–2002 (NRS-2002) scoring scale is commonly used in clinical practice.

The NRS-2002 rating scale is a scale used to screen adult hospitalized patients for nutritional assessment launched at the European Society of Parenteral and Enteral Nutrition in 2002. The scale is divided into a preliminary screening table and a final screening table. The assessment contents are shown in Table 11.1.

11.2.1.1 NRS-2002 Assessment Scale for Reduced Nutritional Status Score and Its Definition

1) 0 score: Definition – normal nutritional status.
2) Mild (1 score): 5% weight loss within 3 months or 50%–75% of normal requirements for food intake.
3) Moderate (2 scores): 5% weight loss within 2 months or 25%–50% of normal food intake requirements in the previous week.
4) Severe (3 scores): 5% weight loss within 1 month (15% weight loss within 3 months) or BMI < 18.5 or 0%–25% of normal requirements for food intake in the previous week.

Note: If only one of the three problems is consistent, the degree of severity will be evaluated according to its score, and if several problems are evaluated according to the highest score.

11.2.1.2 NRS-2002 Assessment Scale for the Severity of Disease and Its Definition

1) 1 score: Patients with chronic diseases who have been hospitalized due to complications. The patient is weak but does not need to stay in bed. Oral supplements to compensate for a slight increase in protein requirements.
2) 2 scores: Patients who need to stay in bed. For example, after major abdominal surgery, the protein requirements increase correspondingly, but most of them can still recover through parenteral or enteral nutrition support.
3) 3 scores: The patient is supported by mechanical ventilation in the intensive ward, and the increased protein requirements cannot be compensated by parenteral or enteral nutrition support; however, protein decomposition and nitrogen loss can be significantly reduced through parenteral or enteral nutrition support.

11.2.1.3 Relationship between the NRS-2002 Assessment Scale Score Results and Nutrition Risk

1) The total score of ≥ 3 (or pleural fluid, ascites, edema, and serum protein < 35 g/L) indicates that the patient is malnourished or at risk of nutrition, so nutritional support should be used.

TABLE 11.1   NRS-2002 RATING SCALE

Evaluation Index	Score	If "yes", please tick "√"
Disease States		
Patients with pelvic fractures or chronic diseases with the following diseases: liver cirrhosis, chronic obstructive pulmonary disease, long-term hemodialysis, diabetes, and tumors.	1	☐
Major abdominal surgery, stroke, severe pneumonia, or blood system tumor.	2	☐
Patients with craniocerebral injury, bone marrow suppression, or ICU (APACHE II score > 10 scores)	3	☐
Total		
Nutritional Status		
Normal nutritional status	0	☐
Weight loss > 5% within 3 months or food intake in the last week (compared to the required amount) reduced by 20%–50 %.	1	☐
Weight loss > 5% within 2 months, BMI 18.5–20.5 kg/m² , or food intake in the last week (compared to the required amount) reduced by 50%–75%.	2	☐
Weight loss > 5% within 1 month (or > 15% loss within 3 months), BMI < 18.5 kg/m² (or human serum albumin < 35 g/L), or food intake in the last week (compared to the required amount) reduced by 70%–100%	3	☐
Total		
Age		
≥ 70 years old	1	☐
Evaluation: The total score of the above three parts is less than 3 points, there is no nutritional risk; 3–5 < scores, there is nutritional risk; ≥5 points, there is high nutritional risk.		

Note: NRS-2002 score refers to nutrition risk screening 2002 score; ICU is the intensive care unit; APACHE II score is the acute physiological and chronic health evaluation score; BMI is body mass index.

2) The total score of < 3 indicates that nutrition should be evaluated weekly. If the result of the subsequent review is ≥ 3 scores, the patient will enter the nutrition support program.
3) If the patient plans to undergo major abdominal surgery, the new score (2 scores) will be scored at the first assessment, and the new total score will be used to determine whether nutritional support is required (≥ 3 scores).

One of the advantages of NRS-2002 rating scale is that it can predict the potential risk of malnutrition and dynamically judge the changes in patients' nutritional status. Additionally, doctors and nurses can operate this scale in the clinic, which is easy to operate and easy for patients to accept.

11.2.1.4 NRS-2002 Score Significance for COVID-19 Patients

If the NRS-2002 score is ≥ 3 scores, it indicates that patients have malnutrition risk, and nutrition intervention is required; if the NRs-2002 score is ≥ 5 scores, it indicates that patients are a high malnutrition risk, and nutrition treatment should be given as soon as possible; malnutrition risk assessment should be performed for all severe COVID-19 patients in ICU as early as possible.

11.2.2 Commonly Used Nutritional Status Evaluation Indicators for Nutritional Assessment

Anthropometric indicators (such as calf circumference, subcutaneous fold thickness, etc.), fat-free mass (FFM), fat mass (FM), degree of weight loss, and whether there are other causes of anorexia (such as disease, drugs, age, etc.), biochemical indicators (albumin, etc.) are some of the commonly used nutritional status evaluation indicators.

11.2.2.1 Nutrition History

Recording the patient's eating log (such as a 3–7-day dietary intake record) helps assess nutritional status. Also, asking the patient to recall what they ate the day before can also assist in the assessment.

11.2.2.2 Anthropometry

11.2.2.2.1 Weight and BMI

Weight and BMI are the simplest, most direct and reliable indicators in nutritional assessment that can reflect the human body's nutritional status as a whole. A short period of weight loss is an important predictor of acute deterioration and the need for mechanical ventilation.

Assessment criteria: Malnutrition can be diagnosed as long as it meets any of the following conditions.

1) BMI < 18.5 kg/m².
2) In a definite time period, the weight loss due to non-human factors > 10%, or the weight loss within 3 months > 5%. On this basis, the diagnosis can be made according to one of the following two points:
   a. BMI < 20 kg/m² (age < 70 years old) or BMI < 22 kg/m² (age ≥ 70 years old).
   b. FFMI < 15 kg/m² (female) or FFMI < 17 kg/m² (male).

11.2.2.2.2 Triceps Skinfold Thickness (TSF)

The normal reference value for this test is 8.3mm for males and 15.3mm for females. It is normal that the measured value is more than 90% of the normal value, 80%–90% is mild malnutrition, 60%–80% is moderate malnutrition, and < 60% is severe malnutrition.

11.2.2.2.3 Arm Muscle Circle (AMC)

$$\text{AMC} = \text{arm circumference (cm)} \left[\text{TSF (mm)} \times 0.314\right]$$

If the measured value of the upper arm muscle circumference is more than 90% of the normal value the patient is normal, 80%–90% indicates mild malnutrition, 60%–80% indicates moderate malnutrition, and < 60% indicates severe malnutrition.

11.2.2.2.4 Body Composition Measurement Method

This measurement includes the bioelectrical impedance method and dual-energy X-ray absorption measurement method.

1) At present, the bioelectrical impedance method has become a widely used method for measuring and assessing the composition of the human body. This method is noninvasive easy to operate. By passing a weak AC (alternating current)signal into the human body and measuring the current impedance to analyze the body's composition, the body fat content and muscle mass of the body can be assessed.
   a. Measurement method: The tester turns on the power and inputs relevant information about the subject. The subject stands on the test bench, holds the two handles with both hands, and opens them to the side of the tester respectively, at about a 30° angle from the body. The tester then clicks the test.
   b. Observation indicators: Total water content, protein, inorganic salt, body weight (kg), body fat (BF), body fat ratio, ratio of fat distribution in waist and hip, skeletal muscle (kg), fat-free body weight, muscle mass index (BMI).

c. Advantages: Short detection time, simple operation and noninvasive. The displayed malnutrition and electrolyte changes must precede the weight change or blood biochemical change, which provides the first opportunity for clinical treatment and improves the patient's rescue ability. At the same time, bioelectrical impedance measurement can also estimate the volume and distribution of stagnated fluid and then assess the heart, lung, and kidney systems' functional status.

2) The dual-energy X-ray absorptiometry can accurately determine the human adipose tissue, muscle tissue, and bone density of the whole body through low-dose X-rays. This test is used for a highly accurate determination of skeletal muscle mass of limbs.

a. Measurement method: The subject must remove all metal objects on the body, lie on the measuring bed, stretch the upper limbs and lay flat on both sides of the body, with the feet slightly joined and toes pointing upward.

b. Observation indicators: Total body and bone mineral salt content, total body fat content, lean tissue content, waist and abdomen area fat content, hip area fat content, total body fat percentage, waist and abdomen area fat percentage, hip area fat percentage, waist and abdomen area fat ratio to that of the hip area. The height and weight of the subject are also measured, and BMI is calculated.

c. Advantages: Safe, convenient, low radiation absorption dose, short inspection time, etc.

11.2.2.3 Laboratory Investigations

11.2.2.3.1 Determination of Serum Protein Level

This method of measurement includes albumin, transferrin, and retinol-binding protein. The persistent presence of hypoproteinemia in patients is a reliable indicator of malnutrition, which generally reflects the nutritional status in the last 2–3 weeks. The initial measurement value of albumin below 25 g/L indicates a poor prognosis; however, due to the long half-life of albumin, it cannot be used for continuous monitoring. In contrast, the half-life of prealbumin and binding protein is short, which is better for the dynamic assessment of nutritional status and nutritional treatment efficacy. Indicators related to the nutritional status of patients with severe COVID-19 are often reduced to varying degrees. For example, the serum prealbumin level of severe COVID-19 patients is often lower than 100 g/L, and some critically severe patients are even lower than 70 g/L or even below 50 g/L.

11.2.2.3.2 Creatinine–Height Index (CHI)

CHI varies with the protein intake level and can be used to monitor the body's nutritional status as long as the daily intake of protein is stable. CHI can reflect protein intake and the state of protein synthesis and decomposition in the body. It is closely related to total muscle mass, body surface area, and body weight and is not affected by edema and other complications. CHI of 60%–80% indicates mild protein deficiency, 40%–59% indicates moderate protein deficiency, and < 40% indicates a severe protein deficiency. Therefore, CHI can be used as a laboratory indicator for nutritional assessment in patients with normal renal function.

11.2.2.3.3 Serum Amino Acid Ratio
Serum amino acid ratio = Gly(glycine) + Ser(serine) + Glu(glutamic acid) + Leu (**leucine**)+Iso(isoleucine) + Met (methionine)+ Val(methionine) > 3 indicates malnutrition.

11.2.2.3.4 Immune Function Indicators
Indicators of immune function include the total number of lymphocytes and delayed type hypersensitivity. The total number of lymphocytes is susceptible to multiple factors, such as virus infection, immunosuppression, and hypersplenism, so it cannot accurately reflect patients' nutritional status.

11.3 NUTRITIONAL SUPPORT THERAPY

Currently, there is a lack of highly effective antiviral drugs for COVID-19 patients. In addition to effective respiratory and circulatory support for severe and critically severe patients, nutritional support treatment is of great significance for improving patients' immune function, shortening the course of the disease, and reducing the mortality of patients. Based on the *Rapid Recommended Guideline for COVID-19 Diagnosis and Treatment (Standard Edition)*, Dynamic assessment of patients' nutritional risks and timely nutritional support. Those who can eat by mouth recommend a diet with high protein and carbohydrate. Enteral nutrition should be opened as soon as possible for those who can't eat orally and have no contraindication of enteral nutrition. Those who cannot open enteral nutrition should be given parenteral nutrition in time, and strive to reach the target energy as soon as possible.

After the patient's nutritional status is fully assessed, a nutritional plan should be formulated for the patient's nutritional needs to maintain the patient's nutritional status at a normal level. Nutritional support includes enteral nutrition and parenteral nutrition, and the main nutrients used in nutritional therapy include carbohydrates, proteins, fats, electrolytes, vitamins, water, etc.

11.3.1 Medical and Nutritional Treatment Recommendations for COVID-19 Patients

The expert group of Enteral and Parenteral Nutrition Society, Chinese Medical Association has made the following recommendations regarding the medical and nutritional treatment of COVID-19 patients:

1) Principles: Nutritional therapy is a necessary treatment method and one of the core components of comprehensive treatment measures for COVID-19 patients. Nutritional therapy should be based on the nutritional diagnosis.
2) Methods: Nutrition treatment, dietary and nutrition education, oral nutrition supplement (ONS), tube feeding, supplementary parenteral nutrition (SPN), and total parenteral nutrition (TPN) are carried out according to the five-step method.
3) Energy: A supply of 20–30 kcal/ (kg·d) is recommended, according to the disease's severity.
4) Protein: Patients' demand for protein increases. It is recommended to increase the supply of branched-chain amino acids according to the supply of 1.0–2.0g/ (kg·d).
5) Fat: Prioritize medium and long-chain fatty acids, and increase the proportion of n-3 fatty acids and n-9 fatty acids.
6) Nonprotein energy supply ratio: The ratio of glucose to fat milk is (50–70)%: (30–50)%. The ratio of nonprotein thermal calorie (kcal) to nitrogen content (g) is (100–150): 1.
7) Fluid volume: Pay attention to maintaining fluid balance. For patients with a large area of lung consolidation and elderly patients, it is recommended to control the volume of intravenous infusion.
8) Micronutrients: Supplements, such as multivitamins and minerals, should be given regularly.
9) Immunonutrients: Pay attention to weighing the advantages and disadvantages and master the indications.
10) Monitoring: Closely observe the adverse reactions, assess the therapeutic effect, dynamically adjust the treatment plan, and pay attention to individual differences.

11.3.2 Nutritional Treatment Plan for COVID-19 Patients

11.3.2.1 Purpose of Nutritional Therapy

Nutritional therapy aims to reduce the weight loss of patients and the decomposition of body protein and increase body weight and body protein. For patients with chronic respiratory insufficiency, nutritional therapy aims to gradually correct their malnutrition and negative nitrogen balance, improve muscle protein synthesis, and reduce respiratory muscle fatigue.

11.3.2.2 General Principles of Nutritional Therapy

For most COVID-19 patients, the general principles of nutritional therapy are recommended as follows:

1) Give a high-protein, high-fat, low-carbohydrate diet or parenteral nutrition.
2) The proportion of calories of protein, fat, and carbohydrates is 20%, 20%–30%, 50%–60%.
3) The daily protein supply should be 1.0–1.5 g/kg, and for critically severe patients, it should be increased to 1.5–2.0 g/kg.
4) Supplement various vitamins and trace elements in appropriate amounts every day, adjust the number of electrolytes according to the clinical situations, and especially supplement potassium, magnesium, phosphorus, and other trace elements that affect respiratory muscle function.

11.3.2.3 Nutritional Treatment Approaches for COVID-19 Patients

According to the *Expert Recommendations on Medical Nutrition Therapy for Patients with COVID-19* by Enteral and Parenteral Nutrition Society, Chinese Medical Association, the five-step method is recommended for nutritional therapy: dietary and nutrition education, ONS, tube feeding, enteral nutrition, SPN, and TPN. Patients with COVID-19 should choose a proper nutritional feeding route based on the disease's severity, gastrointestinal function, and respiratory support.

1) Oral intake or oral enteral nutrition is preferred for patients with mild symptoms who can eat autonomously. If they cannot eat on their own, it is recommended to activate enteral nutrition within 48 hours.
2) Severe patients are often in a state of high catabolism due to severe infections, and together with weakened anabolism, low immune function, and insufficient intake, they are prone to malnutrition. If nutrition is not supplemented in time, it will increase protein consumption and affect the organs' structure and function, resulting in organ failure and increased mortality. Enteral nutrition is preferred if the structure and function of the patient's gastrointestinal tract are not damaged. Because food stimulates the intestinal nerve, it can activate the intestinal neuroendocrine-immune system, which helps maintain the intestinal immune function and prevent intestinal infection. If patients cannot

eat after endotracheal intubation, food can be given through the naso-gastric tube. Enteral nutrition should be postponed in severe patients with uncontrolled shock, severe hypoxemia, severe acidosis, upper gastrointestinal bleeding, gastric residual volume > 500 mL/6 h, intestinal ischemia, intestinal obstruction, and abdominal compartment syndrome. For patients with oral or enteral nutrition contraindications, parenteral nutrition should be activated within 3–7 days. Combining parenteral nutrition in the case of insufficient enteral nutrition intake can avoid the risk of increased blood sugar and blood lipid, which may result from insufficient energy intake and total parenteral nutrition. At the same time, to avoid overfeeding, enteral nutrition, and parenteral nutrition of critically severe patients should gradually reach the target amount of feeding within 3–7 days.

3) Patients with noninvasive ventilation are recommended to change to a nasal mask or temporarily switch to transnasal hyperflow oxygen therapy when eating to reduce the risk of hypoxemia during eating. The "button-type" mask is preferred for patients with noninvasive ventilation because the gastric tube outlet is installed on the mask, which does not affect the efficiency of noninvasive ventilation and is more conducive to the smooth implementation of enteral nutrition. Postpyloric feeding is recommended in patients with severe gastric bloating.

4) For patients with invasive mechanical ventilation or patients receiving extracorporeal membrane oxygenation (ECMO), if there is no contraindicated enteral nutrition, it is recommended to use tube feeding enteral nutrition as soon as possible. Transgastric tube feeding is the preferred feeding channel. In case of gastric retention, erythromycin (100–250mg) can be used three times a day to promote gastrointestinal motility or metoclopramide (10 mg) three times a day, and the amount should be reduced to one-third after 72 hours. If it still cannot be relieved, postpyloric feeding can be selected. If the patient has high aspiration risk, such as loss of airway protection ability, age > 70 years old, decreased level of consciousness, poor oral care, prone position, gastroesophageal reflux, and single load, postpyloric feeding can be the first choice for enteral nutrition. In view of the pandemic's current severity and the relatively insufficient nursing power, postpyloric feeding may be a better way of providing nutrition.

11.3.2.4 Amount of Nutritional Feeding for COVID-19 Patients

According to the severity of the patient's case of COVID-19, domestic and international guidelines recommended supplying 20–30kcal/ (kg·d) and reach the target energy as soon as possible. For severe patients, 25–30kcal/ (kg·d) is recommended, and feeding should start at a low dose. If feeding intolerance occurs, healthy feeding can be considered infusion speed: 10–20 kcal/h or 10–20 mL/h. It is necessary to strengthen protein supply and increase protein intake. According to the *Diagnosis and Treatment Plan for Severe and Critically Severe COVID-19 Patients (2nd Trial Edition)* by the National Health Commission (NHC), it is recommended to provide 1.5–2.0 g/(kg·d) [nitrogen 0.25–0.33 g/(kg·d)] to improve the supply of branched-chain amino acids to promote the synthesis of protein. When protein intake is insufficient, it is suggested to add protein powder based on standard whole protein preparation to improve respiratory muscle function and immune function. Patients with severe COVID-19 complicated with ARDS should reduce their sugar intake. Glucose is a commonly used energy substance to supplement, but a high concentration of glucose will increase carbon dioxide production, aggravating the burden of breathing and ventilation, thus exacerbating respiratory failure. Reducing sugar intake can reduce the burden on patients' lungs. When some patients with severe COVID-19 develop intolerance after enteral nutrition treatment, they need to actively improve their body position, and the infusion speed needs to be decreased. The following types of nutritional preparations can also be selected:

Choose hypotonic or isotonic formulations.

Choose a fat combination that is easy to digest and absorb, such as adding medium-chain fatty acid (MCT) and particular nutrients, such as L-carnitine, that are conducive to digestion and absorption of long-chain fatty acid (LCT); give priority to medium long-chain fatty acids, and increase the proportion of n-3 fatty acid and n-9 fatty acid.

Choose a formulation containing soluble dietary fiber, such as FOS. When receiving enteral or parenteral nutrition therapy, patients' serum electrolytes, especially the level of phosphorus, should be continuously monitored for those with severe COVID-19 with a BMI < 14 kg/m^2, a weight loss of 20% in the past 3–6 months, or a significant reduction in nutritional intake for more than 15 days. If there is a significant decrease in serum phosphorus levels, the refeeding syndrome may be indicated. To avoid the refeeding syndrome during the feeding process, it is recommended to slowly increase enteral nutritional caloric intake, reach 80% of the target caloric intake after 5 days, and supplement with phosphate or high dose (> 100 mg or 200 mg) thiamine.

11.3.2.5 Recommended Intake of Special Nutrients for Severe COVID-19 Patients

1) Fish oil components: Both ESPEN (European Society for Parenteral and Enteral Nutrition) Guidelines for Critical Care Nutrition from the European Society of Clinical Nutrition and Metabolism and

ASPEN/SCCM* Guidelines for Critical Care Nutrition from the American Society of Parenteral Enteral Nutrition and the American Society of Critical Care recommend that severe patients with respiratory failure use enteral and/or parenteral nutrition supplemented with fish oil nutritional formula, but enteral nutrition is limited to 500 mg EPA (Eicosapentaenoic Acid) + DHA (docosahexenoic acid) daily. Fish oil supplementation higher than 3–7 times is harmful. Parenteral nutrition can give fish oil at 0.1–0.2 g/(kg·d).

2) Micronutrients: Trace elements and vitamins are essential nutrient substrates for carbohydrate, protein, and lipid metabolism. They play an important role in improving immune function and antioxidation and regulating the endocrine, DNA synthesis, DNA repair, and cell signaling. For severe and critically severe patients, monitoring the serum micronutrient concentration dynamically and giving normal dietary intake supplementation is recommended. As critically severe patients who use proton pump inhibitors are very likely to have vitamin B12 malabsorption, attention should be paid to vitamin B12 supplementation for such patients. If the serum level of 25-hydroxy-vitamin D in patients with severe COVID-19 is lower than 12.5 ng/mL or 50 nmol/L, a large dose of 500,000 IU (international unit) of vitamin D3 should be supplemented within a week. In the diagnosis and treatment of patients with severe COVID-19 complicated with acute respiratory failure, due to the increase of oxidative stress response and the decrease of the patient's vitamin C intake, the dose of vitamin C can be increased during the treatment, which can be increased to 6 g/d. Therefore, it is necessary to strictly pay attention to vitamin B1, vitamin C, folic acid, vitamin D, and other supplements for high-risk patients. Scientific and reasonable nutritional treatment is of vital importance for the recovery and prognosis of patients with severe COVID-19, and attention should be paid to the core status of nutritional therapy in the treatment of severe patients.

11.4 DIETARY GUIDANCE

The Chinese Nutrition Society, in conjunction with the Chinese Medical Doctor Association, and the Parenteral and Enteral Nutrition Society, Chinese Medical Association, aiming at the characteristics of the prevention, control, and treatment of COVID-19, and following the *Chinese Residents'*

---

* ASPEN (American Society for Parenteral and Enteral Nutrition)/SCCM (Society of Critical Care Medicine).

Dietary Guidelines (2016 Edition) and the *Diagnosis and Treatment Plan for COVID-19 (4th Trial Edition)* issued by the NHC, study and propose the guidance for dietary nutrition.

11.4.1 Dietary Guidance for Different Populations of COVID-19

11.4.1.1 Nutritional Diet for Ordinary or Convalescent Patients

1) Sufficient energy: Every day, 250–400 g of cereals and potato food can be consumed, including rice, flour, miscellaneous grains, potatoes, etc. To ensure adequate protein intake, provide mainly high-quality protein food (150–200 g per day), such as lean meat, fish, shrimp, eggs, and soybeans, etc. If possible, try to ensure patients eat an egg a day, 300 g of milk or dairy products (yogurt can provide intestinal probiotics, and can be chosen more). To increase the intake of essential fatty acids (EFA), use a variety of cooking oils, especially vegetable oil with monounsaturated fatty acids, with the total fat energy supply ratio reaching 25%–30% of the total dietary energy.

2) Give more fresh vegetables and fruits: Patients should eat more than 500 g of vegetables and 200–350 g of fruits every day. It is recommended to choose more dark fruits and vegetables.

3) Ensure adequate drinking water: Patients should drink 1500–2000 mL per day, with small amounts given over the course of the day, mainly drinking plain, boiled water or light tea. Vegetable soup, fish soup, chicken soup, etc., before and after a meal, are good choices.

4) Resolutely prohibit the consumption of wild animals and less spicy food.

5) For people with poor appetite and insufficient food intake, the elderly, and patients with chronic diseases, they can supplement protein and micronutrients such as B vitamins, vitamin A, vitamin C, and vitamin D in an appropriate amount through nutritionally fortified food, formula food for particular medical purposes, or nutrient supplements.

6) Ensure adequate sleep and moderate physical activity, with no less than 30 minutes of daily physical activity time. Increase time patients can spend in the sunshine appropriately.

11.4.1.2 Nutritional Treatment for Patients with Severe Syndrome

Severe patients are often accompanied by decreased appetite and insufficient food intake, making the original weak resistance even worse. Attention should be paid to the nutritional treatment of critically severe patients. For this reason, the principle of sequential nutritional support treatment is proposed.

1) Provide a small number of multiple meals. Give liquid foods that are good for swallowing and digestion six to seven times a day, mainly including eggs, soybeans and their products, milk and its products, fruit juice, vegetable juice, rice noodles, and other ingredients. Ensure that patients receive an adequate amount of high-quality protein supplement. During the disease's gradual remission, patients can take in semiliquid foods that are easy to chew and digest and gradually transition to an ordinary diet as the disease improves.

2) If the food fails to meet nutritional requirements, enteral nutrition preparations (formula foods for particular medical purposes) can be used correctly under the guidance of a doctor or clinical dietitian. For critically severe patients who cannot eat through the mouth normally, a nasogastric tube or nasojejunal tube can be placed, and the nutrient solution can be pumped by gravity drip or enteral nutrition infusion pump.

3) Parenteral nutrition should be adopted to maintain basic nutritional requirements for patients with severe gastrointestinal dysfunction in the case of insufficient or inadequate food and enteral nutrition. In the early stage, it can reach 60%–80% of the nutritional intake. After the disease is alleviated, the energy and nutrients can be gradually supplemented to reach the full amount.

4) The patient's nutritional regimen should be formulated according to the body's overall condition, the amount of access, liver and kidney function, and glucose and lipid metabolism.

11.4.1.3 Nutritional Dietary Guidance for Frontline Workers

According to the principles of a balanced diet, frontline workers' nutritional diet should include the following aspects.

1) Ensure enough energy intake every day. The recommended energy intake is 2,400–2,700 kcal/d for men and 2,100–2,300 kcal/d for women.

2) Ensure daily intake of high-quality protein, such as eggs, milk, livestock, poultry, fish, shrimp, soybeans, etc.

3) The diet should be light and avoid greasy food and natural spices can be used for seasoning to increase medical staff's appetite.

4) Eat more food rich in B vitamins, vitamin C, minerals, and dietary fiber. Match reasonably with rice noodles, vegetables, fruits, etc., and choose more rape, spinach, celery, purple cabbage, carrots, tomatoes, oranges, tangerines, apples, kiwi fruit, other dark vegetables and fruits, mushrooms, agaric, kelp, and other bacteria and algae food.

5) Try to drink 1,500–2,000 mL of water per day.

6) In case of a busy workload and insufficient ordinary dietary intake, enteral nutrition preparations (formula foods for particular medical purposes), milk powder, and nutrient supplements can be used as supplements. An additional oral nutrition supplement of 400–600 kcal per day can ensure nutritional requirements.

7) Separate meals should be adopted to avoid mixing meals and reduce the risk of infection during eating.

8) Hospitals are in charge of the leadership, nutrition department, dietary management department, etc. They should take measures according to local conditions and promptly design reasonable meals according to frontline staff's physical conditions to ensure nutrition.

11.4.1.4 Nutritional Dietary Guidance for Prevention and Control among the General Population

1) Eat a variety of foods, mainly cereals. The daily diet should include cereals and potatoes, vegetables and fruits, livestock, poultry, fish, eggs, milk, soybeans, nuts, and other foods. Pay attention to the choice of whole grains, miscellaneous beans, and potatoes.

2) Eat more fruits and vegetables, milk, and soybeans. Make sure that vegetables are included in, and eat fruits every day. Choose dark fruits and vegetables instead of fruit juice. Eat a variety of milk and its products, especially yogurt, consuming an equivalent to 300 grams of liquid milk per day. Eat soy products regularly and nuts in moderation.

3) Eat fish, poultry, eggs, and lean meat in moderation. Eat less fatty, smoked, and cured meat products. Never eat wild animals.

4) Consume less salt and oil, control sugar, and limit alcohol. Eat fewer salty and fried foods. Drink seven to eight cups (1,500–1,700 mL) of water per day for adults. Drinking boiled water and tea is recommended, and avoid or limit sugary drinks. For adults, the amount of alcohol consumed per day should not exceed 25 g for men and 15 g for women.

5) Eat a balanced diet to maintain a healthy weight. Exercise every day at home to maintain a healthy weight. Avoid overeating, control total energy intake, and maintain energy balance. Reduce sedentary time and get up and move every hour.

6) Cherish food and prepare meals as needed. Separating meals and using public chopsticks and spoons are advocated. Choose fresh, safe food, and appropriate cooking methods. Separate the raw and cooked foods and heat the cooked food thoroughly. Learn to read food labels and choose foods reasonably.

11.4.2 TCM Diet Guidance

TCM is a traditional treasure of our country. In order to consolidate the foundation and strengthen the body, according to the Theory of Traditional Chinese Medicine Preventive Treatment of Disease, experts of Guangdong Hospital of Traditional Chinese Medicine have formulated a medicine and food homology program for COVID-19 patients. The three-course therapeutic diet and its decoction method are as follows:

11.4.2.1 First Prescription

1) Applicable people: This is suitable for people with moderate physical condition (normally healthy, without apparent cold or heat bias).
2) Composition (for three people): 50 g soybeans, 50 g black beans, 15 g northern almonds (crushed), 250 g lean meat, 1 slice of tangerine peel, 30 g ginger, 10 g perilla leaves.
3) Decoction method: Soak beans in water for 30 minutes; wash the lean pork and cut it into minced meat for later use; add 2,000–3,000 mL of water for various ingredients other than lean meat and perilla leaves; boil over high heat and turn to low heat and cook for 40 minutes; add minced meat and perilla leaves, and cook for another 5–10 minutes; add appropriate amount of salt to taste and then eat.
4) Method of taking: Make soup and take it warm 1 hour after meals. It can be taken for 3 consecutive days a week or once every 2–3 days.

11.4.2.2 Second Prescription

1) Applicable people: This is suitable for people with weak constitutions and of a wet type (usually afraid of cold and wind, cold limbs, cold intolerance, poor appetite, loose stools).
2) Composition (for three people): 50 g black beans, 50 g soybeans, 15 g perilla leaves (fresh ones are better, dried ones are also acceptable), three to four green onions (white part of southern spring onion, including beard and root), 50 g ginger (sliced), 30 g stir-fried white lentil, 10 g tangerine peel, about 25 g red dates, 10 g raw licorice.
3) Decoction method: Soak beans in water for 30 minutes; add 1,500 mL of water to all ingredients, boil over high heat, and turn to a low heat to cook for 40 minutes, about 800 mL.
4) Method of taking: Take 150–200 mL daily for people 7–17 years old, 200–300 mL daily for people 18 years old and above. Take it warm 1 hour after meals. It can be taken for 3 consecutive days a week or once every 2–3 days.

11.4.2.3 Third Prescription

1) Applicable people: This is suitable for people with solid constitution and of damp-heat type (usually dry and bitter mouth, dry or sticky stool, greasy face, prone to sore throats and mouth ulcers).
2) Composition (for three people): 50 g soybeans, 15 g north almonds (peeled bitter almond, smashed), 30 g ginger (sliced), 15 g coix seed, 15 g light tempeh, 10 g green peel, 5 g tangerine peel, 20 g pueraria, 10 g dandelion, 10 g raw licorice.
3) Decoction method: Soak soybeans and coix seeds in water for 30 minutes; add 1500 mL of water to all ingredients. After boiling, turn to low heat and cook for 40 minutes, until there is about 800 mL.
4) Method of taking: Take 150–200 mL daily for people 7–17 years old, and 200–300 mL daily for people 18 years old and above. Take it warm 1 hour after meals, and it can be taken for 3 consecutive days.

Note: For patients with hyperuricemia and gout, please remove soybeans from the prescription and add 15–20 g reed rhizome instead. Pregnant women should use the third prescription with caution.

BIBLIOGRAPHY

1. National Health Commission. *Nutritional and Dietary Guidance for Prevention and Treatment of Pneumonia Caused by COVID-19 Infection [EB/OL]*. China. [2020-02-18].
2. Yu Kaiying, Shi Hanping. Interpretation of expert recommendations on medical nutritional therapy for patients with COVID-19 (English Edition) [J]. *Chinese Medical Journal*, 2020, *100* (10): 724–728.
3. Expert Group of the Chinese Medical Association Enteral and Parenteral Nutrition Branch. Expert advice on medical nutrition therapy for patients with COVID-19 (Electronic Version) [J/CD]. *Chinese Journal of General Surgery*, 2020, *14* (1): 1.
4. Pierre Singer, Annika Reintam Blaser, Mette M. Berger, Waleed Alhazzani, Philip C. Calder, Michael Casaer, Michael Hiesmayr, Konstantin Mayer, Juan Carlos Montejo, Claude Pichard, Jean-Charles Preiser, Arthur R.H. van Zanten, Simon Oczkowski, Stephan C. Bischoff. ESPEN guideline on clinical nutrition in the intensive care unit [J]. *Clinical Nutrition*, 2018, *38* (1): 48–79.
5. Dou Zulin. *Evaluation and Treatment of Dysphagia [M]*. Beijing: People's Medical Publishing House, 2009.
6. Shi Hanping, Zhao Qingchuan. Three-level diagnosis of malnutrition [J]. *Electronic Journal of Tumor Metabolism and Nutrition*, 2015, *2* (2): 31–36.
7. Meng Shen, Chen Siyuan. *Pulmonary Rehabilitation [M]*. Beijing: People's Medical Publishing House, 2007.

8. Shi Hanping, Xu Hongxia, Li Suyi, et al. Five-step treatment of malnutrition [J]. *Electronic Journal of Tumor Metabolism and Nutrition*, 2015, *2* (1): 29–33.

9. Branch of Parenteral and Enteral Nutrition of Chinese Medical Association. Expert consensus on oral nutritional supplements for adults [J]. *Chinese Journal of Gastrointestinal Surgery*, 2017, *20* (4): 361–365.

10. Liu Jia, Huang Hua. Research progress in evaluation methods of malnutrition in liver cirrhosis [J]. *Modern Medicine and Health*, 2020, *36* (2): 532–535.

11. J Kondrup, HH Rasmussen, O Hamberg, et al. Nutritional risk screening (NRS 2002): A new method based on an analysis of controlled clinical trials [J]. *Clinical Nutrition*, 2003, *22* (3): 321–336.

12. Yinghui Jin, Lin Cai, Zhenshun Cheng, et al. Guidelines for rapid advice on diagnosis and treatment of Pneumonia infected by novel coronavirus (2019-nCoV) (Standard Edition) [J]. *Journal of Chinese PLA Medicine*, 2020, *45* (01): 1–20.

13. Expert advice on medical nutrition treatment for patients with novel coronavirus [EB/OL], issued by the Branch of Extraintestinal and Enteral Nutrition of Chinese Medical Association and the Branch of Extraintestinal and Enteral Nutrition of Chinese Medical Association (CSPEN). (January 30, 2020) [February 5, 2020].

14. Diagnosis and treatment scheme of severe and critical cases in novel coronavirus (trial 2nd edition) [J]. *Chinese Journal of Virology*, 2020, *10* (03): 161–163.

15. Beth E. Taylor, Stephen A. McClave, Robert G. Martindale, Malissa M. Warren, Debbie R. Johnson, Carol Braunschweig, Mary S. McCarthy, Evangelia Davanos, Todd W. Rice, Gail A. Cresci, Jane M. Gervasio, Gordon S. Sacks, Pamela R. Roberts, Charlene Compher. Guidelines for the provision and assessment of nutrition support therapy in the adult critically ill patient: Society of Critical Care Medicine (SCCM) and American Society for Parenteral and Enteral Nutrition (A.S.P.E.N.). JPEN, 2016, *44* (2): 390–438.

16. Yuexin Yang, Huanmei Zhang. Introduction to dietary guidelines for Chinese residents (2016) [J]. *Journal of Nutrition*, 2016, *38* (03): 209–217.

17. Novel coronavirus pneumonia diagnosis and treatment plan (trial version fifth) [J]. *Chinese Medicine*, 2020, *52* (02): 96+95.

18. Cheng Song, Junjun Liu, Shiwen Yao, et al. Screening and preventing novel coronavirus's "medicine and food homology" based on the theory of "preventing disease" [J]. *Asia Pacific Traditional Medicine*, 2020, *16* (11): 18–21.

Chapter 12

Community- and Home-Based Rehabilitation of COVID-19

Upon being approved for discharge, COVID-19 patients have many physical dysfunctions, such as shortness of breath, weakness, and palpitations as well as psychological, daily life, and social participation dysfunction. Hospital rehabilitation is only a short process; after discharge, patients should be further rehabilitated in the community and family, helping them to gradually return to everyday life.

Unlike hospital rehabilitation, community rehabilitation can better integrate and utilize social resources and mobilize COVID-19 patients' enthusiasm. Appropriate community-based rehabilitation interventions are an important part of the layered and refined management of COVID-19 patients. According to the different needs of patients, the community should be equipped with basic management, guidance, and rehabilitation intervention capabilities to improve the overall functional status of patients, promote the overall improvement of their quality of life, and finally return to the family and society.

Home-based rehabilitation means that rehabilitation and related medical personnel go to the streets or homes to provide professional and continuous comprehensive guidance, such as rehabilitation, medication, and nursing for patients with functional disorders in need. Home-based rehabilitation is mainly evaluated based on the people in need (including living environment, physical function, and mental state) to make corresponding plans and provide guidance. Patients' self-rehabilitation management is also an essential part of home rehabilitation.

12.1 COMMUNITY-BASED REHABILITATION

Community-based rehabilitation, a concept put forward by the World Health Organization in 1976, is an economical, effective practical and convenient way to provide rehabilitation services. It can expand the coverage of rehabilitation services and enable disabled people in developing countries to enjoy rehabilitation services. Telemedicine and internet therapy have been gradually carried out in China, which provide convenience for the further development of community-based rehabilitation and home-based rehabilitation. As the pandemic is nearing its end, treatment of newly diagnosed COVID-19 patients is mainly focused on patient rehabilitation. Many patients left with respiratory and physical dysfunction can be treated according to their own needs. Community rehabilitation is the link between hospital rehabilitation and home-based rehabilitation, which complement and permeate each other.

12.1.1 Dysfunction Requiring Rehabilitation Treatment

12.1.1.1 Dysfunction of Daily Living Ability and Social Participation

The Barthel Index is used to assess daily living abilities, which includes the ability to defecate, urinate, use the toilet, eat, transfer beds and chairs, walk, dress, go upstairs and downstairs, and bathe independently. Communication with the outside world is an essential human survival ability, while social participation manifests comprehensive ability. Clinically, it has been found that some patients are unable to achieve regular interpersonal communication and return to work due to their long medical treatment, which requires a more extended period of rehabilitation and more help from society.

12.1.1.2 Respiratory Dysfunction

Respiratory dysfunction is the residual symptom after lung injury, mainly including cough, sputum, dyspnea, and shortness of breath after activity and may be accompanied by respiratory muscle weakness and impaired lung function. Currently, there are not enough statistics on the duration of patients' respiratory dysfunction. Some patients have been discharged from the hospital for more than 2 months and their daily living ability assessed by Barthel Index has reached 100 points. However, the above respiratory dysfunction still exists, which seriously affects patients' quality of life, so community rehabilitation should be given as soon as possible.

12.1.1.3 Physical Dysfunction

Physical dysfunction's main symptoms are lack of power, easy fatigue, and muscle ache and can be accompanied by muscle atrophy, decreased muscle strength, etc. This is mainly due to the decreased oxygen uptake capacity of the body caused by lung tissue damage. In the early stage of treatment, especially in severe and critically severe patients, taking breaks and resting are adopted to reduce oxygen consumption, causing muscle tissue atrophy. Some hospitals carry out convalescent hospital rehabilitation, but for some patients who have not received hospital rehabilitation, physical dysfunction will be more obvious and will need attention.

12.1.1.4 Psychological Dysfunction

Most COVID-19 patients have psychological dysfunction, the duration and severity of which vary from person to person. Psychological dysfunction may cause somatization symptoms, so most of the psychological dysfunction is accompanied by physical dysfunction. Symptoms of simple mental dysfunction include emotional problems, such as fear, anger, anxiety, and depression. Short-term emotional problems are conducive to the regulation and release of pressure. After a long treatment and isolation in an unfamiliar medical environment, some patients with poor emotional regulation ability will become ill and need drug control. Even for people with psychological dysfunction who need drug control, community-based rehabilitation is more appropriate.

12.1.2 Goals of Rehabilitation

1) Improve and eliminate patients' dysfunction.
2) Improve the patient's muscle strength, endurance, physical strength, and respiratory function.
3) Prevention of complications and sequelae.
4) Regulate patients' bad emotions and restore normal psychological conditions.
5) Improve the patient's daily living activities and social adaptation skills so that the patient can return to the family and society.

12.1.3 Process of Rehabilitation

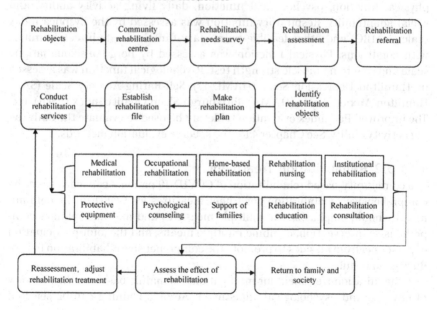

12.1.4 Implementation of Rehabilitation Treatment

According to the medical level and resource condition of different communities, rehabilitation treatment should be different, including but not limited to community health service centers, nursing homes, recuperation centers, family, etc. Thanks to the internet and social communication methods, some rehabilitation treatment can take place with patients' families through communication methods such as QQ group, WeChat group, and video conference, and social software can also be used as a community rehabilitation management platform.

Community rehabilitation members include community organizers and leaders, community rehabilitation physicians, rehabilitation therapists, rehabilitation nurses, community volunteers, patients, and their families. All the members put the patient at the center, the community acts as the foundation, the family as the support, and the patient's functional status and rehabilitation needs as the guidance. These members use the internet to share resources and form the community rehabilitation training service network to provide the patients with nearby convenient, timely, and effective rehabilitation training and services.

12.1.5 Content of Rehabilitation

12.1.5.1 Rehabilitation Evaluation

Rehabilitation evaluation mainly includes assessing respiratory function, physical function, psychological function, daily living activity ability, and social adaptability. Respiratory function was assessed by the dyspnea index scale (mMRC) and other feasible pulmonary function tests in communities with conditions. Physical function was assessed by Borg conscious fatigue scale and free-hand muscle strength test. Psychological function was assessed by Hamilton Depression Scale (HAMD-17), Self-Rating Anxiety Scale (SAS), Hamilton Anxiety Scale (HAMA), Pittsburgh Sleep Quality Index (PSQI), etc. The improved Pap index evaluation table can be used to evaluate the daily living activity ability. See Chapter 4 for the specific evaluation methods.

12.1.5.2 Rehabilitation Treatment

The community-based rehabilitation of COVID-19 patients can learn from the comprehensive rehabilitation treatment measures for COPD in the community. It should emphasize the multiple measures and multidisciplinary comprehensive intervention, combine multiple means, and the joint participation of personnel from all sides to promote the comprehensive rehabilitation to produce good results.

Rehabilitation treatment for mild patients is mainly based on the recovery of physical and psychological adjustment. Aerobic training can be selected step by step according to the patient's past exercise habits and hobbies, and the activity ability before the onset of the disease can be gradually restored. Some critically severe patients may suffer from fatigue, shortness of breath, muscle atrophy, and some psychological problems for some time after discharge. According to patients' evaluation results, we can formulate the corresponding rehabilitation plan and help patients recover their function through a variety of physical factors, rehabilitation equipment, functional training, other modern rehabilitation treatment technologies, and traditional Chinese medicine (TCM) or proprietary Chinese medicine, traditional Chinese medicine rehabilitation techniques such as external treatment techniques and traditional techniques. The specific rehabilitation technology can be seen in Chapters 5 and 6.

12.1.5.2.1 Guidance of Rehabilitation Training

This includes guiding the patient to master the correct training methods, such as appropriate posture placement and effective breathing patterns to improve the patient's respiratory function. Selecting the appropriate movement and physical exercise methods for the patient, such as baduanjin, tai chi chuan, and other traditional exercises, to improve the patient's muscle strength and muscle endurance and enhance immunity. Rehabilitation training also guides patients to carry out physical activities, such as self-massage, exercise with equipment, medical gymnastics, walking training, and so on, to promote their recovery.

12.1.5.2.2 Psychological Intervention

Patients' bad emotions and psychological status can be adjusted by understanding, supporting, encouraging, persuading, and using other psychological interventions or professional psychological counseling. Refer to Chapter 10 for specific methods of psychological rehabilitation.

12.1.5.2.3

Other treatments include exercise therapy, oxygen therapy, nutrition guidance, music therapy, patient education and social and behavioral interventions, improvement of living environment, etc.

12.1.5.2.4

Referral: Patients with severe adverse reactions and symptoms should be referred to a psychology professional promptly.

12.1.5.3 Configuration and Use of Auxiliary Appliances

Common assistance devices include vibration massage (vibration sputum removal), dumbbells, barbells, elastic belt, treadmill (endurance training), other sports equipment (muscle strength training), etc.

1) Training community-based rehabilitation personnel
   Community rehabilitation personnel are required to receive training on assistive devices, including the type, purpose, function, access, and

use of assistive devices. Proper information, referrals, and education for COVID-19 patients are also needed.

2) Build capacity of personnel and family

Community rehabilitation personnel should help COVID-19 patients and their families know the types of assistive devices and how to use them correctly and safely.

3) Deal with environmental barriers

Community-based rehabilitation personnel should understand the environmental barriers to the use of assistive devices and work with COVID-19 patients and the community to identify and respond.

4) Health education

Under the professional guidance of community-based rehabilitation personnel, the community can make full use of broadcasting, WeChat, QQ group, and other means to actively carry out targeted publicity of COVID-19 protection knowledge. We can also actively adopt online services and online counseling and provide online guidance to patients in home exercise, dietary hygiene, and mental health.

a. During rehabilitation and exercise, patients should still take effective isolation measures to avoid entering or leaving crowded places.

b. The rehabilitation physician team should guide the patients and their families to adopt an effective rehabilitation exercise program, mainly aerobic exercise, reasonable diet, and regular rest.

c. Patients and their families should do a good job of health protection, regular disinfection, and pay attention to the prevention of other infectious diseases.

d. Patients and their families should pay close attention to patients' common psychological problems such as depression, anxiety, and self-cognition deviation. The online questionnaire and scale can be used for evaluation, and timely psychological intervention and counseling can be conducted.

e. Local governments and education departments can be contacted to organize professional vocational education rehabilitation.

f. The functional status of patients should be checked regularly.

12.2 HOME-BASED REHABILITATION

Rehabilitation at home is convenient and beneficial to the patients. Online diagnosis and treatment or professional personnel go deep into the family to provide convenient rehabilitation guidance for most residents. Simple appliances in the home can be used to complete rehabilitation training. The patients themselves mainly complete rehabilitation treatment. Rehabilitation personnel regularly carry out a systematic evaluation on the patients and adjust the rehabilitation treatment prescription based on their physical condition. Patients' self-rehabilitation management mainly improves lung function, restores physical strength, and improves living ability through traditional exercises, respiratory rehabilitation techniques, physical rehabilitation techniques, and activities of daily living (ADL) intervention. It is supplemented by psychological and dietary adjustment to promote comprehensive rehabilitation of patients. The techniques of respiratory and physical rehabilitation have been introduced in detail in other chapters. This chapter focuses on rehabilitation exercises that are easy for patients to recover at home and manage themselves.

12.2.1 Traditional Methods

By reviewing the research on Traditional Chinese mind and body exercises (TCMBE) in regulating the body immunity, improving cardiopulmonary function, improving the quality of life, and improving bad emotions, under the guidance of professional rehabilitation doctors, COVID-19 patients selected appropriate traditional techniques, such as baduanjin, tai ji chuan, five-animal exercise, and yi jin jing, etc., according to their recovery condition. Traditional exercises are selected based on the patient's preference and acceptance level. They can finish one set at a time, one to two times a day.

12.2.1.1 Baduanjin

QR code for Baduanjin exercise video

There are 10 postures including preparation and closing postures. Refer to Chapter 6.

1) Hold the hands high with palms up to regulate the internal organs.
   a. Cross your hands in front of the lower abdomen, turn your palms up and lift them up, leave your palms apart like a cloud and mist, hold the sample with your hands, and return to the original posture. Walk slowly with the breath, breathe in one cycle, stop for a moment when you exhale, and become natural with the breath (Figure 12.1).

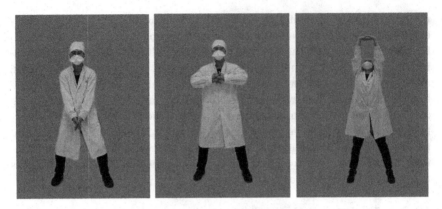

Figure 12.1   Two hands hold up the heavens to regulate sanjiao (triple burner meridian). Cross your hands, turn the palms outward, raise your hands from the lower abdomen to the top of the head.

2) Pose as an archer shooting both left- and right-handed.
   a.   Squat down steadily, crossing your hands to your left chest, pushing your right hand with your left hand to pull like archery, and changing your posture to the right with your waist. Cross your hands to your right chest, pushing your left hand with your right hand to pull, pointing at you, and taking your hands back (Figure 12.2).

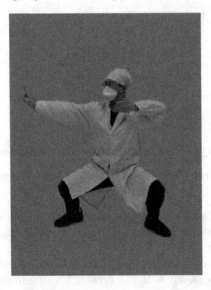

Figure 12.2   Draw the bow to shoot the eagle. Squat down in a lower horse stance and imitate the action of drawing a bow to either side.

3) Hold one arm aloft to regulate the functions of the spleen and stomach.
   a. Overlapping hands with palms up, right palm up and left palm down, holding round with both arms, supporting right palm with spiral arms up, turning left palm down to spleen position, both palms walking along stomach meridian, changing arms to support and pressing for one cycle, breathing out and sucking feet without exertion, and retracting both palms back to Dantian (Figure 12.3).
4) Look backward to prevent sickness and strain.
   a. Holding both hands as if holding a tray, turning over the palm and pressing the inner rotation of the arm, the head should turn left with the hand, bleed qi down to Yongquan, calm and relax when exhaling, take back the palm with both arms, continue to run into the right type, and lift the qi back to Dantian Figure 12.4).
5) Swing the head and lower the body to relieve stress.
   a. You can choose your own stance, with your hands on your knees. On the top, your head should turn to the left as you exhale, but your eyes should look at the right toe. When you inhale, you can restore the right style, and turn your head to look at the left toe obliquely. You should not be impetuous and concentrate (Figure 12.5).

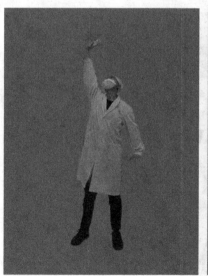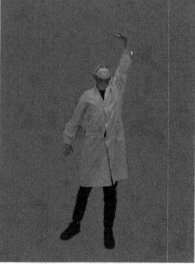

Figure 12.3 Raise single arm up to regulate the spleen and stomach. Turn the palms upward, raise the right hand with the palm facing upward while pushing the left palm downward. Then repeat this exercise with the left hand.

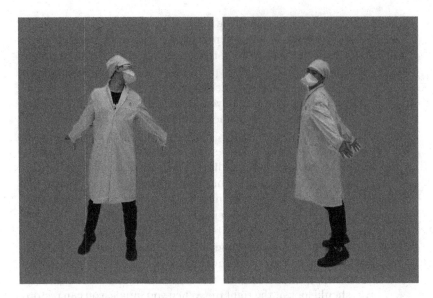

Figure 12.4 Look backward to eliminate five strains and seven impairments. Stretch your arms with palms facing upward behind the back, rotate the head to the left and look backward, adjust your breath, then switch to the right side.

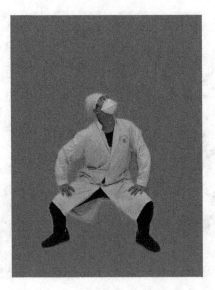

Figure 12.5 Swing the head and buttocks to expel heart fire. Squat down in a lower horse stance, put your hands on your knees, and turn your head from left to right with your body.

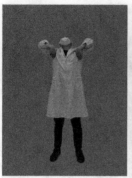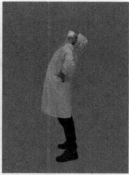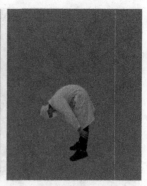

Figure 12.6 Pull toes with both hands to reinforce the kidney and lower back. Stand straight with feet apart, place two hands on both sides of the body, and then bend forward to touch the legs from top to lower legs on both sides.

6) Move the hands down the body and legs, and touch the feet to strengthen the kidneys.
   a. Open your feet one step wide, hold your hands flat in front of your lower abdomen, and turn back with your hands equally left and right. When inhaling, hide your waist and support your back, and set the depth with your breath. When exhaling, bend over and form a circle with your feet. Don't use force when guiding with gestures, and relax your waist and accept your abdomen to keep Yongquan (Figure 12.6).
7) Thrust the fists and make the eyes glare to enhance strength.
   a. Squat down with eyes wide open, with fists in your chest, with fists leading your inner qi to turn around with your waist, swing your arms back and forth, inhale, draw in and exhale, rotate your eyes from right to left, hold your fists in front of your chest, and take back your feet, press your hands down, and return to the original position (Figure 12.7).
8) Raise and lower the heels to cure diseases.
   a. Legs stand side by side, leaving the toes. The toes force the heels to hang in the air, the body tops when exhaling, the hands press down. Exhale when the feet fall. This is a cycle. Repeat seven times, the qi of whole body goes back to Dantian, relaxed and shook, and breath naturally (Figure 12.8).

12.2.1.2 Simplified Tai Chi Chuan

Simplified tai chi chuan is also called 24 style simplified tai chi chuan. Its concise content was compiled by the General Administration of Sport of China in

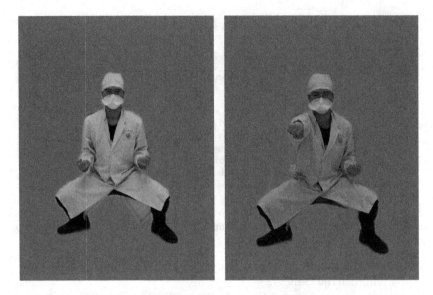

Figure 12.7 Clench the fists and glare fiercely to increase strength. Squat down in a lower horse stance with eyes wide open and fists clenched. Then extend the left fist first and then the right fist.

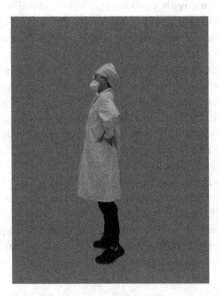

Figure 12.8 Shake the back seven times to prevent illness. Stand straight with heels together, place both hands behind the waist, stand on tiptoe and then lower the heels. Repeat this seven times with balanced breathing.

1956 and it takes the essence of Yang's taijiquan. It fully reflects the characteristics of tai chi chuan. Tai chi chuan movements are slow and steady and pay attention to breathing and movements' coordination. When the movement rises, the arm bends, draws in, and holds the strength, all while inhaling; exhalation occurs when squatting, stretching, kicking, and reaching out the arm for strength.

There are 24 styles of simplified tai chi chuan, the same as Chapter 6, for which there are many training videos.

12.2.1.3 Five-Animal Exercise

In this exercise, you should pay attention to the relaxing of the whole body, and pay attention to Dantian, breathe evenly to achieve the appearance and spirit like the five animals. It can achieve the state of external dynamic but internal static. Pursue static in the dynamic state, and make the balance of gentleness and rigidity both inside and outside.

1) Bear exercise
   a. Imitate manner: Act like a bear – vigorous and composed, in a gentle and calm manner, heavy and flexible.
   b. Bear paw: Press your thumb on your index finger, bend the rest of your fingers, and keep the circle between your thumb and index finger.
   c. Movement: The body stands naturally, the feet are parallel and shoulder-width apart, the arms are naturally drooping, the eyes look out in front. Bend your right leg first and turn your body slightly to the right. At the same time, move your right shoulder forward and downward, and lower your right arm. Then extend your left shoulder outward and raise your left arm slightly. Then bend your left leg and move the rest of the motion opposite the top and left. Repeat and shake an unlimited number of times (Figure 12.9).

2) Crane exercise
   a. Imitate manner: Imitating its high-spirited, upright and carefree attitude, it shows bright wings, light flying, wild goose and independence.
   b. Bird wing: Hold all five fingers together, straight, and down.
   c. Action: Stand with the feet stand parallel. The arms hang naturally, and the eyes look out in front. The left form is as follows, the right form is the same as the left form, but the left form is opposite.
      (i) Take a step forward with your left foot and follow with your right foot for half a step. At the same time, lift your arms up slowly from the front of your body, palms up, and your shoulders with your left and right arms up, then inhale deeply.

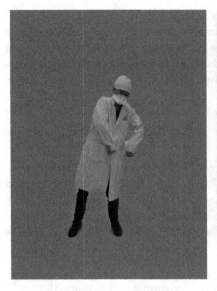
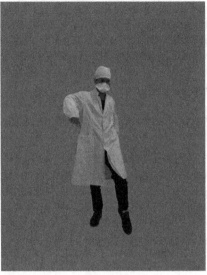

Figure 12.9   Bear exercise.

(ii)   With your right foot forward or parallel with the left foot, let your arms fall to your sides with the palms down. Squat down at the same time, and place both arms under the knee intersection, palms up, then exhale deeply (Figure 12.10).

3) Deer exercise

a.   Imitate manner: Act like a deer – the heart is quiet, the body is relaxed, the posture is stretched; show the attitude of leaning forward, lifting neck, running and looking back.

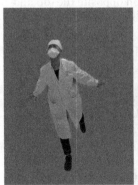
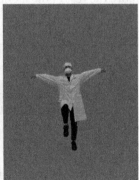
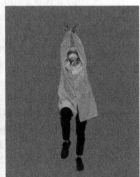

Figure 12.10   Crane exercise.

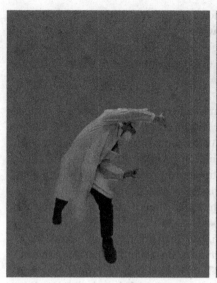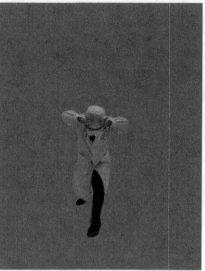

Figure 12.11   Deer exercise.

   b. Antler: Make the thumb, index finger, and little finger straight, and the middle finger and ring finger are curved inward bending fingertip contact forms a ring.

   c. Movement: The body stands up naturally, the arms hang naturally, and the eyes look out in front. The left and right forms are as follows, the right and left forms are the same, but the left and right are opposite, and the direction of rotation around the ring is also different.

      (i) Bend the right leg, sit back, extend the left leg forward, slightly bend the left knee, and step on the left foot. Extend your left hand forward and bend your left arm slightly. Put the palm of your left hand to the right and place your right hand inside your left elbow, with palm of your right hand to the left.

    (ii) Both arms should rotate counterclockwise in front of the body at the same time. The left hand should circle the ring larger than the right hand. Simultaneously, pay attention to the counterclockwise rotation of the waist and the coccygeal and the coccygeal parts (Figure 12.11).

4) Tiger exercise

   a. Imitate manner: Intense eyes, wagging tail, flapping, turning to fight and other movements to show the tiger's fierce, firm, and powerful manner

b. Round between thumb and forefinger, five fingers open, first and second knuckles bent like claws.

c. Action: The heel draws close to establish a positive posture, the arms hang naturally, and the eyes look out in front. Divide into left and right forms.

Left form

   i. Bend your knees, move your weight to your right leg, step on the left foot, point the ball of your foot on the ground, lean on the inside ankle of your right foot. At the same time, lift your fist to both sides of your waist, your heart upward, and look to the front left.

  ii. The left foot leans forward further, the right foot follows half a step, the center of gravity sits on the right leg. The left palm touches the ground slightly. At the same time, two fists are lifted up along the chest, and the boxing heart is backward. When lifted to the front of the mouth, two fists are relatively turned over, and the palm is pressed forward. The height is equal to the chest, and the palm is forward. The position between the thumb and forefinger of the two palms is opposite. Look at the left hand.

Right form

   i. Take half a step forward with your left foot, then follow your right foot to the left medial ankle, sit with your weight on your left leg, step by step on the sole of your right foot, bend your knees. At the same time, pull your two palms back to the sides of your waist, look at the front right.

  ii. It is the same as the Left 2, but the left and right are opposite. Repeat the tiger exercises an unlimited number of times (Figure. 12.12).

5) Ape exercise

a. Imitation manner: Imitate the monkey – nimble, active, showjumping along a mountain stream, climbing a tree and pushing off branches, picking peaches, and offering fruit.

b. Ape hook: Hold all five fingers together and flex the wrist.

c. Action: The heel draws close to establish a positive posture, the arms hang naturally, and your eyes look out in front. Divide left and right form; the right and left form actions are the same, but the left and right are the opposite.

   i. Bend your knees and step forward with your left foot. At the same time, keep your left hand along the front of your chest to the level of your mouth. When you reach the finish line, your fingers pinch together, your wrists droop naturally, and the whole hand is like a hook.

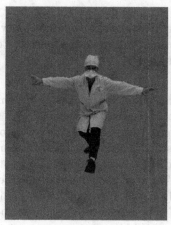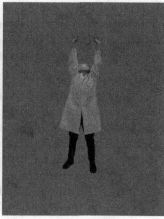

Figure 12.12   Tiger exercise.

  ii. The right foot steps forward lightly, and the left foot follows
      the right foot to the medial ankle, placing the sole of the foot
      on the ground. At the same time, when the right hand goes
      along the chest to the mouth level, it will lean forward like tak-
      ing samples. When the end point is reached, the palm will be
      pinched like a hook, and the left hand will be collected under
      the left rib at the same time.
 iii. The left foot rears back, then the right foot rears back to the left
      medial malleolus, placing the sole of the foot on the ground. At
      the same time, the left hand moves forward along the chest to
      the level of the mouth. Finally, a hook-like hand is formed, and
      the right hand is retracted under the right rib (Figure 12.13).

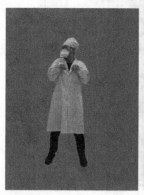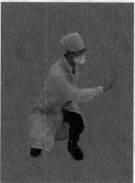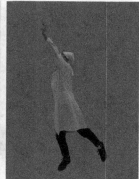

Figure 12.13   Ape exercise.

12.2.1.4 Yi Jin Jing

This exercise consists of 12 forms. It requires relaxation of mind, unity of form and spirit, natural breathing, hardness and softness, step-by-step. Complete one set each time, one to two times a day.

1) Wei Tuo offers a pestle
   a. Form: Trunk straight, ring arch hands in the chest, gas calm god all collect, the clear heart appearance is also beneficial.
   b. Natural breathing, legs straight, two heel with the inside of the contact, Tippy toes outward, stand at attention, the trunk upright, the head of Baihui point and the crotch under the long, strong point to form a straight line. The arms hang naturally on the side of the body. Eyes are level and focused. Then, both hands point forward, stop at the "Danzhong" acupoint on the chest, after about a minute of static standing (Figure 12.14).
2) Cross bear dropping magic pestle
   a. Form: Feet hang on the ground, the hands are open flat. Heart flat, breath quiet, Eyes wide open, head up: Breathe naturally. Bring both palms from the chest to the side of the body placing them flat, palms up. The arms are open in a line. At the same time, two feet heel up, Tippy toes touchdown, eyes staring straights straight ahead. Calmly, stand still for half a minute (Figure. 12.15).

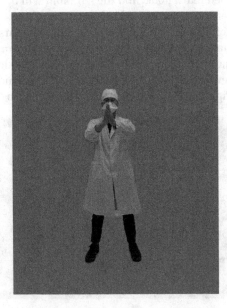

Figure 12.14   Wei Tuo offers a pestle.

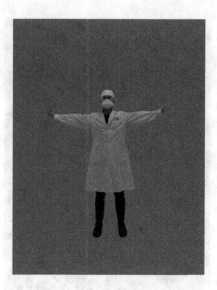

Figure 12.15   Yi Jin Jing cross bear dropping magic pestle.

3) Holding the door in the palm

   a. Form: Palms hold the Tianmen meridians eyes look up. Stand straight on your toes, the legs strong like a plant. The tongue produces fluid and licks the jaw, clenched teeth do not relax. The nose adjusts the breath and makes people feel at ease. The tongue can produce saliva to the palate, and the nose can regulate the rest of the mind. Pull both fists back slowly. At the same time of closing the fist, the heel falls slowly with the momentum. When the fist reaches the waist, the heel just falls to the ground.

   b. Follow the moves above: Lift the palms of your hands up until your arms are u-shaped. Bend your elbows slightly, palms up, and try to lift them up. At the same time place the tongue against the roof of the mouth. Let the breath be full of mind. Stand still for about half a minute (Figure 12.16).

4) Reach the star and change the bucket

   a. Form: One hand against the sky, palm covers the head, eyes look at the palm, constantly adjust the breath. The left and right eyes are retracted inward alternately.

   b. Right: Follow the actions above; against the breath only inhale not exhale, both heels on the ground, land on the balls of your feet. Put your left palm behind you, palm down, and press as hard as you can. At the same time, reverse your neck and look at your right palm. After the end of the breath to the chest, the nose takes a deep breath.

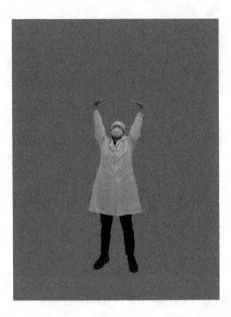

Figure 12.16   Holding the door in the palm.

    c.   Left action: Left and right hand gestures interchange, right palm drops behind your back, palms down, press as hard as you can. At the same time the left palm self after the sky, twist your neck and look at your left palm. After the end, against the breath only inhale not exhale. Stand still for about half a minute (Figure 12.17).

5) Backward drag nine oxtail style

    a.   Form: The two legs stretch back and bend forward, the lower abdomen is relaxed, the strength lies in the two arms, and the two pupils should be focused when watching boxing.

    b.   Right: Step forward with your right foot to make a right lunge. At the same time, change your right palm from the back to the front of your body and make a clenched fist. Turn your wrist and raise it. The left palm becomes a fist, keep your fist up behind your body. Both elbows are slightly bent inward, and both arms are hard. Eyes on the right fist. Stand for half a minute.

    c.   Left: The left and right legs should be exchanged, the left leg should kick, the body should move forward, the weight should be on the right leg, then the left foot should be raised and stepped forward, and the left fist should be lifted from the body to the body, and the right fist should be rolled from the front to the body, and the left hand should be rolled from the front to the body, change to the left move. Stand still for about half a minute (Figure. 12.18).

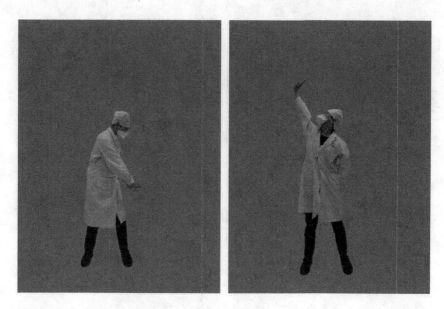

Figure 12.17 Reach the star and change the bucket.

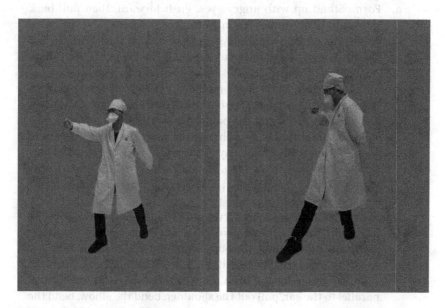

Figure. 12.18 Backward drag nine oxtail style.

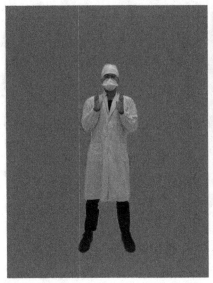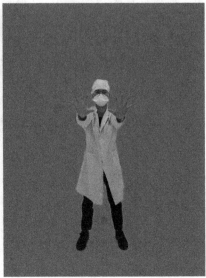

Figure 12.19 Flapping claw type.

6) Flapping claw type
   a. Form: Stand up with angry eyes. Push forward, then pull back forcefully, to do 7 times is complete.
   b. Follow the previous action. Against the breath, push with the left leg, lift the left foot, and place it on the inside of the right foot. At the same time, the two fists are at the waist, and the heart is up. Then breathe in through your nose, body straight, eyes glaring. Both fists become upright palms. Push forward towards the body, The palms are forward, the palms are straightened as far as possible. Exhale with the nose, change the two palms into fists again, recover from the original way to the waist, with the heart of fists upward; inhale with the nose, change the two fists into two palms forward, repeat seven times; the idea is in Tianmen (Figure 12.19).

7) Nine ghosts saber drawing style
   a. Form: Side head bent humerus, hold the top and neck; from the beginning to return to the original position, the force is fierce; alternate left and right, the body is straight and the Qi is still.
   b. Right: Follow the upper position; follow the breathing; turn the right fist into palm and lift it up from the waist, with the big arm parallel to the ear, pull out the shoulder, bend the elbow, bend the waist, twist the neck, and stop the right palm inward in front of the left side, like holding the head; at the same time, turn the left

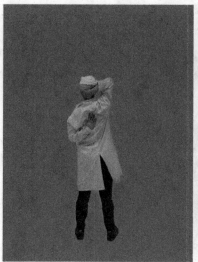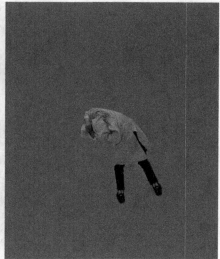

Figure. 12.20 Nine ghosts saber drawing style.

fist into palm, return to the back of the body, and try to lift it up. After setting the formula, stand still for about half a minute.

c. Left-hand gesture: The left-hand gesture is exchanged, the left arm is unbent, the left palm is lifted from the back to the side of the body. At the same time, the right arm is unbent, the right palm is lowered from the head to the side of the body, and the left-hand gesture is formed, standing for about half a minute after the fixed gesture (Figure 12.20).

8) Three-plate floor style

a. Form: Hold tongue firmly against the palate. Open your eyes and bite your gums; open your legs with your feet and squat, and press your hands as hard as you can. Turn your palms together, like holding a thousand pounds. Keep your eyes open and keep your mouth shut, and stand upright without inclination.

b. Follow the actions above. Natural breathing; when the left foot falls, the right palm is lifted from the back of the body to the front of the body. When both of the palms meet in front of the chest, then continue to separate outwards. With the elbows slightly bent and the palms facing down. The palm press the force on the outside in front of both knees. Press the tongue against the palate, stare, pay attention to the teeth, squat about half a minute to a minute. Then stand on both legs, palms turned up. Raising slowly upwards as if lifting a weight. When it is raised to chest level, turn it over to palm

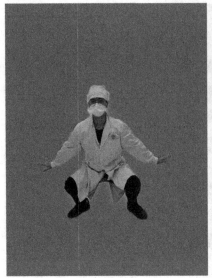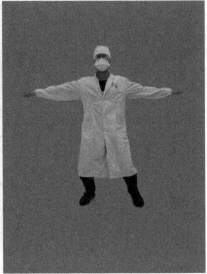

Figure 12.21   Three-plate floor style.

down, change its stance, and then form it. Repeat for three times, squat down and stand still for 1.5–3 minutes (Figure 12.21).

9) Green dragon claw

   a. Mouth: Qinglong explores claws, from left to right. The friar imitates it, and his palm is flat; force through the shoulder and back; binocular head-up, calm.

   b. Right formula: Continued formula; breathe smoothly; the eyes are straight up, and the left foot is closed inside the right foot to establish a positive posture; exhale through nose, the left palm changes fist from chest to waist, the right palm changes claw from chest, the five fingers bend slightly, force through shoulder and back, and extend claw to the left.

   c. Left type: The left and right gestures are exchanged, inhaling through the nose, bending over, bending the waist forward, and the right paw passes through the knee from left to right; exhale through the nose, straighten up, change your fist to stop at the waist, change your left fist to claw, and extend your claw from the waist to the right. The right and left positions should be repeated three times (Figure 12.22).

10) Tiger eating style

   a. Mouth: The feet are separated and the body leans forward slightly, and the left leg bends forward and the right leg stretches back;

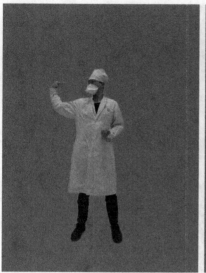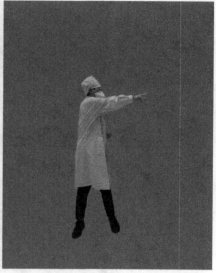

Figure 12.22   Green dragon claw.

raise your head and stand your chest as if you were leaning forward, and your back is still flat; breathe and adjust your breath,
and lean on the ground with your fingertips as a support.

b.   Right formula: Continued formula; at present, they are looking
straight up, and the upper knot type is double fists, stopping at the
waist. Take a big step forward with your right foot. Raise the left
heel and land on tiptoe in a right lunge. At the same time bending
over, pulling out the ridge, arching the back, heading up, two arms
in front of the body vertical, two palm ten fingers to support the
ground, aiming at the fingertips. Stand still for about half a minute.

c.   Left type: Stand up, and move the left foot forward one big step
to become a left lunge. Make the gesture of a reclining tiger at its
prey. When the action is reversed, exchange with respect to the
left and right sides, after making sure, stand still for half a minute
(Figure 12.23).

11) A bow type

a.   Form: Hold the head with both hands. Bend your waist to your
knees, head down to crotch. Head down near the crotch, biting the
jaw; cover your ears, and adjust your qi; the tip of the tongue is still
on the palate, and the force is on the elbows.

b.   Follow the actions above; feet open, toe buckled, slowly lift your
palms from left to right, squeeze the back of your head. Moments

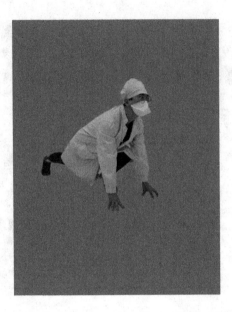

Figure 12.23   Tiger eating style.

after the finger clicks on the cerebellum, with the breathing do flexion body movement. As you inhale, keep your body straight, eyes forward, and it's like having an object on your head. As you exhale, bend at the waist, keeping the knees straight, and push your head between your knees. Do not lift your heels off the ground. Repeat 8–20 times according to physical strength (Figure. 12.24).

12) Tail off type

    a.   Form: Knees straight, push hands from the ground; stare and hold your head high; gather your spirit in one place. Get up and stamp your feet 21 times. Stretch your arms left and right, seven times, then practice sitting, cross legs and vertical canthus. What you want to say in your mouth is meditated in your heart, and your interest is adjusted to your nose; mind stability to get up.

    b.   Follow the pattern, follow the breath, straighten your knees, ten toes on the ground, hands down, a little bend, the two attached. Support the floor with palms, and stare at the end of the nose, head up, arch the back lamented ridge, collect the will of the mind. When the posture is fixed, the heels fall to the ground, lift again, and repeat three times, then stretch the elbow once. Both heels touch the ground 21 times, stretch out arms seven times, then stand up in a straight pose (Figure 12.25).

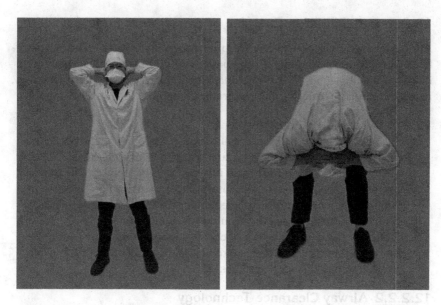

Figure. 12.24   Yi Jin Jing – bow type.

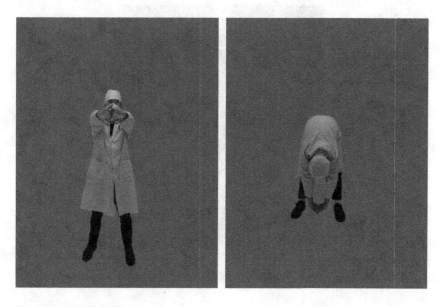

Figure 12.25   Tail off type.

12.2.2 Rehabilitation Exercise of Respiratory Function

After discharge, if the patient has symptoms such as shortness of breath or difficulty in sputum excretion, etc., the patient can take training without auxiliary equipment, such as position management, airway clearance technology, respiratory muscle training, and respiratory rehabilitation exercise.

12.2.2.1 Position Management

- Sitting at 60° on the bed: Place a pillow under the knees, slightly bend the hips and knees, lean on the back, and lower body forward (Figure 12.26).
- Sitting position: Lean your torso forward 20°–45° and sit at a table or in front of a bed. Two quilts or four pillows are placed on the table or bed. The patient's arms are placed under the quilt or pillow to fix the shoulder strap and relax the shoulder strap muscles.
- Standing: Use a walking stick or cart to support and secure your chest for relaxation. This position can reduce the work of breathing and can be used by patients with dyspnea.

12.2.2.2 Airway Clearance Technology

The patients can use position drainage, tapping, breathing methods to help expel phlegm.

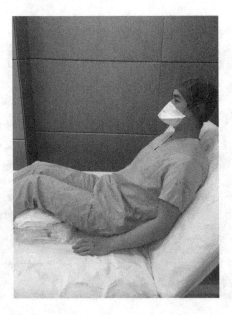

Figure 12.26   Body position management.

Self-cough training: Lean forward a little, take a deep breath slowly, hold your breath, contract your abdominal muscles, adduct your abdominal wall, open your mouth, and cough three times. When coughing up sputum, use closed plastic bags. If sputum aspiration is needed, use larger closed plastic bags to prevent the spread of the virus.

12.2.2.3 Respiratory Muscle Training

1) Contracted lip breathing

   Relax in a comfortable position, do not speak, inhale through the nose, shrink the lips into the shape of a whistling mouth, slowly exhale for 4–5 seconds. The inspiratory and expiratory time ratio was 1:2, gradually reaching the target ratio of 1:5 (Figure 12.27).

2) Controlled deep breathing

   You can consciously control the frequency, depth, and location of your breath. Take slow, deep breaths, and pause for 1–3 seconds at the end of your inhalation. Try to slow down your breathing rate, increase your inspiratory capacity, and extend your exhalation time.

3) Anti-breathing training

   When lying down, you can put sandbags or other heavy objects on top of the chest to increase the resistance when inhaling. Use convenient tools at home to blow air, such as candles or toilet paper, and repeat (Figure 12.28).

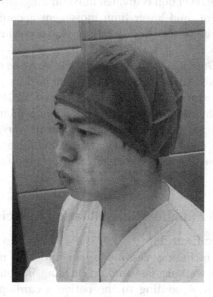

Figure 12.27   Contracted lip breathing.

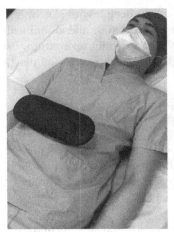 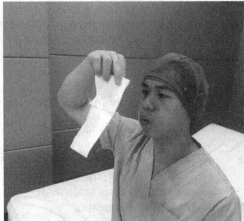

Figure 12.28   Anti-respiratory training.

4) Respiratory rehabilitation exercise

Refer to the teaching video of *Guidance for Respiratory Rehabilitation of COVID-19 Patients* compiled by experts organized by the Respiratory Rehabilitation Professional Committee of the Chinese Rehabilitation Medical Association. This video is divided into two versions: mild and severe. Each version is divided into standing, sitting, lying, upper limb movement, and lower limb movement according to exercise. Patients can choose the appropriate version according to their physical conditions.

The video *Guidance for Respiratory Rehabilitation of Mild COVID-19 Patients* includes three positions: the lying position, the sitting position, and the standing position, also known as "Trinity breathing exercise". Each breathing exercise lasts about 8–15 minutes. Patients recovering at home can choose the standing version for exercise. Patients with good physical strength can complete the whole set, and patients with weak physical strength should use only the lying position.

12.2.3 Physical Function Rehabilitation Exercises

12.2.3.1 Aerobic Exercise

Aerobic exercise, including continuous or indirect marching in place (Figure. 12.29), slow walking, fast walking, jogging, jumping rope, indoor and outdoor bicycle, etc. According to the patient's cardiopulmonary exercise

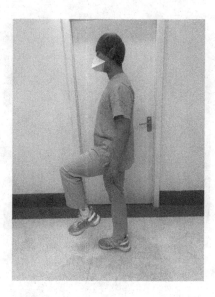

Figure 12.29   Marking time.

function, they can adjust exercise intensity step by step, three to five times per week. The time is mainly 10–30 minutes per time. The first 3 minutes are the warm-up stage, and the last 5 minutes are the finishing stage. If an intermittent motion is used, the cumulative time of motion is calculated. When doing aerobic exercise at home, it is normal to have moderate fatigue, to wheeze, sweat, and experience muscle pain. If there is chest pain, severe dyspnea, muscular fatigue, head dizziness, or nausea, the patient should stop exercise.

12.2.3.2 Strength Training

The patient can make use of the progressive resistance training methods. Books, water bottles, elastic belts, dumbbells, and other items or types of equipment can be used as auxiliary instruments. Exercise three to five times a week for 15–30 minutes each time. Do it gradually and continuously. High intensity produces more excellent physiological benefits than low intensity. Therefore, the exercise intensity can be appropriately high within the range of the body, and the "difficulty in breathing" during exercise can also be used as an alternative index to determine the exercise intensity.

   1) Upper limb strength training
      a. Flexion and extension of both arms: The patient holds the dumbbell and curls the arm to the shoulder six to ten times for each arm as a group. Patients should complete do one to three groups (Figure 12.30).

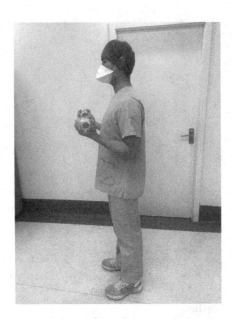

Figure 12.30   Strength training – upper limb strength training.

    b. Putting stress on the shoulders: The patient can choose to sit or stand and hold dumbbell in hands and lift it up, keeping the whole arm straight, six to ten times for a group. Patients should complete three groups (Figure 12.31).

    c. Pushing the wall: The patient should stand, lean against the wall, and then push away from the wall six to ten times as a group. Patients should do one to three groups, keeping the distance of their feet from the wall fixed (Figure 12.32).

    d. Bench press: The patient is in the recumbent position, the patient pushes the dumbbell up to the arm extension six to ten times for one group. Patients should do three groups (Figure 12.33).

2) Lower limb strength training

    a. Kick training: The patients sit and stretch their legs until their knees are flat six to ten times one group. Patients should do three groups (Figure. 12.34).

    b. Bounce training: The patients step off the ground for six to ten times for one group. Patients should do one to three groups. Dumbbells can also be used for hand training (Figure 12.35).

    c. Lunge: Take a big step forward with one foot and bend your legs until your thighs are parallel to the ground. 6–10 times as a group, do three groups (Figure 12.36).

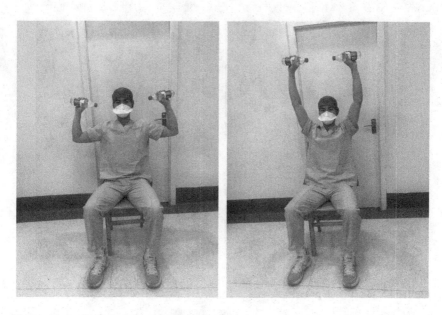

Figure 12.31   Putting stress on the shoulders.

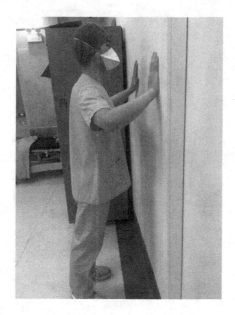

Figure 12.32   Pushing the wall.

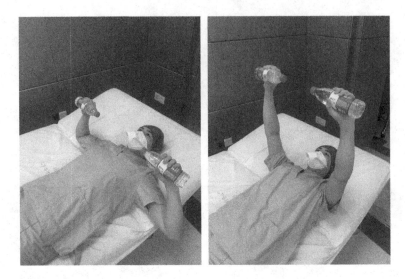

Figure 12.33   Bench press.

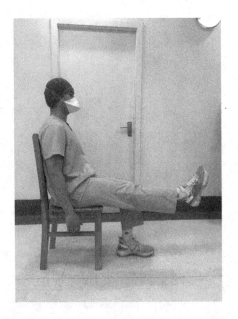

Figure. 12.34   Kick training.

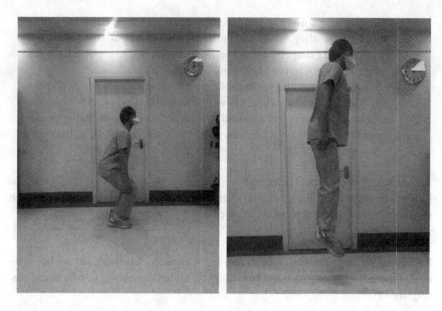

Figure 12.35   Bounce training.

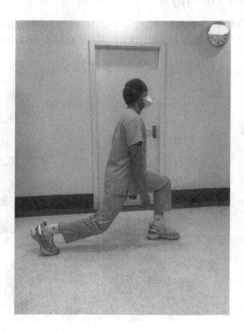

Figure 12.36   Lunge.

    d. Sitting and standing practice: The patients sit on the edge of the chair, then they stand up. Patients should repeat this six to ten times for a group. Patients should complete three groups. Patients should try not to use their arms (Figure 12.37).

    e. Squat training: The patients stand with feet shoulder-width apart and squat, bending their knees not more than 90°, six to ten times for one group. Patients should complete three groups. Patients can hold dumbbells or other heavy objects while completing this exercise (Figure 12.38).

12.2.3.3 Flexibility Training

Flexibility training is mainly to stretch the main body muscle group, prevent sports injury, relieve muscle fatigue, etc.

12.2.3.4 Balance Training

Patients with balance dysfunction can train kneeling position, sitting balance and standing on one foot on the training bed under the care of family members (Figure 12.39).

12.2.4 Oxygen Therapy

If the symptoms of shortness of breath, polypnea, and fatigue are obvious and cannot be relieved in a short time, the patient can take advantage of oxygen

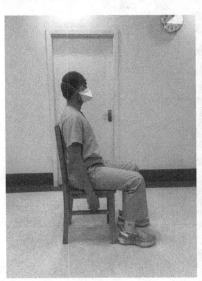
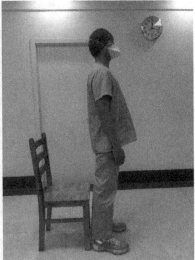

Figure 12.37   Sitting and standing exercise.

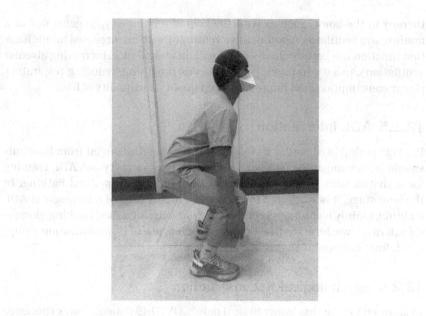

Figure 12.38   Squat training.

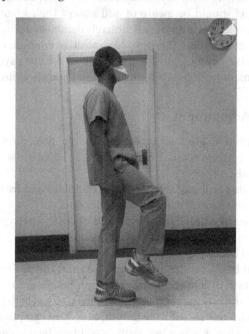

Figure 12.39   Standing on one leg.

therapy in the home, such as with the help of a home oxygen generator or a noninvasive ventilator. A noninvasive ventilator with an increased humidification function has better tolerance and patient compliance, increasing alveolar ventilation capacity, improving spontaneous breathing, reducing respiratory power consumption, and improving sleep quality and quality of life.

12.2.5 ADL Intervention

Patients with ADL disorder 2–4 weeks after being discharged from hospitals should be accompanied by their family members to carry out ADL training for activities such as transfer, modification, toilet flushing, and bathing. In the later stage, it is suggested to carry out a higher level of instrumental ADL training, mainly including shopping, outdoor activities, food cooking, domestic activities, washing clothes, taking medicine, use of communication equipment, financial processing ability, and so on.

12.2.6 Psychological Reconstruction

In addition to suffering from physical pain, COVID-19 patients may experience varying degrees of long-term psychological stress. After being discharged from hospitals, patients should be aware of and accept their emotional reactions, properly vent their negative emotions, actively establish a connection with the outside world, and stimulate their internal positive emotions. In case of deterioration of adverse psychological state, seek and receive psychological counseling and treatment from psychological professionals in time.

12.2.7 Diet Adjustment

1) Eat high-protein food every day, including fish, meat, eggs, milk, beans, nuts, etc. Increase the amount on the usual basis and do not eat wild animals.
2) Take vitamins properly and eat fresh vegetables and fruits every day.
3) Drink no less than 1,500 mL of water per day.
4) Ensure adequate nutrition, enrich and diversify the types and colors of food. Don't be picky eaters, do not diet, and balance portions of vegetables and meat.
5) Select food based on the food properties and the patient's condition. For patients with cold and stomach symptoms, ginger, onion, mustard, coriander, and other spicy foods can be used to warm the stomach. For patients with dry throat, dry mouth, boredom symptoms, and other symptoms, choose green tea, fermented black beans, carambola, and other heat-clearing *yin* food. For patients with symptoms such as cough

and phlegm, choose pears, lily, groundnut, almond, ginkgo, plum, Chinese cabbage, orange peel, perilla, and other cough- and asthma-clearing food. For patients with loss of appetite, abdominal distention, and other symptoms of temper weakness, choose hawthorn, Chinese yam, white lentil, poria, pueraria, semen raphani, Arenicola, and other spleen-invigorating and digestive food. For patients with constipation and other symptoms, choose honey, bananas, sesame seeds, and other moist laxative foods. For patients with symptoms such as insomnia, choose jujube kernel, cypress kernel, and other food that helps induce sleeping.

12.3 CONTRAINDICATIONS AND PRECAUTIONS

12.3.1 Contraindications

1) If the patient has any of the following conditions, it is not recommended to carry out the above rehabilitation treatment.
   a. Resting heart rate > 100 beats/min.
   b. Blood pressure < 90/60 mmHg or > 140/90mmHg, or blood pressure fluctuation exceeding 20 mmHg of baseline, accompanied by obvious uncomfortable symptoms such as dizziness and headache.
   c. Blood oxygen saturation ≤ 95%.
   d. Other diseases that are unsuitable for exercise are combined.
2) When the patient has the following conditions during the treatment, the above rehabilitation treatment should be stopped, and the treatment plan should be reassessed and adjusted.
   a. Obvious fatigue and cannot be relieved after rest.
   b. Chest tightness, chest pain, dyspnea, severe cough, dizziness, headache, blurred vision, palpitations, sweating, and standing instability.
   c. When there are pain symptoms of the musculoskeletal system, the doctor should be consulted to adjust the exercise prescription according to the circumstances, and the exercise intensity should increase gradually to avoid the occurrence of excessive fatigue, leading to a relapse of the illness or an aggravated illness.

12.3.2 Precautions

1. Patients with pulmonary hypertension, congestive heart failure, deep venous thrombosis, unstable fractures, and other diseases should

consult with a specialist before starting respiratory rehabilitation therapy.

2. Elderly patients are often accompanied by various basic diseases, with poor physical conditions and poor tolerance to rehabilitation training. A comprehensive evaluation should be conducted before rehabilitation treatment, and rehabilitation training should start from a small dose and proceed step by step to avoid training injuries and other serious complications.

3. Community-based rehabilitation applies to mild and ordinary patients. Severe and critically severe patients can be rehabilitated after discharging from hospitals in designated rehabilitation medical institutions and primary medical and health institutions.

4. Discharged patients should be isolated at home for 14 days to avoid reinfection and to pay close attention to whether symptoms reoccur, at which point the patient would take a nucleic acid test to check for reinfection.

5. Pay attention to protection in daily life to avoid cross-infection. Wash your hands frequently, wear a mask, develop good hygiene habits, and try to avoid going to crowded places.

BIBLIOGRAPHY

1. General Office of National Health and Wellness Committee, State Administration of Traditional Chinese Medicine Office. Novel Coronavirus Diagnosis and Treatment Program (Trial Seventh Edition). [2020-03-04] http://www.nhc.gov.cn/yzygj/s7653p/202003/46c9294a7dfe4cef80dc7f5912eb1989.shtml.

2. General Office of the National Health and Health Commission. Notice of the General Office of the National Health and Health Commission on Printing and Distributing Rehabilitation Program for Pneumonia Discharged Patients in COVID-19. [2020-03-04]. http://www.gov.cn/zhengce/zhengceku/2020-03/05/content-5487160.htm.

3. General Office of the National Health and Health Commission. Notice of the General Office of the National Health and Health Commission on Printing and Distributing the Prevention and Control Program of Pneumonia Infected in Novel Coronavirus (Third Edition). [2020-01-28] http://www.gov.cn/zhengce/zhengceku/2020-01/29/content_5472893.htm.

4. Wang Gang. *Community Rehabilitation*. 2nd Edition. Beijing: People's Health Publishing House, 2018: 165–176.

5. Liu Xiaodan, Li Liu, Lu Yunfei, Feng Ling, Zhao Feiran, Wu Xubo, Qi Tang Kai, Zhao Jingjun, Xiao Lu, Xu Shufu, Yang Liu, Shen Yanan, Liu Yijie, Lu Hongzhou, Shan Chunlei. Guidance on rehabilitation training of integrated traditional Chinese and western medicine for patients with functional recovery in novel coronavirus. *Shanghai Journal of Traditional Chinese Medicine*, 2020, 54 (3): 9–13.

6. State Administration of Traditional Chinese Medicine Office. Notice on Printing and Distributing the Guiding Suggestions of TCM Rehabilitation in Recovery Period in Novel Coronavirus. [2020-02-23] .http://yzs.satcm.gov.cn/zhengcewenjian/2020-02-23/13319.html.

7. Li Xiaodong, Liu Baoyan, Wang Yi, Guan Ling, Li Guangxi, Wang Hua, Wang Jian, Weng Changshui, Xiao Mingzhong, Tong Xiaolin. Interpretation of Covid-19 Guidance and Suggestions for Traditional Chinese Medicine Rehabilitation in Convalescence (Trial) [J]. Journal of Traditional Chinese Medicine, 2020, 61 (11): 928–934.

8. Guo Guangxin, Cao Ben, Zhu Qingguang, Zhang Shuaipan, Zhou Xin, Lu Zhizhen, Wu Zhiwei, Xu Shanda, Kong Lingjun, Sun Wuquan, Cheng Yanbin, Fang Min. Discussion on the application of traditional chinese medicine in the prevention and treatment of novel coronavirus. *Shanghai Journal of Traditional Chinese Medicine*, 2020, 54 (05): 28–31.

9. Twelve-formula diagram of Dharma Yijinjing. [2018-07-10] https://jingyan.baidu.com/article/20095761655216cb0721b4a9.html.

10. Tian Wei, Liu Geng, Zhang Xiaoying, Liu Qingquan, Lei Yan, Zhao Hongmei, Gong Weijun, Wang Minghang, Bing Lin, Wang Peng, Shu Yan, Cheng Xiankuan, Yang Aoran. Novel Coronavirus Respiratory Rehabilitation Program of Integrated Traditional Chinese and Western Medicine (Draft). *Chinese Journal of Traditional Chinese Medicine Information*, 2020, 27(08): 1–7.

11. China Rehabilitation Medical Association. Notice on Printing and Distributing 2019 Novel Coronavirus Respiratory Rehabilitation Guidance (First Edition). [2020-02-03] http://www.carm.org.cn/Home/Article/detail/id/2524.html.

12. Respiratory Rehabilitation Professional Committee of Chinese Rehabilitation Medical Association. Respiratory Rehabilitation Guidance for Severe Upper Limb novel coronavirus. [2020-03-05]. http://health.gmw.cn/2020-03/05/content_33621595.htm.

13. 2019 Novel Coronavirus Respiratory Rehabilitation Guidance (2nd Edition). *Chinese Journal of Tuberculosis and Respiratory Medicine*, 2020 (04): 308–314.

14. National Health and Wellness Committee. Nutritional Dietary Guidelines for Prevention and Treatment of Infected Pneumonia in Novel Coronavirus. [2020-02-08]   http://www.nhc.gov.cn/xcs/fkdt/202002/a69fd36d54514c5a9a3f456188cbc428.shtml.

Appendices: Related Rating Scales

APPENDIX 1: BORG DYSPNEA ASSESSMENT SCALE

Level	Assessment of the Severity of Dyspnea
0 score	I do not feel any dyspnea or fatigue.
0.5 score	Very slight dyspnea or fatigue, almost imperceptible.
1 score	Very mild dyspnea or fatigue.
2 score	Mild dyspnea or fatigue.
3 score	Moderate dyspnea or fatigue.
4 score	Slightly severe dyspnea or fatigue.
5 score	Severe dyspnea or fatigue.
6–8 score	Very severe dyspnea or fatigue.
9 score	Extreme dyspnea or fatigue.
10 score	Intolerable and needs medical help. Dyspnea or fatigue reaching to the limit.

This scale is generally applied in conjunction with the 6-minute walking test. Before starting the 6-minute walking test, patients should read the scale and report their the level of dyspnea. The level of dyspnea is reassessed after exercise.

APPENDIX 2: 6-MINUTE WALK TEST

Bed Number	Name	Admission Number	Date
Gender	Age	Diagnosis	
Medication before test	Yes/No		
Oxygen before test	Yes/No		
Time	Pre-experiment	Post-experiment	
Heart rate (beat/minute)			
Blood pressure (mmHg)			
Blood sugar (mmol/L)			
SPO_2 (%)			
Dyspnea			
Stop halfway	Yes/No		
Other discomforts	Yes/No	Angina	Dizziness
Number of back and forth		Number of incomplete circles	Total distance
Results of the analysis			

Patients are asked to walk as fast as possible in a straight corridor to measure a 6-minute walk distance, and minimum back and forth distance $\geq$ 30 m. It measures the patient's physiological response to increased oxygen demand. There are four classes based on the 6-minute walking distance: Level 1 is less than 300m, Level 2 is 300–375 m, Level 3 is 375–450 m, and Level 4 is over 450m. The Borg Fatigue rating (RPE) was used to evaluate the patients' fatigue and the main reason for not being able to walk further after the trial.

APPENDIX 3: MODIFIED MEDICAL RESEARCH COUNCIL SCALE

Level	Assessment of the Severity of Dyspnea
0	I have dyspnea only during strenuous exercise.
1	I get shortness of breath when I jog or walk up a hill.
2	Because of my shortness of breath, I walk more slowly than my peers or need to stop to rest.
3	I walk on flat ground for about 100 meters or a few minutes before I needed to stop and catch my breath.
4	I have so much trouble breathing that I could not leave home, or I have dyspnea while putting on clothing or undressing.

Dyspnea is classified into 0–4 levels according to patients' activity level when they have shortness of breath. Level 4 indicates dyspnea occurring at the slightest activity.

APPENDIX 4: 2-MINUTE MARKING TIME TEST

Test Facilities	Stopwatch, tape, or a 76 cm long rope, marker bar, counter
Exercise Test	On the day of the test, the minimum height that the knee-joint should achieve for marking is set for each subject, i.e. it should be the midpoint of the connecting line between the knee and anterior superior iliac spine. The tape can be used to measure, or a rope can be used from knee to anterior superior iliac spine, then folded equally, and the marker bar is used to stick the folded points onto the thigh.
Test Method	1. Subjects can stand by the wall, a doorway, or a high-backed chair and transfer the marks on their thighs to the corresponding spots on the wall or chair. If the subject is tall enough, books can also be stacked on a small table as a marker. 2. Start the timing after signaling to the patient to start the test. 3. Use a counter to record the number of times the knee reaches the specified height within 2 minutes. 4. When the subject cannot reach the specified height, they are required to slow down or rest until they can reach the appropriate height again, during which time the scoring will continue. The score is based on the steps completed within 2 minutes (e.g., the number of times the right knee has reached the specified height).

Safety tips:

1. Subjects with balance disorders should stand against the wall or between the arms of chairs for support in case of loss of balance. It also requires careful observation.
2. Monitor subjects for signs of overexertion.
3. After the test, subjects were asked to walk slowly for several minutes to relax.
4. If subjects stomp their feet during the test, they should be encouraged to lower their feet gently so as not to injure their knees.

APPENDIX 5: 3-MINUTE STEP TEST

Test Facilities	Steps (30 cm for male; 25 cm for female)
Test Method	1. Step rhythm is 30 beats per minute (up and down) for 3 minutes. You can ask your partner to use a metronome (set to 60 beats per minute, with one step per beep) or voice prompt to help you keep the proper rhythm. Therefore, you need to step up and down once in 2 seconds. During the test, you should rotate your legs from side to side. After each step up and down, your upper body and legs must be straight without bending your knees.
	2. After the test, you should sit down immediately, and your partner will help you record and measure your heart rate during the three convalescent periods: 1–1.5 minutes, 2–2.5 minutes, and 3–3.5 minutes.
	3. The cardiopulmonary adaptation was evaluated according to the evaluation index, which was equal to time of stair climbing exercise (s) ×100/2× (the sum of the three heart rates during convalescent period).

Evaluation Index of 3-Minute Step Test

Level of Adaptability	Male	Female
1 score (poor)	45.0–48.5	44.6–48.5
2 score (inferior)	48.6–53.5	48.6–53.2
3 score (average)	53.6–62.4	53.3–62.4
4 score (good)	62.5–70.8	62.5–70.2
5 score (excellent)	>70.9	>70.3

Note: 1 or 2 score – the cardiopulmonary adaptation level is lower than average, which is poor or inferior.

4 score – the level of cardiopulmonary adaptation is higher than the average level of people in the same gender and age group, which is relatively good.

5 score – the cardiopulmonary level adaptation is in the top 15% for people of the same age group are excellent.

APPENDIX 6: 30-SECOND CHAIR STANDING EXPERIMENT

Test Facilities	A standard 43-cm straight-back chair, stopwatch.
Test Method	1. Make the subject sit in a standard 43-cm straight-back chair, placed against a wall, with the back upright, feet flat on the floor, arms and wrists crossed and held in front of the chest.
	2. Let the subjects stand one or two times to get familiar with the experiment.
	3. Start the time after signaling the patient to start the experiment.;
	4. The subjects are in a full standing position, then sit down, and touch the chair seat, and then repeat the above actions as much as possible within 30 seconds.
	5. Count the number of times the subjects stand. For each count, the subject must complete all the actions.
	6. Encourage subjects when they maintain good movement.

APPENDIX 7: 30-SECOND ARM FLEXION TEST

Test facilities	A standard 43-cm straight-back chair, a 5-pound hand dumbbell for women, an 8-pound hand dumbbell for men, a stopwatch.
Test Method	1. Subjects should sit in a chair with their backs straight and their feet flat on the floor. The hand dumbbells should be held in the handshake position by the dominant hand; elbows should be fully extended; arms should be perpendicular to the ground; palms should be toward the inside of the body.
	2. Subjects should squat on the side of the subject's dominant hand, place one hand behind the subject's triceps to stabilize the upper arm to prevent the elbow from moving backward (flexing). And they can place one finger in the elbow to prevent the arm from moving forward, and touch the forearm to ensure complete buckling action.
	a. Starting position: The examiner places his hands in front of and behind the elbow to prevent arm movement.
	b. Subject's arm flexes inward to complete the arm retraction motion, with the palm facing upward at the end.
	3. Subjects are asked to do one of two exercises to familiarize themselves with the test.
	4. Start the time after signaling the patient to begin.
	5. Subjects complete the buckling action by elbow rotation and returning to the starting position.
	6. Subjects will complete as many flexion movements as possible within 30 seconds.
	7. Encourage participants when they maintain good movement.

Safety tip: Some researchers assess strength by lifting the heaviest objects, but this is controversial, and these tests carry a risk of injury to older people.

APPENDIX 8: CHAIR-STRETCHING FORWARD TEST

Test Facilities	A standard 43-cm straight-back chair and a ruler (about 45.7cm)
Test Method	1. Subjects are asked to sit in a chair, bending their body forward and downward.
	2. Demonstrate standard body positions and movements to the subjects.
	3. Subject are asked to bend the left leg and place the left foot flat on the ground, extend the right leg completely so that the knee is straight, the heel is on the ground, and the ankle is bent to 90°.
	4. Let the subjects straighten their arms, with dominant hands on the top, fingers straight forward and down, slide their hands down along the ruler, raise their heads as much as possible, and hold their chest out.
	5. Subjects must push forward through their fingertips and try to push through their toes.
	6. Remind subjects to keep breathing smoothly, move their fingers slowly, and do not reach the maximum stretch all at once during the experiment.
	7. During the experiment, the knee must be straight. If the knee is bent, the subject should be asked to do the experiment again.
	8. It takes at least 2 seconds for the finger to reach its maximum point to count as a forward extension.
	9. Subjects need to conduct two preliminary experiments followed by two formal experiments.
	10. Replace the left leg and repeat the above experiment.
	11. Record the distance between the middle finger and the tip of subject's foot. If the front extension fails to pass the tip of the subject's foot, the distance will be a negative number. If the front extension passes the tip of subject's foot, subjects can get a positive number. Record the best result from both measurements.

APPENDIX 9: BACK-SCRATCHING EXPERIMENT

Test Facilities	A Ruler
Test Method	1. Demonstrate to the subject before the experiment begins.
	2. Subjects stand with their backs straight.
	3. Place the right hand over the right shoulder on the back with the palm facing the back. Then place the left hand on the lower back with the back of hand facing the back.
	4. Subjects should extend their hands as far as possible along the spine in both directions, and try to make their fingers touch or pass each other.
	5. The stretch is not valid until the subject can hold it for more than 2 seconds.
	6. Subjects should conduct two formal experiments after two preliminary experiments.
	7. Repeat the experiment by changing the left side and the position of the hand.
	8. Use a ruler to record the distance between the fingertips of the middle fingers. If the fingers of both hands cannot touch each other, write down a negative number; if the fingers pass each other, write a positive number. Record the best result from both tests.

APPENDIX 10: MODIFIED BODY ROTATION TEST

Test Facilities	Meter ruler, tape, cavities band, or other types of markers
Test Method	1. Demonstrate the standard position and form for the subjects before the experiment begins.
	2. At the beginning of the test, subjects should stand with their shoulders perpendicular to the wall, and they should stand perpendicular to the straight line made of tape, with their toes just touching the straight line. A ruler should be placed on the subject's shoulder level, and their toes should be aligned with the scale of 30 cm on meter ruler.
	3. Rotate the subject's body backward and extend it forward as far as possible along the scale.
	4. Performance will be assessed by measuring how long the subject's knuckle of middle finger can extend along the ruler, which is relative to the scale of 30 cm on meter ruler; for example, if the subject's knuckle of middle finger reached 58.4 cm, the extension would be 28.4 cm, i.e., 58.4 cm minus 30 cm.
	5. Subjects should conduct three experiments for the best results.

APPENDIX 11: SINGLE-LEG UPRIGHT BALANCE TEST

Single-leg upright balance test originated in 1965 and has become a commonly used method to test balance ability in clinical practice. This method is not only an experimental method to test postural stability, but also a training method to prevent falling in clinic. The experiment was divided into two methods: eye-opening method and eye-closing method, among which the eye-closing method was obviously more difficult than the eye-opening method.

Test Facilities	Stopwatch, a wall on which there is a reference mark for visual reference of subjects
Test Method	1. Subjects are asked to stand at the position that is three steps (1 m) away from the wall or visual reference point. Subjects should stand with both feet together and both arms at their sides.
	2. Demonstrate to subjects prior to the test.
	3. Subjects are asked to bend a knee, allow the foot to lift 15–20 cm from the ground, both legs separate slightly without touching each other, and keep both hands naturally at their sides.
	4. Start timing by the stopwatch after subjects complete the single-leg upright action.
	5. Subjects shall stand on a single leg as long as possible, with eyes watching the reference mark, keeping the standing lower limb perpendicular to the ground. both arms at their sides, and the lifted foot in position. Subjects are allowed to pre-test two times before collecting data.
	6. When the subject's arms deviate from both sides of body, the standing lower limb deviates from original position, or the lifted leg comes in contact with the ground, stop the test immediately.
	7. If the subject's single-leg upright duration exceeds 60 s, the subject's balance function is considered as good. The subjects are then asked to repeat the test with their eyes closed.

APPENDIX 12: FUNCTIONAL FORWARD EXTENSION TEST

The functional forward extension test, which is used to assess balance in older people, has proven to be a very effective method. The test is simple and measured as far forward as the subject could reach while maintaining a stable position that supported the body. The results of this method are highly correlated with those measured by classical pressure sensors (r = 0.83) and can be sensitive to age-related changes in balance.

Test Facilities	1. A 100-cm meter ruler 2. Stick the ruler on the wall with tape 3. An assistant
Test Method	1. Ask the subjects to take off their shoes and socks and stand relaxed with their right shoulder perpendicular to the wall. 2. Demonstrate standard actions to the subjects before the test begins. 3. Stick the ruler parallel to the ground on the wall at the level of the subject's right acromion. 4. One tester should stand in front of the subject so that they can read the scale easily. The other tester should stand behind the subject to see if the subject's heel is on the ground and watch the process of subject's knuckle of middle finger moving forward along the ruler. 5. Let the subject extend the right upper limb horizontally (at an angle close to 90° from the shoulder joint) and make a fist with the right hand so that the knuckle of middle finger is facing forward to measure the original measurement value at the length of the upper limb). 6. Let the subjects lean forward as far as possible while maintaining their balance. 7. There is no special requirement for the completion of this experiment. The experiment should be stopped immediately when the subject's feet are lifted off the ground. 8. Let the subjects conduct two pre-tests before the formal start of the test to familiarize themselves with the test procedures. Then assess the balance ability of the subjects during the formal experiment. 9. The result of the functional forward stretch test is the maximum distance that can be achieved minus the original measured value. 10. Two tests are needed to get the best result.

APPENDIX 13: 2.4-M STANDING UP AND WALKING TEST

The 2.4-meter standing up and walking experiment, also known as standing up and walking experiment, is the most common and reliable test method in the literature for muscle strength and muscle adaptability.

Experimental Facilities	1. A standard seat with an upright back, which is 43 cm from the ground 2. A cone-shaped marker 3. A stopwatch
Experimental Method	1. Lean the chair against the wall and place a marker 2.4 m away from the leading edge of the chair. 2. Let the subjects sit on the chairs with hands on their thighs, their back on the back of the chair, one foot slightly in front of them and their torso slightly forward. 3. Demonstrate to the subjects that at least one foot should always be on the ground (i.e., walking, not running); 4. Start the stopwatch after signaling to the patients to begin. 5. The subjects will immediately get up from their chairs (with the help of their arms), walk around the marked points, and then return to their chairs and sit in their original positions. 6. Let the subjects conduct one pre-test and two formal experiments. Record the best score of the two experiments as the experimental result.

APPENDIX 14: BARTHEL INDEX EVALUATION SCALE

Parameter	Scoring Criteria	Month Day
1. Defecation	0 = Incontinence or in a coma 5 = Occasional incontinence < 1 per week 10 = Controlled	
2. Urination	0 = Incontinence or in a coma or needs others to help them urinate 5 = Occasional incontinence < 1 time every 24 hours, a week > 1 time 10 = Controlled	
3. Modification	0 = Needs help 5 = Wash, comb, brush, and shave independently	

Parameter	Scoring Criteria	Month Day
4. Using toilet	0 = Dependent on others 5 = Needs some help 10 = Self-care	
5. Having meals	0 = Dependent on others 5 = Needs some help with cooking, filling, and cutting bread 10 = Complete self-care	
6. Transferring from chair to bed or bed to chair	0 = Totally dependent on someone else; cannot sit 5 = Needs a lot of help (two people); can sit 10 = A small amount of help or guidance is required (1 person) 15 = Self-care	
7. Activity is walking in and around the ward, which does not include long walks.	0 = Cannot move 5 = Can move independently in a wheelchair 10 = One person is required to help walk physically or by oral instruction 15 = Independent walking with assistance	
8. Dressing	0 = Dependent on others 5 = Needs more help during dressing 10 = Self-fastening/unbuttoning, closing/ unzipping and wearing shoes	
9. Up and down the stairs with a walking stick are also independent.	0 = Fails to accomplish 5 = Needs help with physical or verbal instruction 10 = Self-care	
10. Bathing	0 = Dependent on others 5 = Self-care	

ADL capability defect degree:

0–20 score represents very serious functional defects.

25–45 score represents serious functional defects.

50–70 score represents moderate functional defects.

75–90 score represents mild functional defects.

100 score represents self-care.

ADL self-care degree:

0–35 score represents basically complete assistance.

35–80 score represents wheelchair life; needs some assistance.

80 score represents level of wheelchair self-care.

80–100 score represents self-care for most ADL.

100 score represents complete self-care for ADL.

APPENDIX 15: SELF-RATING DEPRESSION SCALE (SDS)

Notes for filling in this form: Please read each parameter carefully to clearly understand the meaning of the question. Put a $\sqrt{}$ in the appropriate box according to your actual situation in the latest week.

	Occasionally A	Sometimes B	Often C	Continuously D
1. I feel blue and depressed.				
2. I think the morning is the best part of the day.				
3. I burst into tears or want to cry.				
4. I do not sleep well at night.				
5. My appetite is the same as before.				
6. I am as happy with the opposite sex as I was before.				
7. I find myself losing weight.				
8. I have trouble with constipation.				
9. My heart is beating faster than usual.				
10. I feel tired without any reason.				
11. My mind is clear as ever.				
12. I do not find it difficult to do what I often do.				
13. I feel uneasy and can hardly calm down.				
14. I'm hopeful about the future.				
15. I get angry more easily than before.				

	Occasionally A	Sometimes B	Often C	Continuously D
16. I think it is easy to decide what to do.				
17. I think I am a useful person and someone needs me.				
18. My life is very interesting.				
19. Others will be better off if I die.				
20. I am interested in things that I used to interested.				

Rating method: SDS uses four levels to evaluate the frequency of symptoms, i.e., occasionally (less than once a week), sometimes (one to two times a week), often (three to four times a week), and continuously (almost daily).

Scoring: Questions A, B, C, and D are based on a 1, 2, 3, and 4 score. The reverse score is based on 4, 3, 2, and 1.

Reverse scorecard number: 2, 5, 6, 11, 12, 14, 16, 17, 18, and 20. The standard score is obtained by multiplying the total score by 1.25 to an integer.

According to the Chinese norm, the threshold for SDS standard score is 53, in which 53–62 is mild depression, 63–72 is moderate depression, 72 or above is severe depression, and lower than 53 is considered normal.

APPENDIX 16: SELF-RATING ANXIETY SCALE (SAS)

Notes for filling in the form: There are 20 sentences below. Please read each one carefully to clearly understand the meaning. Then, according to your actual feelings from the past week, circle the number from 1 to 4 that is most suitable for your situation. Please choose the frequency of symptoms to assess the present mental and physical status by yourself.

Evaluated Project	Seldom	Sometimes	Often	Usually
1. I feel more nervous or anxious than usual.	1	2	3	4
2. I feel afraid for no reason.	1	2	3	4
3. I tend to get upset or scared.	1	2	3	4

Evaluated Project	Seldom	Sometimes	Often	Usually
4. I think I might go crazy.	1	2	3	4
*5. I think everything is fine and nothing bad will happen.	4	3	2	1
6. My hands and feet tremble.	1	2	3	4
7. I am troubled with headache, neck pain, and backache.	1	2	3	4
8. I feel weak and tire easily.	1	2	3	4
*9. I feel calm and find it easy to sit quietly.	4	3	2	1
10. I feel my heart beating faster.	1	2	3	4
11. I am troubled by bouts of dizziness.	1	2	3	4
12. I fainted before or feel like I am about to faint.	1	2	3	4
*13. I find it easy to breathe in and out.	4	3	2	1
14. I have numbness and tingling in my hands and feet.	1	2	3	4
15. I am troubled with stomachache and indigestion.	1	2	3	4
16. I often have to urinate.	1	2	3	4
*17. My hands and feet are often dry and warm.	4	3	2	1
18. I blush and burn.	1	2	3	4
*19. I fell asleep easily and sleep soundly all night.	4	3	2	1
20. I have nightmares.	1	2	3	4

Rating method: SAS uses four levels to evaluate the frequency of symptoms, i.e., 1 indicates never or seldom, 2 indicates sometimes, 3 indicates often; 4 indicates usually. 15 of the 20 parameters are stated with negative words and are scored in the order of 1 to 4 above. The remaining five parameters (Parameter 5, 9, 13, 17, 19) marked with * are stated with positive words and scored in reverse order from 4 to 1.

Analysis index: The main statistical index of SAS is the total score. Add up the score for each of the 20 parameters and you get a raw score. If you multiply the raw score by 1.25 and take the integral part, you get the standard score, or you can look up the table and do the same conversion.

Results interpretation: According to Chinese norm results, the threshold for SAS standard score is 50, in which 50–59 is mild anxiety, 60–69 is moderate anxiety, and above 70 is severe anxiety.

APPENDIX 17: HAMILTON DEPRESSION SCALE (HAMD17)

Parameter	Scoring Criteria	Score
1. Depressed mood	0 = Absent 1 = Tell only when they are asked 2 = Express spontaneously in the conversation 3 = Show this feeling from expression, posture, voice, or not smiling without words 4 = Almost show this feeling by verbal and nonverbal words (expression, actions)	
2. Feelings of guilt	0 = Absent 1 = Self-reproach, feel they have let people down 2 = Ideas of guilt or rumination over past errors or sinful deeds 3 = Present illness is punishment 4 = Delusions of guilt are accompanied by accusatory or threatening hallucinations	
3. Suicide	0 = Absent 1 = Thinks there is no meaning in living 2 = Wishes to be dead, or always thinking of something to do with death 3 = Negative thoughts (suicide) 4 = Serious suicide	
4. Insomnia [early]	0 = Absent 1 = Difficulty falling asleep, that is, not being able to fall asleep 30 minutes after going to bed 2 = Difficulty falling asleep every night	
5. Insomnia [middle]	0 = Absent 1 = Light sleep, nightmares 2 = Woke up in the middle of the night (before 12 a.m.) (not including going to the bathroom)	
6. Insomnia [late]	0 = Absent 1 = Wakes up early, wakes up 1 hour earlier than usual, but can return to sleep 2 = Wakes up early and cannot get back to sleep	

Parameter	Scoring Criteria	Score
7. Work and activities	0 = Absent 1 = Tell only when they are asked 2 = Spontaneously express, directly or indirectly, a loss of interest in activities, work, or study, such as feeling listless, indecisive, unable to insist, or forced to work or study 3 = Activity time is reduced or efficiency is reduced, hospitalized patients participate in hospital labor or recreation less than 3 hours per day 4 = As a result of the current illness, the inpatient is unable to carry out the daily routine of the hospital without taking part in any activities or without the assistance of others	
8. Retardation (slowness of thought and speech; impaired ability to concentrate)	0 = Absent 1 = Slight retardation at mental examination 2 = Obvious retardation at mental examination 3 = Difficulty during mental examination 4 = Completely unable to answer questions (stupor)	
9. Agitation	0 = Absent 1 = Distracted during examination 2 = Obviously distracted or more petty actions 3 = Can hardly sit still, standing up during exanimation 4 = Hand rubbing, nail biting, hair pulling, and lip biting	
10. Psychogenic anxiety	0 = Absent 1 = Tell when they are asked 2 = Spontaneous expression 3 = Obvious anxiety by expression and words 4 = Obviously scared	
11. Somatic anxiety (physical, including dry mouth, bloating, diarrhea, burps, abdominal cramps, palpitations, headaches, excessive breathing and sighing, as well as frequent urination and sweating)	0 = Absent 1 = Mild 2 = Moderate, with the certain symptoms 3 = Severe, the above symptoms are serious, affecting life and need to be treated 4 = Seriously affect life and activities	

Parameter	Scoring Criteria	Score
12. Gastrointestinal symptom	0 = Absent 1 = Loss of appetite but will eat without encouragement 2 = Take food at the urging or request of others and use laxatives or digestants	
13. Physical symptoms [general]	0 = Absent 1 = Heaviness in limbs, back or neck, back pain, headache, muscle pain, general fatigue or tiredness 2 = Obvious symptoms	
14. Genital symptoms (decreased libido, menstrual disorder, etc.)	0 = Absent 1 = Mild 2 = Severe 3 = Not sure, or not suitable for the respondent (not included in the total score)	
15. Hypochondriasis	0 = Absent 1 = Overly concern about body 2 = Mull over health issues 3 = Hypochondriac delusion 4 = Hypochondriac delusion accompanied by hallucinations	
16. Loss of weight	0 = Weight recorded; less than 0.5 kg in 1 week 1 = Weight records show a loss of more than 0.5 kg within 1 week 2 = Weight records show a loss of more than 1 kg in 1 week	
17. Insight	0 = Know that they are sick, showing depression 1 = Know that they are sick, but blaming poor food, environmental problems, overwork, virus infection, need for rest, etc. 2 = Completely deny illness	

Scoring criteria: If total score is more than 24, it may be severe depression. If the score is 18–24, it may be moderate depression. If the score is 8–17, it may be mild depression. If the score is less than 8, it is normal.

APPENDIX 18: HAMILTON ANXIETY SCALE (HAMA)

Parameter	Content	Select the Score That Best Suits the Patient's Condition					Score
Anxious mood	Worried, and feeling that the worst is about to happen, and is easily provoked	0	1	2	3	4	
Nervousness	Nervousness, fatigue, inability to relax, emotional reactions, crying easily, trembling, feeling uneasy	0	1	2	3	4	
Fear	Fear of the dark, strangers, solitude, animals, cars or traveling, and large crowds	0	1	2	3	4	
Insomnia	Difficulty falling asleep, waking up easily, not sleeping deeply, many dreams, nightmares, night terrors, and feeling tired after waking up	0	1	2	3	4	
Cognitive function	Also called memory and attention disorders. Poor concentration and memory	0	1	2	3	4	
Depressed mood	Loss of interest, lack of pleasure in past hobbies, depression, early awakening, these symptoms worsen at day and relieve at night	0	1	2	3	4	
Muscular system symptoms of somatic anxiety	Muscle soreness, immobility, muscle twitching, limb twitching, teeth chattering, voice shaking	0	1	2	3	4	
Physical anxiety sensory system symptoms	Blurred vision, chills, fever, weakness, tingling all over	0	1	2	3	4	
Cardiovascular symptoms	Tachycardia, palpitation, chest pain, pulsating blood vessels, fainting, cardiac leakage	0	1	2	3	4	
Respiratory symptoms	Chest tightness, feeling of suffocation, sighing, dyspnea	0	1	2	3	4	

Parameter	Content	Select the Score That Best Suits the Patient's Condition					Score
Gastrointestinal symptoms	Dysphagia, belching, dyspepsia (abdominal pain after eating, burning pain in the stomach, bloating, nausea, a feeling of fullness in the stomach), bowel movements, bowel noise, diarrhea, weight loss, constipation	0	1	2	3	4	
Genitourinary symptoms	Frequent urination, urgent urination, menopause, sexual apathy, premature ejaculation, premature ejaculation, impotence	0	1	2	3	4	
Autonomic nervous system symptoms	Dry mouth, flush, pale, easy to sweat, easy to get "goose bumps", tension headache, hair standing up	0	1	2	3	4	
Behavior during the interview	General symptoms: Nervousness, inability to relax, butterflies in one's stomach, finger biting, clenching fists, touching handkerchief, facial muscles twitching, stomping, shaking hands, frowning, stiff expression, high muscle tension, sighing breathing, pallor Physiological symptoms: Swallowing, burping, fast heart rate, fast breathing when quiet (more than 20 times/min), tendon hyperreflexia, tremor, dilated pupils, pulsating eyelids, easy to sweat, protruding eyes.	0	1	2	3	4	
Total Score							

0: normal, 1: mild, 2: moderate, 3: moderately severe, 4: severe.

Scoring criteria: If total score is over 29, it may be severe anxiety. If the score is more than 21, it means you have obvious anxiety. If the score is over 14, it means you have anxiety. If the score is over 7, you may have anxiety. If the score is less than 7, it is normal.

APPENDIX 19: GENERALIZED ANXIETY SCALE (GAD-7)

In the past 2 weeks, how much of the time have you felt the following:					
S/N	Parameter	Completely No (0)	A few Days (1)	More Than Half the Time (2)	Almost Every Day (3)
1	Feel nervous or anxious				
2	Cannot stop or control worrying				
3	Worry too much about all kinds of things				
4	Hard to relax				
5	Unable to sit still because of uneasiness				
6	Become easily annoyed or irritable				
7	Feel afraid, as if something terrible is going to happen				
Total Score					

Scoring criteria: There is 0–3 score for each parameter. The total score is the sum of the seven parameters. The total score ranges from 0–21.

- 0–4   =   no GAD
- 5–9   =   mild GAD
- 10–14 =   moderate GAD
- 15–21 =   severe GAD

APPENDIX 20: SOCIAL READJUSTMENT RATING SCALE (ADULTS)

S/N	Life Events	Life Change Unit
1	Death of spouse	100
2	Divorce	73
3	Separation	65
4	Been in prison	63
5	A close family member died	63
6	Have been hurt or sick	53
7	Got married	50
8	Got fired	47
9	Rekindled your relationship with your spouse	45
10	Retired	45
11	Changes in the health status of family members	44
12	Pregnancy	40
13	Sexual dysfunction	39
14	Added a new member to the family	39
15	Job readjustment	39
16	Change in income and expenditure	38
17	Death of a close friend	37
18	Change of your profession	36
19	Changes in the number of arguments with your spouse	35
20	Massive debt	32
21	Foreclosure or loan of valuable property that cannot be recovered	30
22	Job responsibilities changed	29
23	Children leaving home	29
24	Disputes between in-laws	29
25	Outstanding personal achievements	28
26	Spouses started or stopped working	26
27	Beginning or ending education	26
28	Changes in living conditions	25
29	Change of personal habits	24
30	Not getting along with your boss	23

S/N	Life Events	Life Change Unit
31	A change in working hours or conditions	20
32	Moved house	20
33	Changed school	20
34	Changes in entertainment	19
35	Changes in church activities	19
36	Changes in social activities	18
37	Took out small mortgages or loans	17
38	Changes in sleep habits	16
39	Changes in the number of family reunions	15
40	Changes in eating habits	15
41	Went on holiday	13
42	Christmas	12
43	Committed minor offense	11

Scoring criteria:

- 0–149 score   = No major problems
- 150–199 score   = Minor health risk (33% chance of getting sick)
- 200–299 score   = Moderate health risk (50% chance of disease)
- Above 300 score = Serious health risk (80% chance of disease)

APPENDIX 21: SOCIAL READJUSTMENT RATING SCALE (JUVENILE)

S/N	Life Events	Life Change Unit
1	Father or mother dies	100
2	Unwanted pregnancy or miscarriage	100
3	Got married	95
4	Parents divorced	90
5	Produce visible deformities	80
6	Being a father or mother to your children	70
7	Your father or mother was jailed for more than a year	70
8	Parents separated	69
9	Brothers and sisters died	68
10	Changes in acceptance by peers	67

S/N	Life Events	Life Change Unit
11	Your sister is pregnant unplanned	64
12	Found out you were adopted	63
13	Your father or mother remarried	63
14	Death of a close friend	63
15	You have a visible congenital malformation	62
16	You have had serious illnesses requiring hospitalization	58
17	Failed in school	56
18	Did not participate in extracurricular activities	55
19	Either father or mother was hospitalized	55
20	Your father or mother was jailed for more than 30 days	53
21	Broke up with your boyfriend (girlfriend)	53
22	Fell in love	51
23	Dropped out of school	50
24	Started using drugs or alcohol	50
25	A younger brother or sister was born	50
26	The number of arguments with parents increased	47
27	Your father or mother lost their job	46
28	Outstanding personal achievements	46
29	Changes in parents' balance of payments	45
30	Went to college	43
31	Went to high school	42
32	A sibling was hospitalized	41
33	Increased time spent away from home	38
34	Brothers and sisters left the family	37
35	Families have grown with adults other than parents	34
36	Become a full member of the church	31
37	Fewer arguments between parents	27
38	Fewer arguments with parents	26
39	Mother or father started to work	26

Scoring criteria:

- 0–149 score = No major problems
- 150–199 score = Minor health risk (33% chance of getting sick)
- 200–299 score = Moderate health risk (50% chance of disease)
- Above 300 score = Serious health risk (80% chance of disease)

APPENDIX 22: MENTAL HEALTH SELF-ASSESSMENT QUESTIONNAIRE (SRQ)

1. All 20 parameters are scored as 0 or 1.
2. 1 indicates the presence of symptoms in the past month.
3. 0 indicates the absence of symptoms.
4. The highest total score is 20, and the threshold value is 7 or 8.
5. A positive result indicates that the subject has emotional pain and needs mental health help.

Contents	Yes	No
1. Do you often have headaches?	1	0
2. Do you have a poor appetite?	1	0
3. Do you have poor sleep?	1	0
4. Are you easily frightened?	1	0
5. Are your hands shaking?	1	0
6. Are you feeling nervous or worried?	1	0
7. Do you have indigestion?	1	0
8. Are you not thinking clearly?	1	0
9. Are you not feeling well?	1	0
10. Do you cry more than before?	1	0
11. Do you find it difficult to derive pleasure from your daily activities?	1	0
12. Do you find it difficult to make decisions?	1	0
13. Do you suffer from routine work?	1	0
14. Are you unable to play a role in your life?	1	0
15. Have you lost interest in things?	1	0
16. Do you feel like a worthless person?	1	0
17. Have you ever thought of ending your life?	1	0
18. Do you get tired at any time?	1	0
19. Do you feel sick to your stomach?	1	0
20. Do you get tired easily?	1	0

APPENDIX 23: PITTSBURGH SLEEP QUALITY INDEX (PSQI)

The following questions are about your sleep situation in the last month. Please choose the answer that best fits your actual situation in the last month. Please answer the following questions:

1. For nearly a month, I usually go to bed at night at (_____) o 'clock.		
2. In the last month, it usually takes (_____) minutes from going to bed to falling asleep.		
3. For nearly a month, I usually get up at (_____) am.		
4. I usually sleep (_____) hours per night for nearly 1 month (not equal to bedtime).		
5. In the last 1 month, I have had trouble sleeping due to the following conditions	a. Difficulty falling asleep (inability to fall asleep within 30 minutes) (1) No (2) < 1 time per week (3) 1–2 times per week (4) ≥ 3 times per week	
	b. Easily wake up in the middle of the night or too early (1) No (2) < 1 time per week (3) 1–2 times per week (4) ≥ 3 times per week	
	c. Go to the bathroom at night (1) No (2) < 1 time per week (3) 1–2 times per week (4) ≥ 3 times per week	
	d. Disturbance in respiration (1) No (2) < 1 time per week (3) 1–2 times per week (4) ≥ 3 times per week	
	e. Cough or snore loudly (1) No (2) < 1 time per week (3) 1–2 times per week (4) ≥ 3 times per week	
	f. Feel cold (1) No (2) < 1 time per week (3) 1–2 times per week (4) ≥ 3 times per week	
	g. Feel hot (1) No (2) < 1 time per week (3) 1–2 times per week (4) ≥ 3 times per week	
	h. Nightmares (1) No (2) < 1 time per week (3) 1–2 times per week (4) ≥ 3 times per week	
	i. Pain and discomfort (1) No (2) < 1 time per week (3) 1–2 times per week (4) ≥ 3 times per week	

j. Other things that interfere with sleep (1) No (2) < 1 time per week (3) 1–2 times per week (4) ≥ 3 times per week	
If yes, please explain:	
6. In the last month, in general, what do you think of your sleep quality? (1) Very good (2) Good (3) Bad (4) Very Bad	
7. How often do you use sleeping pills in the past month? (1) No (2) < Once/week (3) 1–2 times/ week (4) ≥ 3 times/week	
8. How often have you felt sleepy in the past month? (1) No (2) < 1 time/week (3) 1–2 times/ week (4) ≥ 3 times/week	
9. Have you been lacking energy in the past month? (1) No (2) Occasionally (3) Sometimes (4) Often	

- Sleep quality score ( )
- Sleep time score ( )
- Sleep time score ( )
- Sleep efficiency score ( )
- Sleep disorder score ( )
- Hypnotic drug score ( )
- Daytime dysfunction score ( )
- Total PSQI score ( )

Tested by:

Note: PSQI is used to evaluate the sleep quality of the subjects in the last 1 month. It is composed of 19 evaluation parameters and five other evaluation parameters, among which the first evaluation parameter and five other evaluation parameters do not participate in the scoring. Only 18 evaluation parameters that participate in the scoring are introduced here (see the attached questionnaire for details). The 18 parameters comprise seven components, and each component is scored on a scale of 0 to 3. The cumulative score of each component is the total score of PSQI, which ranges from 0–21. The higher the score, the worse the sleep quality. It took 5–10 minutes for the subjects to complete the test. The meaning and scoring method of each component are as follows:

A. Sleep quality: 1 score for good, 2 score for poor, and 3 score for very poor according to the response to Parameter 6.

B. Bedtime

B.1. The score for Parameter 2: A score of 0 is assigned for ≤ 15, a score of 1 is assigned for 16–30, a score of 2 is assigned for 31–60, and a score of 3 is assigned for ≥ 60.

B.2. The score for Parameter 5a: if it is absent, a score of 0 is assigned, a score of 1 is assigned for < 1 week/time, and a score of 2 is assigned for 1–2 weeks/time, and a score of 3 is assigned for ≥ 3 weeks/time.

B.3. Score for Parameters 2 and 5a are accumulated, if the accumulated score is 0, 0 score is assigned; if it is 1–2, a score of 1 is assigned; if it is 3–4, a score of 2 is assigned; if it is 5–6, a score of 3 is assigned.

C. Sleep time: Score according to the response to Parameter 4. A score of 0 is assigned for > 7 hours; a score of 1 is assigned for 6–7 hours; a score of 2 is assigned for 5–6 hours; and a score of 3 is assigned for < 5 hours.

D. Sleep efficiency

D.1. Bedtime = Parameter 3 (wake-up time) — Parameter 1 (bedtime).

D.2. Sleep efficiency = Parameter 4 (sleep time)/time in bed ×100%.

D.3. Component D scoring position: A score of 0 is assigned if sleep efficiency > 85%; a score of 1 is assigned if 75%–84%; a score of 2 is assigned if 65%–74%; a score of 3 is assigned if <65%.

E. Sleep disorders: Score according to Parameters 5b to 5j. A score of 0 is assigned if it is absent; a score of 1 is assigned if it is < 1 week/time; a score of 2 is assigned if it is 1–2 weeks/time; a score of 3 is assigned if it is ≥ 3 weeks/time. Score for Parameters 5b to 5j are accumulated; if the accumulated score is 0, a score of 0 is assigned for Component E; if it is 1–9, a score of 1 is assigned; if it is 10–18, a score of 2 is assigned; if it is 19–27, a score of 3 is assigned.

F. Hypnotic drugs: Score according to the response to Parameter 7. A score of 0 is assigned if it is absent; a score of 1 is assigned if it is < 1 week/time; a score of 2 is assigned if it is 1–2 weeks/time; a score of 3 is assigned if it is ≥ 3 weeks/time.

G. Daytime dysfunction

G1. Score according to the response to Parameter 7. A score of 0 is assigned if it is absent; a score of 1 is assigned if it is < 1 week/time; a score of 2 is assigned if it is 1–2 weeks/time; a score of 3 is assigned if it is ≥ 3 weeks/time.

G2. Score according to the response to Parameter 7. A score of 0 is assigned if it is absent; a score of 1 is assigned if it is occasionally; a score of 2 is assigned if it is sometimes; a score of 3 is assigned if it is frequently.

G3. Score for Parameters 8 and 9 are accumulated; if the accumulated score is 0, a score of 0 is assigned for Component G; if it is 1–2, a score of 1 is assigned; if it is 3–4, a score of 2 is assigned; if it is 5–6, a score of 3 is assigned.

Total Score of PSQI = Component A + Component B + Component C + Component D + Component E + Component F + Component G

Scoring criteria:

- 0–5 score   = Very good sleep quality
- 6–10 score   = Good sleep quality
- 11–15 score = Moderate sleep quality
- 16–21 score = Poor sleep quality

APPENDIX 24: LIST OF RELEVANT ACUPUNCTURE POINTS

Head and Face

Temple	It is located on the head, between the tip of the eyebrow and the outer canthus, in a depression about one finger back.
Dazhui	First sit up and lower head (both vertebras can separate when lowering head, and protruding spinous process can be touched), the depression below the highest point of the neck (the seventh cervical vertebra) is dazhui, which is between the two vertebrae, the upper one is the cervical vertebra and the lower one is the thoracic vertebra. If the protruding bones are not too obvious, allow the patient to move the neck, and the immobile bone is the first thoracic vertebra, which is about level with shoulder.
Fengfu	It is located in the posterior cervical region, the exoccipital bulge is convex and straight down, and in the concavity of the quality control of the oblique muscles on both sides.
Fengchi	It is located in the posterior region of the neck, below the occipital bone, in the depression between the upper end of the sternocleidomastoid muscle and the upper end of the trapezius muscle.

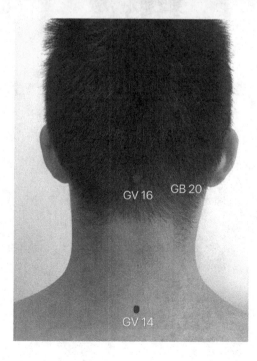

Back

Dingchuan	It is located on the back of the forehead, 0.5 cun from the midpoint of the inferior border of the seventh cervical spine.
Fengmen	It is located in the spinal region, below the second thoracic spine and 1.5 cun away from the median line.
Feishu	It is located on the back, inferior of the third thoracic spine, 1.5 cun away from the median line.
Pishu	It is located on the back, below the eleventh thoracic spine, about 1.5 cun wide beside the middle of the spine (governor channel). The acupuncture point is taken in the prone position.
Shenshu	It is located in the lumbar region, below the second lumbar spinous process away from the median line. In the sitting or standing position, have the patient cross his/her hands and find the highest point of the iliac bone on both sides of the body; the intersection of the two points and the lumbar vertebrae is the fourth lumbar spine, counting upward two, is the second lumbar spine, 1.5 cun from the lower side.

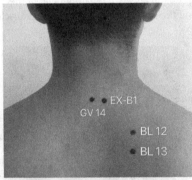

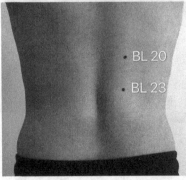

Abdomen

Qihai	At supine position, guanyuan is at four transverse fingers below umbilicus, and qihai is at midpoint of the connecting line between guanyuan and umbilicus. There is an obvious feeling of acid distension when it is pressed.
Guanyuan	It is located at the lower abdomen, above anterior median line, 3 cun from middle-lower umbilicus.

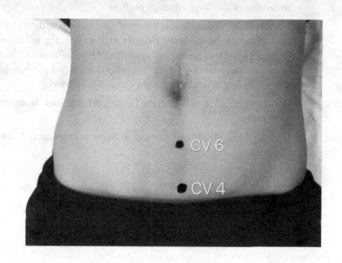

Upper Limbs

Quchi	It is located at the tip of transverse striation of elbow when bending the elbow; there is a feeling of acid distension when it is pressed.
Chize	It is located in the transverse ridge of the elbow and the depression of the radial side of the biceps tendon.
Taiyuan	It is located in the anterior region of the wrist, between the radial styloid process and the scaphoid bone, in the ulnar depression of the tendon of the long extensor pollicis.
Hegu	Open one hand naturally and hold out your thumb with the other hand. Place the horizontal stripe of the thumb on the junction of the thumb and index finger of the opened hand. Press the thumb down, and the point below the fingertip is hegu point. There is an obvious feeling of acid distension when it is pressed.
Shaoshang	It is located at radial side of distal thumb, 0.1 cun away from the root of the nail.
Shangyang	It is located radial side of distal index finger, 0.1 cun away from the root of nail.

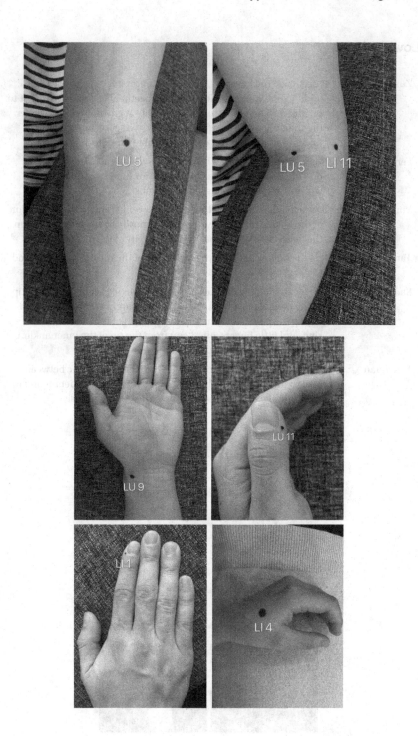

Lower Limbs

Zusanli	It is outside the lower leg, 3 cun from outer knee eyes (index, middle, ring, and little fingers close together, it should be subject to proximal transverse striation of median segment of middle finger, the transverse distance for four fingers is 3 cun), one transverse finger from the anterior edge of the tibia (middle finger)
Fenglong	It is on the anterolateral leg, 8 cun above lateral malleolus tip, outside tiaokou, distance from anterior margin of tibia is the width of transverse lines of two thumbs.
Yinlingquan	It is located in the medial side of the lower leg and in the depression of the medial tibia below the knee, opposite to zusanli point (or in the depression of the posterior lower part of the medial tibia).
Taixi	It is the hollow between the inner side of the medial malleolus and the heel tendon.
Sanyinjiao	It is located on the medial side of the lower leg, 3 cun above the tip of the medial malleolus, the posterior margin of the tibia. When taking the point, with the transverse lines of the index, middle, ring, and little fingers, it is 3 cun from the tip of the inner ankle, on the posterior border of the tibia.
Yongquan	Yongquan acupoint is located at the upper third of line between heel to the junction of the second and third toes, or depression in the front of planta pedis when bending toes vigorously.

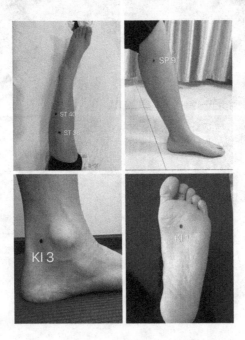

Auricular

Lung	It is located around the auricular center.
Chest	It is located in the middle two-fifths of the anterior part of anthelix.
Trachea	It is located in the cavity of auricular concha, between the heart area and the external auricle gate.
Kidney	It is located lower bifurcation of upper and lower crus of helix.
Sympathetic	It is located at the junction between the lower crus of helix and inner side of helix.
Shenmen	It is located at the upper third part behind the triangle fossa.
Spleen	It is located at the posterior upper part of the cavity of auricular concha, i.e., Area 13 of auricular concha.
Stomach	It is located at the area there is no crus of helix, i.e., Area 4 of auricular concha.
Endocrine	It is located in the interscreen notch, the anterior lower part of the cavity of auricular concha, i.e., Area 18 of auricular concha.

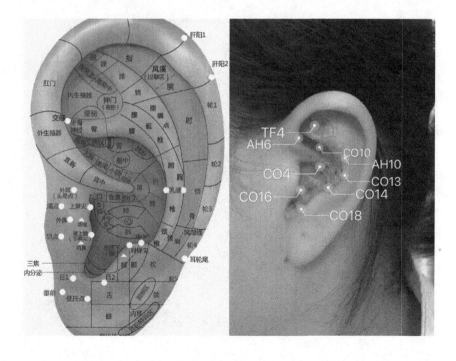

Index

Abdomen, acupuncture points in, 331
Abdominal breathing exercises, 69
Abdominal breath training, 179–180
Abnormal blood gas, 38
ACBTs, *see* Active cycle of breathing
techniques
Acceptability, principle of, 138
ACE2, *see* Angiotensin-converting
enzyme 2
ACT, *see* Airway clearance technique
Active cycle of breathing techniques
(ACBTs), 65–66
precautions for, 74
Activities of daily living (ADL)
assessment, 59
dysfunction, 48
intervention, 296
training, 86
BADL training (*see* Basic
activities of daily living
training)
instrumental activities of daily
living (IADL), 89
Acupoint application therapy, 119
operation method
composition and production of
drugs, 121–122
operation steps, 122
selection of acupoints, 121
treatment mechanism
immune mechanism, effects of,
120–121
inflammatory mechanisms, effects
of, 121
long-term acupoint
stimulation, 120
medicine acts on pathogen, 119
regulate the body as a whole, 120

Acupoint (meridian) massage
therapy, 115
contraindications, 118–119
location of acupoints, 117
operation method, 118
operation precautions, 118
principles of treatment, 116
selection of points, 116
main points, 116
match acupoints with symptoms,
116–117
treatment mechanism, 116
Acupuncture points
in abdomen, 331
in auricular, 335
in back, 330
in head and face, 329
in lower limb, 334
in upper limb, 332–333
Acupuncture therapy, 107
choice of acupoints
clinical treatment period, 110
convalescent period, 111
medical observation period, 110
contraindication to acupuncture, 112
location of points, 111–112
mechanism of treatment
dredging the meridian, 110
harmonizing yin and yang,
108–109
nourishing good and dispel
evil, 109
operation method, 112
principles of treatment, 108
Acute respiratory distress syndrome
(ARDS), 23, 61
posture management for patients
with, 64

and respiratory failure, 40–41
Adjustment disorder, 46
ADL, *see* Activities of daily living
Aerobic exercise, 75–77, 288–289
Aerosol transmission, 3
Air disinfection, 172–173
Airway clearance technique (ACT), 38, 61,
    64, 286–287
    active cycle of breathing techniques
        (ACBTs), 65–66
    chest physical therapy techniques,
        67–68
    effective cough, 65
    high-frequency chest wall oscillation
        (HFCWO), 67
    oscillating positive expiratory
        pressure (OPEP), 67
    postural drainage techniques, 67
AIS, *see* Athens insomnia scale
AMC, *see* Arm muscle circle
Anger therapy, 136
Angiotensin-converting enzyme 2
    (ACE2), 1, 4
Anthropometry
    arm muscle circle (AMC), 245
    body composition measurement
        method, 245–246
    triceps skinfold thickness (TSF), 245
    weight and BMI, 244–245
Anti-breathing training, 287–288
Ape exercise, 274–275
ARDS, *see* Acute respiratory distress
    syndrome
Arm muscle circle (AMC), 245
Athens insomnia scale (AIS), 59
Auricular acupoint pressing therapy,
    122, 335
    auricular point positioning, 123–124
    auricular point selection, 123
    contraindications, 124
    operation method, 124
    treatment mechanism, 122–123
Auxiliary examination, of COVID-19
    chest imaging, 20
    laboratory examination
        etiological, 19–20
        routine examination, 19
        serological examination, 20

Back, acupuncture points in, 330
Back-scratching experiment, 307
Back-scratch test, 57
BADL training, *see* Basic activities of
    daily living training
Baduanjin, 132, 265–269
Balance, assessment of, 57
    functional reach test, 57
    one-leg standing balance test, 57
    timed up and go test (TUG), 57
Balance training, 83, 294
    for patients who can barely get up, 84
    for patients who can stand on a flat
        surface for a certain time, 84
    for patients who can't stand, 84
Barthel Index, 260
    evaluation scale, 310–311
Basic activities of daily living (BADL)
    training, 86
    bathing, 88
    brushing teeth, 88
    dressing, 87–88
    eating, 88–89
    putting on shoes, 88
    sitting up, 87
    standing up, 87
    turning over, 86
    walking, 87
    washing face, 88
Bat SARS-like coronavirus (bat-SL-
    CoVZC45), 1
BC technique, *see* Breathing control
    technique
Bear exercise, 271
Behavior therapy, 94, 229–230
    aversion therapy, 94–95
    behavior-shaping method, 95
    relaxation response training, 95
    systematic desensitization, 94
    token economy, 95
Bereavement and mourning reaction, 47
Biofeedback therapy, 232
Bloodletting therapy, 129
    contraindications, 131
    location of acupoints, 131
    operation method, 131
    selection of acupoints, 131
    treatment mechanism, 130–131

Blood purification treatment, 25
Blood vessels, 7
Body composition measurement method,
    245–246
Body-weight assessment of
    cardiopulmonary function, 56
Bone marrow, 6–7
Borg Dyspnea Assessment Scale, 301
Brain imaging technology, 222
Breathing, difficulty in, 85
Breathing control (BC) technique, 62, 65
Breathing exercises, 72–73
Breathing training, 68
    local dilation breathing training, 71
    relaxation training, 71
    respiratory pattern training, 69
        abdominal breathing exercises, 69
        breathing rhythm adjusting
            training, 70
        pursed-lip breathing training, 69
    rhythm adjusting training, 70
Bronchiectasis, 38

Cardiopulmonary exercise test
    (CPET), 56
Cardiopulmonary function, safe
    and effective improvement
    of, 195
Catheter-related bloodstream infection,
    prevention of, 28
Chair-stretching forward test, 306
Chest CT examination
    advantages and characteristics,
        11–12
    stages of chest CT manifestations,
        12–13
Chest imaging, 20
Chest X-ray, 11
CHI, see Creatinine–height index
Chlorine-containing disinfectant,
    precautions for using, 175
Chrysanthemum bat, 1
Circulation support, 24
Clinical classification, of COVID-19, 17
    critically severe, 18
    mild, 17
    moderate, 17
    severe cases, 17–18

Clinical manifestations, of COVID-19, 7
    clinical outcome, 9
    epidemiological characteristic, 8
    respiratory system signs, 8
    symptoms, 8
Clinical outcomes, of COVID-19, 9
Clinical rehabilitation of COVID-
        19; see also Treatment, of
        COVID-19
    connotation of rehabilitation
        intervention
    activity/physical strength,
        enhancement of, 196
    cardiopulmonary function,
        enhancement of, 196
    health education, 196–197
    psychological treatment, 197
    for discharged patients, 209
        mild/moderate discharged
            patients, 210–211
        severe/critically severe disease,
            patients with, 211–214
    guiding principles of rehabilitation
        cardiopulmonary function,
            improvement of, 195
        physical fitness, improvement
            of, 196
        whole-course psychological
            intervention, 195
    home rehabilitation procedures, 202
    hospitalized patients, 203
        mild patients, 203–205
        moderate patients, 205–207
        severe/critically severe patients,
            207–209
    in-hospital rehabilitation
        procedures, 200
    outpatient rehabilitation
        procedures, 201
    process management, 197
        diagnosis and treatment
            procedures, 199
        job description, 198–199
        overall objective, 198
        precautions, 199
        prerequisites for intervention,
            199–201
        safety precautions, 198

suspension and withdrawal of
rehabilitation treatment,
202–203
working principle, 197–198
relevant policies and basis in
rehabilitation diagnosis and
treatment, 197
Clinical treatment, of COVID-19, 21, 26
discharge criteria, 30
general treatment, 22–23
management measures, 31
precautions after being discharged
from hospitals, 30
and prevention
of catheter-related bloodstream
infection, 28
of deep vein thrombosis, 28
of ICU-related complications, 29
of stress ulcers, 28
of ventilator-associated
pneumonia, 28
re-positive nucleic acid conversion,
analysis of, 30
re-positive nucleic acid tests
infectivity of patients with, 31
treatment measures for patients
with, 31
of severe and critically severe cases
blood purification treatment, 25
circulation support, 24
immunotherapy, 26
principles of treatment, 23
psychotherapy, 27
recovered patients' plasma
therapy, 25
rehabilitation treatment, 26
renal failure and renal
replacement therapy, 24
respiratory support, 23–24
Traditional Chinese Medicine
treatment, 29
clinical treatment, 29
medication observation, 29
treatment place determination
according to patients'
condition, 21
Close contact transmission, 3

Cognition therapy, 228–229
Cognitive problems, 27
Cognitive therapy, 92
main strategies of, 92–93
methods for, 93–94
Community-based rehabilitation, 259
dysfunction of daily living ability and
social participation, 260
goals of rehabilitation, 261
implementation of rehabilitation
treatment, 262
physical dysfunction, 260
process of rehabilitation, 261
psychological dysfunction, 261
rehabilitation evaluation, 262
respiratory dysfunction, 260
treatment, 262
auxiliary appliances,
configuration and use of,
263–264
guidance of rehabilitation
training, 263
psychological intervention, 263
Confidentiality, principle of, 139
Continuous Renal Replacement Therapy
(CRRT), 24
Contracted lip breathing, 287
Contraindications, 297
Controlled deep breathing, 287
Convalescent period, 29
Core strength training, 81
Coronaviruses, 1
Cough, effective, 65
nursing guidance and training
techniques for, 182
definition, 182
key points of operation, 182
precautions, 182–183
purpose, 182
COVID-19 rehabilitation unit (CRU), 145
common complications of COVID-19
and their management
disuse muscle weakness and
muscle atrophy, 166–167
disuse osteoporosis, 167–168
joint contracture, 167
malnutrition, 166–167

pressure ulcers (see Pressure
    ulcers)
urinary tract infection, 165–166
vein thromboembolism (VTE),
    161–164
concept of, 145–146
diagnosis and treatment plan
    assessing COVID-19 patients in
        detail, 158
    contents of rehabilitation
        nursing, 158–159
    extended rehabilitation
        therapy, 161
    holding a CRU teamwork group
        meeting, 158
    preventing complications, 160
    rehabilitation therapy, 160
    TCM rehabilitation therapy, 160
    treatment measures, 159
discharge follow-up, 153
discharge plan, 153
dysfunction
    barriers to social participation, 155
    physical dysfunction, 154–155
    psychological dysfunction, 155
    respiratory dysfunction, 154
health education, 152
isolation wards, equipment
        conditions for
    medical personnel, protection of,
        149–150
    prerequisite, 149
    requirements, 149
    site, 149
    strengthening patient
        management, 150
organization and operation of CRU
        ward, 152
principal member of, 150
rehabilitation and treatment areas,
        setting of, 150
    environmental requirements, 150
    training equipment and
        apparatus, 150
responsibilities of, 150–151
role of, 147
significance of, 147

clinical research, conducive to, 148
effective clinical results,
    producing, 147
improving the satisfaction of
    patients and their families,
    147–148
types of
    convalescent period, 148–149
    early period, 148
    ultra-early period, 148
work content of, 151–152
workflow, 156–157
work principles, 156
work requirements, 156
CPET, see Cardiopulmonary exercise test
Crane exercise, 271–272
Creatinine–height index (CHI), 246–247
Critically severe cases
    clinical criteria, 18
    traditional Chinese medicine
        treatment, 29
CRU, see COVID-19 rehabilitation unit
CRRT, see Continuous Renal
        Replacement Therapy
Cupping therapy, 124
    contraindications, 127
    location, 126
    location selection, 126
    operation methods
        bloodletting puncture and
            cupping, 126
        moving cupping, 126
        retaining cupping, 126
    treatment mechanism
        thermothermal effect,
            mechanism of, 126
        traditional Chinese medicine
            (TCM), mechanism of, 125
        Western medicine, mechanisms of,
            125–126
Cytokines, 4, 5
Cytokine storm, 25

Deep vein thrombosis, prevention of, 28
Deep venous thrombosis (DVT), 163–164
Deer exercise, 272–273
Depression in patients with PTSD, 45

Diagnostic criteria, of COVID-19, 15
    auxiliary examination
        chest imaging, 20
        etiological, 19–20
        routine examination, 19
        serological examination, 20
    clinical classification, 17
        critically severe, 18
        mild, 17
        moderate, 17
        severe cases, 17–18
    confirmed cases, 16–17
    differential diagnosis
        non-infectious disease, 20
        upper respiratory disease, 20
        viral and mycoplasma
            pneumonia, 20
    exclusion criteria, 21
    reporting system, 20–21
    suspected cases, 15
        clinical manifestations, 16
        epidemiological history, 15
    warning signals, 18
        adults, 19
        children, 19
Diet adjustment, 296–297
Dietary guidance
    for frontline workers, 254–255
    for ordinary/convalescent
        patients, 253
    for prevention and control among
        general population, 255
    severe syndrome, nutritional
        treatment for patients with,
        253–254
    TCM diet guidance, 256
        first prescription, 256
        second prescription, 256
        third prescription, 256
Differential diagnosis, of COVID-19
    non-infectious disease, 20
    upper respiratory disease, 20
    viral and mycoplasma pneumonia, 20
Discharged patients, rehabilitation
        treatment of COVID-19 patients
        for, 209
    mild/moderate patients

methods, 210–211
    objectives, 210
    severe/critically severe disease,
        patients with
        criteria exclusion and motion
            termination, 211–212
        methods, 212–214
        objectives, 211
Discharge guidance and health
        education
    breathing training and activities,
        adherence to, 192
    diet, attention on, 191
    disease prevention, 192
Disinfection
    air, 172–173
    of articles and ground, 173
    medical fabric washing and, 174
    of reusable instruments and
        articles, 174
    ultraviolet air disinfection,
        precautions for, 174–175
Disuse muscle weakness and muscle
        atrophy, 166–167
Disuse osteoporosis, 167–168
Doubt analysis, therapy of, 191
DVT, see Deep venous thrombosis
Dysfunction, 35
    of daily living ability and social
        participation, 260
    physical dysfunction, 41, 260
        decreased exercise ability and
            tolerance, 42–44
        tachycardias, 41–42
    psychological and social dysfunction
        (see Psychological and social
            dysfunction)
    respiratory dysfunction, 35, 260
        acute respiratory distress
            syndrome (ARDS), 40–41
        dyspnea, 35–38
        hypoxemia, 38–40
Dyspnea, 35, 37
    definition of, 35–36
    mechanism causing, 36
    pathophysiology of, 36–38
Dyspnea scale, 55–56

ECMO, *see* Extracorporeal membrane
        oxygenation
Education and cooperation of
        patients, 181
Emotional problems, 27
Emotion nursing, 190
    calming the mind, therapy of, 191
    doubt analysis, therapy of, 191
    therapy
        of emotion being diverted, 191
        of emotion interresistance, 191
        of emotions and depression
            relieving, 191
Emotions and feelings, assessment of, 222
Emotion therapy of TCM, *see* Traditional
        Chinese medicine, emotion
        therapy of
Energy-saving techniques, 63
Epidemiology, of COVID-19, 8
    mortality rate, 4
    route of transmission, 2–3
        aerosol transmission, 3
        close contact transmission, 3
        fecal–oral transmission, 3
        mother-to-child transmission, 3
        respiratory droplet transmission, 2
    source of infection, 2
    susceptible groups, 3
Etiological and serological examination,
        19–20
Etiology, of COVID-19, 1–2
Evaluation, rehabilitation, 262
Exclusion criteria, of COVID-19, 21
Exercise ability and tolerance, 42
    fatigue, 43
    immobilization syndrome, 43–44
Exercise training, 233
Extracorporeal membrane oxygenation
        (ECMO), 23–24, 40, 250

Face, acupuncture points in, 329
Family psychotherapy, 232
Fatigue, 43, 85
Fecal–oral transmission, 3
FET, *see* Forced expiration technique
Fish oil components, 251–252
Five-animal exercise, 133, 271

ape exercise, 274–275
bear exercise, 271
crane exercise, 271–272
deer exercise, 272–273
tiger exercise, 273–274
Flexibility, assessment of
    back-scratch test, 57
    improved twist test, 57
    sit-and-reach test, 57
Flexibility training, 84, 294
Focus solution mode, 227–228
Forced expiration technique (FET), 66
Forced vital capacity (FVC), 53
Frontline workers, nutritional dietary
        guidance for, 254–255
Functional forward extension test, 311
Functional reach test, 57
FVC, *see* Forced vital capacity

GAD-7, *see* Generalized Anxiety Scale
Gallbladder, 7
Generalized Anxiety Scale (GAD-7), 320
GGO, *see* Ground-glass opacity
GM-CSF, *see* Granulocyte-macrophage
        colony-stimulating factor
Goals of rehabilitation, 261
Granulocyte-macrophage colony-
        stimulating factor (GM-CSF), 4
Grief reaction, 47
Ground-glass opacity (GGO), 11, 20, 37
Group psychotherapy, 231–232

Half-closed lip respiration training, 179
HAMA, *see* Hamilton Anxiety Scale
HAMD17, *see* Hamilton Depression Scale
Hamilton Anxiety Scale (HAMA), 318–319
Hamilton Depression Scale (HAMD17),
        315–317
Head and face, acupuncture points
        in, 329
Health education, 234
Health-Related Quality of Life (HRQL)
        Scale, 59
Heart and blood vessels, 7
Heart rate and oxygen uptake, 42
High-frequency chest wall oscillation
        (HFCWO), 67

precautions for, 74
Hilar lymph nodes, 6–7
Home-based rehabilitation, 264
    ADL intervention, 296
    diet adjustment, 296–297
    oxygen therapy, 294–296
    physical function rehabilitation
        exercise
        aerobic exercise, 288–289
        balance training, 294
        flexibility training, 294
        strength training, 289–294
    psychological reconstruction, 296
    respiratory function, rehabilitation
        exercise of, 286
        airway clearance technology,
            286–287
        position management, 286
        respiratory muscle training, 287–288
    traditional methods, 265
        Baduanjin, 265–269
        five-animal exercise (see Five-
            animal exercise)
        simplified tai chi chuan, 269–271
        Yi Jin Jing (see Yi Jin Jing)
Hospitalized patients with
        COVID-19, 203
    mild patients, 203–205
    moderate patients, 205–207
    severe/critically severe patients,
        207–209
HRQL scale, see Health-Related Quality
        of Life Scale
Hypoventilation, 38–39
Hypoxemia, 5–6, 38
    dead space, increase of, 39
    diffusion impairment, 39
    hypoventilation, 38–39
    local ventilation/blood flow
        disorder, 39
    oxygen-carrying capacity, 39–40
Hypoxia, 5, 6

IADL, see Instrumental activities of daily
        living
ICU-related complications, prevention
        of, 29

IgG antibody, 10, 11
IgM antibody, 10, 11
Immobilization syndrome, 43–44
Immune function indicators, 247
Immunotherapy, 26
Implementation of rehabilitation
        treatment, 262
Improved twist test, 57
Infection, source of, 2
Inflammatory cytokines, 5
Instrumental activities of daily living
        (IADL), 89
Interpersonal problems, 27
Interview, 220
Isolation ward, rehabilitation
    disinfection and isolation
        management in the ward, 172
        air disinfection, 172–173
        chlorine-containing disinfectant,
            precautions for using, 175
        disinfection of articles and
            ground, 173
        disinfection of reusable
            instruments and articles, 174
        medical fabric washing and
            disinfection, 174
        medical waste, treatment of, 174
        ultraviolet air disinfection,
            precautions for, 174–175
    nursing personnel, management
        of, 172
    nursing staff, establishment of, 172
    protection management of medical
        staff, 175
        hand hygiene, 177
        protection classification and
            requirements, 176–177
        rational and scientific layout, 171

Joint contracture, 167
Joy therapy, 137

Kidney, 7

Laboratory examination
    etiological, 19–20
    routine examination, 19

serological examination, 20
Laboratory examination and imaging
        examination, 9
    chest CT examination
        advantages and characteristics,
            11–12
        stages of chest CT manifestations,
            12–13
    chest X-ray, 11
    routine examination, 9
    serological test, 10–11
    virus nucleic acid testing
        false negative results and
            countermeasures, reasons for, 10
        testing methods, 9–10
Laboratory investigation, 221
Laughter therapy, 136
LCU, see Life change unit
Length-tension inappropriateness, 36
LES, see Life Event Scale
Life change unit (LCU), 224
Life Event Scale (LES), 224
Liu zi jue, 134–135
Liver and gallbladder, 7
Lower limb
    acupuncture points in, 334
    strength training, 81–83, 289
Lung auscultation, 8
Lungs, 6–7
Lung signs of COVID-19, 8–9
Lung volume, 52–53

Macrophage colony-stimulating factor
        (M-CSF), 4
Malnutrition, 166, 239
    nutritional screening and assessment
        for COVID-19 patients, 166
    nutritional treatment plan, selection
        of, 166
Maximum ventilatory volume (MVV), 53
McGill Pain Questionnaire (MPQ), 58
MCP-1, see Monocyte chemoattractant
        protein 1
M-CSF, see Macrophage colony-
        stimulating factor
Medical fabric washing and
        disinfection, 174

Medical test
    brain imaging technology, 222
    laboratory investigation, 221
    physical examination, 221
    physiological and psychological
        assessment, 222
Medical waste, treatment of, 174
Mental and psychological state,
        evaluation of, 58
Mental Health Self-Assessment
        Questionnaire (SRQ), 324
MERS-CoV, see Middle East respiratory
        syndrome coronavirus
Micronutrients, 252
Middle East respiratory syndrome
        coronavirus (MERS-CoV),
        1, 40
Mild COVID-19 cases
    clinical classification, 17
    traditional Chinese medicine
        treatment, 29
Moderate COVID-19 cases
    clinical classification, 17
    traditional Chinese medicine
        treatment, 29
Modified body rotation test, 307
Modified medical Research Council
        (mMRC) Scale (mMRC), 302–303
Monocyte chemoattractant protein 1
        (MCP-1), 4
Mortality rate, 4
Mother-to-child transmission, 3
Moxibustion therapy, 112
    acupoints, selection of
        main acupoints, 114
        match acupoints with
            symptoms, 114
    contraindicated area, 115
    contraindicated demographic, 115
    contraindicated existing
        condition, 115
    mechanism of treatment
        moxibustion materials, 112–113
        therapeutic mechanism of
            moxibustion, 113–114
    operation method, 114
    precautions

applied amount of
moxibustion, 115
moxibustion duration, 115
operation order of
moxibustion, 115
posture selection, 114
principles of treatment, 112
MPQ, *see* McGill Pain Questionnaire
Multi-dimensional assessment, 58
Muscle strength, body-weight
assessment of
30-second arm curl test, 57
30-second chair standing test, 56
Muscle strength and endurance,
nursing guidance and training
techniques for enhancing
definition, 185
key points of operation, 186
precautions, 186–187
purpose, 186
Music therapy, 141, 228
MVV, *see* Maximum ventilatory volume

NRS-2002, *see* Nutrition risk
screening-2002
Nursing personnel, management of, 172
Nursing staff, establishment of, 172
Nutritional dietary guidance
for frontline workers, 254–255
for prevention and control among the
general population, 255
Nutritional diet for ordinary/
convalescent patients, 253
Nutritional status evaluation
indicators, 244
anthropometry
arm muscle circle (AMC), 245
body composition measurement
method, 245–246
triceps skinfold thickness
(TSF), 245
weight and BMI, 244–245
laboratory investigation
creatinine–height index (CHI),
246–247
immune function indicators, 247
serum amino acid ratio, 247

serum protein level, determination
of, 246
nutrition history, 244
Nutritional treatment plan for COVID-19
patients, 248
approaches, 249–250
general principles, 249
nutritional feeding, amount of,
250–251
purpose, 248–249
for severe COVID-19 patients, 251–254
Nutrition risk screening-2002 (NRS-
2002), 241
assessment scale
for reduced nutritional status
score and its definition, 242
score results and nutrition risk,
242–244
for the severity of disease and its
definition, 242
rating scale, 243
score significance for COVID-19
patients, 244

Observation, 220
Occupational therapy, 90, 233
One-leg standing balance test, 57
OP, *see* Osteoporosis
Oscillating positive expiratory pressure
(OPEP), 67
Osteoporosis (OP), 167
Oxidative stress, 5
Oxygen-carrying capacity, 39–40
Oxygen therapy, 294–295

Pain, 85
multi-dimensional assessment, 58
single-dimensional assessment, 57
Pain therapy, 136–137
Panting, 85
Pathogenesis, of COVID-19, 4
hypoxemia, 5–6
inflammatory response and cytokine
storm, 4–5
oxidative stress, 5
Pathology, of COVID-19, 6
heart and blood vessels, 7

kidney, 7
liver and gallbladder, 7
lungs, 6–7
spleen, hilar lymph nodes and bone
     marrow, 6–7
PCR, *see* Polymerase chain reaction
PEEP, *see* Positive end-expiratory
     pressure
Peroxidation damage, 5
Pharmacotherapy, 234
Physical dysfunction, 41, 260
  decreased exercise ability and
       tolerance, 42
     fatigue, 43
     immobilization syndrome, 43–44
  tachycardias, 41
     cause of tachycardia, 41–42
     heart rate and oxygen uptake, 42
Physical examination, 221
Physical factor therapy, 233
Physical fitness, gradual and steady
     improvement of, 196
Physical function, assessment of
  balance, assessment of, 57
     functional reach test, 57
     one-leg standing balance test, 57
     timed up and go test (TUG), 57
  flexibility, assessment of
     back-scratch test, 57
     improved twist test, 57
     sit-and-reach test, 57
  muscle strength, body-weight
       assessment of
     30-second arm curl test, 57
     30-second chair stand-test, 56
  pain, assessment of
     multi-dimensional assessment, 58
     single-dimensional assessment, 57
Physical function, rehabilitation
     treatment techniques for, 75
  aerobic exercise, 75–77
  balance training, 83
     for patients who can barely get
          up, 84
     for patients who can stand on
          a flat surface for a certain time,
          84

for patients who can't stand, 84
  flexibility training, 84
  precautions
     difficulty in breathing, 85
     fatigue, 85
     pain, 85
     panting, 85
  strength training, 77
     core strength training, 81
     lower limbs strength training,
          81–83
     upper limbs strength training,
          79–81
Physical function rehabilitation exercise
  aerobic exercise, 288–289
  balance training, 294
  flexibility training, 294
  strength training, 289
     lower limb, 290
     upper limb, 290
Physiological and psychological
     assessment, 222
PiCCO monitoring, *see* Pulse index
          continuous cardiac output
          monitoring
Pittsburgh Sleep Quality Index (PSQI), 59,
     325–328
Plasma therapy, of recovered patients, 25
Polymerase chain reaction (PCR), 6
Position exercise, 181
Position management, 286
Positive end-expiratory pressure
     (PEEP), 73
Post-traumatic stress disorder (PTSD), 44
  clinical symptoms of, 45
  prognosis and influence of, 46
Postural drainage techniques, 67
  nursing guidance and training
          techniques of
     definition, 184
     key points of operation, 184
     precautions, 184–185
     purpose, 184
Posture management, 63
  for patients with ARDS, 64
  for patients with sedation/
          consciousness disorders, 64

Precautions, 297–298
    breathing, difficulty in, 85
    during respiratory function training,
        181–182
    fatigue, 85
    pain, 85
    panting, 85
Pressure ulcers, 164
    stages of, 164
    treatment of
        analgesics, 165
        antibiotics, 165
        debridement, 165
        external antibacterial agents, 165
        external dressings, 165
        general treatment, 164–165
        growth factors, 165
        surgical treatment, 165
Prevalence, of COVID-19, 1
Process of rehabilitation, 261
Protein-deficient malnutrition, 239
PSQI, see Pittsburgh Sleep Quality Index
Psychological and social dysfunction, 44
    activities of daily living (ADL)
        dysfunction, 48
    adjustment disorder, 46
    bereavement and mourning
        reaction, 47
    post-traumatic stress disorder
        (PTSD), 44
        clinical symptoms of, 45
        prognosis and influence of, 46
    sleep disorder, 47
    social engagement dysfunction, 48–49
Psychological assessment method, 219
    emotions and feelings, assessment
        of, 222
    interview, 220
    medical test
        brain imaging technology, 222
        laboratory investigation, 221
        physical examination, 221
        physiological and psychological
            assessment, 222
    observation, 220
    observation and medical testing
        changes in various systems
            throughout the body, 225

general state and behavior, 225
    psychological test, 220
        personality test, 220–221
        rating scale, 221
    stress, assessment of
        evaluation of rating scale, 224
        interview, 223–224
        stress response, 224
    work analysis, 220
Psychological disorder assessments, 217
    appropriate population for
        assessment, 218–219
    prospect, 225
    purpose of, 218
    role of, 218
Psychological dysfunction, 261
Psychological rehabilitation
    objectives of, 226
    objects of, 226
Psychological rehabilitation counseling,
        forms of, 237
Psychological rehabilitation
        nursing, 187
    common methods, 188
    goal, 187–188
    measures, 188
Psychological rehabilitation of
        COVID-19 patients
    cognitive therapy, 92
        main strategies of, 92–93
        methods for, 93–94
    supportive therapy, 90–92
Psychological rehabilitation treatment
    behavior modification therapy,
        229–230
    biofeedback therapy, 232
    cognition therapy, 228–229
    confirmed COVID-19 patients
        initial isolation treatment, 234
        isolation treatment period, 235
    exercise training, 233
    family psychotherapy, 232
    focus solution mode, 227–228
    group psychotherapy,
        231–232
    health education, 234
    medical staff and related
        personnel, 236

mild patients for home isolation
and patients with fever for
treatment, 235
music therapy, 228
occupational therapy, 233
patients with respiratory distress,
extreme restlessness, and
difficulty in expression, 235
people who are in close contact with
patients, 236
people who are reluctant to seek
medical treatment in
public, 236
pharmacotherapy, 234
physical factor therapy, 233
principles of, 226
psychological support therapy,
226–227
relaxation therapy, 231
susceptible groups and the general
public, 236
suspected patients, 235
TCM therapy, 233–234
traditional exercise therapy, 234
Psychological therapy, 89–90
Psychosocial function, assessment for
activities of daily living (ADL),
assessment of, 59
commonly used psychological
assessment scales, 58–59
Health-Related Quality of Life (HRQL)
scale, 59
mental and psychological state,
evaluation of, 58
World Health Organization Quality
of Life–BREF (WHOQOL-
BREF), 60
Psychosocial functional rehabilitation,
treatment techniques of, 85
activities of daily living (ADL)
training, 86
basic activities of daily living
(BADL) training, 86–89
instrumental activities of daily
living (IADL), 89
behavior therapy, 94
aversion therapy, 94–95
behavior-shaping method, 95

relaxation response training, 95
systematic desensitization, 94
token economy, 95
cognitive therapy, 92–94
supportive therapy, 90–92
therapeutic activities, 89
occupational therapy, 90
psychological therapy, 89–90
social therapy, 90
Psychotherapy, 27
PTSD, see Post-traumatic stress disorder
Pulmonary signs of COVID-19, 17
Pulmonary ventilation volume
analysis, 53
Pulse index continuous cardiac output
(PiCCO) monitoring, 24
Pursed-lip breathing training, 69

Qi stagnation, 136

Rational emotive therapy (RET), 93
Reactive oxygen species (ROS), 5
Recovered patients' plasma therapy, 25
Rehabilitation nursing, objective of, 177
Rehabilitation nursing assessment, 177
course of onset and treatment, 178
course of illness, 178
current status, 178
diagnostic and therapeutic
process, 178
relevant medical history, 178
psychosocial data
knowledge about the disease, 178
psychological status, 178
social support systems, 178
Rehabilitation nursing measures, 178
effective cough, nursing guidance
and training techniques
for, 182
definition, 182
key points of operation, 182
precautions, 182–183
purpose, 182
muscle strength and endurance
definition, 185
key points of operation, 186
precautions, 186–187
purpose, 186

nursing guidance and training
      techniques for respiratory
      function
   abdominal breath training,
      179–180
   definition, 179
   education and cooperation of
      patients, 181
   half-closed lip respiration
      training, 179
   position exercise, 181
   precautions during respiratory
      function training, 181–182
   purpose, 179
   respiratory muscle training, 180
postural drainage, nursing guidance
      and training techniques of
   definition, 184
   key points of operation, 184
   precautions, 184–185
   purpose, 184
psychological rehabilitation
      nursing, 187
   common methods of psychological
      rehabilitation therapy, 188
   goal, 187–188
   measures, 188
Relaxation therapy, 231
Relaxation training, 71
Renal failure and renal replacement
      therapy, 24
Repetitive transcranial magnetic
      stimulation (rTMS), 233
Reporting system, of COVID-19, 20–21
Respiratory burst, 5
Respiratory droplet transmission, 2
Respiratory dysfunction, 35, 260
   acute respiratory distress syndrome
      (ARDS) and respiratory failure,
      40–41
   dyspnea, 35
      definition of dyspnea, 35–36
      mechanism that causes
         dyspnea, 36
      pathophysiology of dyspnea, 36–38
   hypoxemia, 38
      decreased oxygen-carrying
         capacity, 39–40

   diffusion impairment, 39
   hypoventilation, 38–39
   increase of dead space, 39
   local ventilation/blood flow
      disorder, 39
Respiratory function, 51
   common assessment of
      body-weight assessment of
         cardiopulmonary function, 56
      cardiopulmonary exercise test
         (CPET), 56
      dyspnea scale, 55–56
   objective examination
      lung volume, 52–53
      pulmonary ventilation volume
         analysis, 53
      respiratory gas analysis, 54
   rehabilitation exercise of, 286
      airway clearance technology,
         286–287
      position management, 286
   respiratory muscle endurance,
      measurement of, 55
   respiratory muscle fatigue,
      measurement of, 55
   respiratory muscle strength,
      measurement of, 55
   small airway function
      examination, 55
   subjective symptoms, 52
Respiratory muscles, 37
Respiratory muscle training (RMT),
      71–72, 180
   anti-breathing training, 287
   contracted lip breathing, 287
   controlled deep breathing, 287
   respiratory rehabilitation
      exercise, 288
Respiratory patterns, 37–38, 69
   abdominal breathing exercises, 69
   breathing rhythm adjusting
      training, 70
   pursed-lip breathing training, 69
Respiratory rehabilitation exercise, 288
Respiratory rehabilitation therapy
      techniques, 62
   airway clearance technique
      (ACT), 64

active cycle of breathing technique
(ACBTs), 65–66
chest physical therapy techniques,
67–68
effective cough, 65
high-frequency chest wall
oscillation (HFCWO), 67
oscillating positive expiratory
pressure (OPEP), 67
postural drainage techniques, 67
breathing exercises, 72–73
breathing training, 68
local dilation breathing
training, 71
relaxation training, 71
respiratory pattern training, 69–70
intervention activities at early
stage, 62
breathing control techniques, 62
energy-saving techniques, 63
posture management, 63
for patients with ARDS, 64
for patients with sedation/
consciousness disorders, 64
respiratory intervention
techniques, 73
active cycle of breathing
techniques (ACBTs),
precautions for, 74
high-frequency chest wall
oscillation (HFCWO),
precautions for, 74
mechanical/artificial dilated
ventilation, 73–74
patients' position, 73
precautions in manual
treatment, 74
sputum suction, 73
respiratory muscle training (RMT),
71–72
techniques implementation,
principles of, 74–75
Respiratory support, 23–24
Respiratory system signs, of COVID-19, 8
RET, see Rational emotive therapy
Reverse therapy, 137
Reverse transcription polymerase chain
reaction (RT-PCR) assays, 38

RMT, see Respiratory muscle training
ROS, see Reactive oxygen species
Routine examination, 9, 19
rTMS, see Repetitive transcranial
magnetic stimulation
RT-PCR assays, see Reverse transcription
polymerase chain reaction
assays

SARS, see Severe acute respiratory
syndrome
SARS-CoV, see Severe acute respiratory
syndrome coronavirus
SAS, see Self-Rating Anxiety Scale
Science, principle of, 139
Scraping therapy, 127
contraindications, 129
location selection, 128
operation method, 129
positioning, 128
treatment mechanism, 127–128
SDS, see Self-Rating Depression scale
Self-Rating Anxiety Scale (SAS), 313–315
Self-Rating Depression Scale (SDS),
312–313
Serological antibody test, 16–17
Serological test, 10–11
Serum amino acid ratio, 247
Serum protein level, determination
of, 246
Severe acute respiratory syndrome
(SARS), 61
Severe acute respiratory syndrome
coronavirus (SARS-CoV), 1, 40
Severe COVID-19 cases
clinical classification, 17–18
nutritional treatment, 253–254
special nutrients for, 251–252
traditional Chinese medicine
treatment, 29
Shame therapy, 137–138
Shock-denial-invasion-constant
correction-end, 44
Simplified tai chi chuan, 269–271
Sincerity, principle of, 138–139
Single-dimensional assessment, 57
Single-leg upright balance test, 310
Sit-and-reach test, 57

6-minute walking test (6MWT), 56, 302
Sleep disorders, 47
    in patients with PTSD, 45
Sleep problems, 27
Social engagement dysfunction, 48–49
Social Readjustment Rating Scale
    adults, 321–322
    juvenile, 322–323
Social therapy, 90
Spike protein (S protein), 2
Spleen, 6–7
Step test, 56
Strength training, 77, 289
    core strength training, 81
    lower limb, 81–83, 290–294
    upper limb, 79–81, 289–290
Stress, assessment of
    evaluation of rating scale, 224
    interview, 223–224
    stress response, 224
Stress ulcers, prevention of, 28
Supportability, principle of, 138
Supportive therapy, 90–92
Susceptible groups, 3
Symptoms, of COVID-19, 1, 8

Tachycardia, 41
    cause of, 41–42
    heart rate and oxygen uptake, 42
Tai chi chuan, 132–133
TCM, see Traditional Chinese medicine
TEE, see Thoracic expansion exercises
Therapeutic activities, 89
    occupational therapy, 90
    psychological therapy, 89–90
    social therapy, 90
30-second arm curl test, 57
30-second arm flexion test, 305
30-second chair standing
    experiment, 305
30-second chair standing test, 56
Thoracic expansion exercises (TEE), 66
3-minute step test, 304
Tiger exercise, 273–274
Timed up and go test (TUG), 57

Traditional Chinese medicine (TCM),
        emotion therapy of, 135
    anger therapy, 136
    joy therapy, 137
    laughter therapy, 136
    major emotion therapies, 139
        emotion interresistance, 139
        speech induction therapy, 140
        therapy to follow one's emotions
            and desires, 140
        transference therapy, 139–140
    pain therapy, 136–137
    precautions
        assessment, 140
        explanation, 140
        understanding, 140
    principles of treatment, 138
        acceptability, principle of, 138
        confidentiality, principle of, 139
        science, principle of, 139
        sincerity, principle of, 138–139
        supportability, principle of, 138
    shame therapy, 137–138
Traditional Chinese medicine (TCM),
        external treatment techniques of
    acupoint application therapy (see
        Acupoint application therapy)
    acupoint (meridian) massage therapy
        (see Acupoint (meridian)
        massage therapy)
    acupuncture therapy (see
        Acupuncture therapy)
    auricular acupoint pressing therapy
        (see Auricular acupoint
        pressing therapy)
    bloodletting therapy (see Bloodletting
        therapy)
    cupping therapy (see Cupping therapy)
    moxibustion therapy (see Moxibustion
        therapy)
    scraping therapy (see Scraping
        therapy)
Traditional Chinese medicine (TCM)
        nursing
    emotion nursing, 190
        calming the mind, therapy of, 191

doubt analysis, therapy of, 191
emotion being diverted, therapy
of, 191
emotion interresistance,
therapy of, 191
emotions and depression relieving,
therapy of, 191
instructions for taking TCM
decoction, 188
techniques
acupoint application, 188–190
auricular plaster therapy, 190
precautions, 190
Traditional Chinese medicine (TCM)
treatment, 29, 99, 233–234
clinical treatment stage, 103
convalescent period, 29, 106–107
critically severe cases, 29, 106
mild cases, 29, 103–104
moderate cases, 29
ordinary cases, 104–105
severe cases, 29, 105–106
medication observation, 29
principles of treatment, 100
stage of medical observation, 103
traditional methods, 265
Baduanjin, 132, 265–269
five-animal exercise (see Five-
animal exercise)
liu zi jue, 134–135
tai chi chuan, 132–133, 269–271
treatment mechanism, 100–103
Yi Jin Jing (see Yi Jin Jing)
Traditional exercise therapy, 234
Transmission, route of, 2–3
aerosol transmission, 3
close contact transmission, 3
fecal–oral transmission, 3
mother-to-child transmission, 3
respiratory droplet transmission, 2
Treatment, rehabilitation, 262
auxiliary appliances, configuration
and use of, 263–264
guidance of rehabilitation
training, 263
psychological intervention, 263

Triceps skinfold thickness (TSF), 245
TUG, see Timed up and go test
2-minute marking time test, 303
2-minute step test, 56
2.4-m standing up and walking test, 310
Type II alveolar epithelial cells, 6

Ultraviolet air disinfection, precautions
for, 174–175
Upper limb
acupuncture points in, 332
strength training, 79–81, 289
Upper respiratory disease, 20
Urinary tract infection, 165–166

VAS, see Visual Analogue Scale
Vein thromboembolism (VTE)
risk assessment, 162
risk factors, 161
VTE prevention advice for inpatients
in CRU ward, 162–163
Ventilation instruction, 36–37
Ventilation resistance, 37
Ventilator-associated pneumonia,
prevention of, 28
Virus nucleic acid testing
reasons for false negative results and
countermeasures, 10
testing methods, 9–10
Visual Analogue Scale (VAS), 57
VTE, see Vein thromboembolism

Warning signals, of COVID-19, 18
adults, 19
children, 19
Weight and BMI, 244–245
Whole-course psychological
intervention, adherence to, 195
Work analysis, 220
World Health Organization Quality of
Life–BREF (WHOQOL-BREF), 60

Yi Jin Jing, 134, 276
backward drag nine oxtail style, 278
bow type, 283–284
cross bear dropping magic pestle, 276

flapping claw type, 280
green dragon claw, 282
holding the door in the palm, 277
nine ghosts saber drawing style,
    280–281

reach and change the star, 277–278
tail off type, 284
three-plate floor style, 281–282
tiger eating style, 282–283
Wei Tuo offers a pestle, 276

Printed in the United States
by Baker & Taylor Publisher Services